The Quality Solution

The Stakeholder's Guide to Improving Health Care

Edited by

David B. Nash, MD, MBA

**The Dr. Raymond C. and Doris N. Grandon Professor of Health Policy
Chairman, Department of Health Policy
Jefferson Medical College**

Neil I. Goldfarb

**Program Director for Research, Department of Health Policy
Jefferson Medical College**

JONES AND BARTLETT PUBLISHERS

Sudbury, Massachusetts

BOSTON   TORONTO   LONDON   SINGAPORE

World Headquarters

Jones and Bartlett Publishers
40 Tall Pine Drive
Sudbury, MA 01776
978-443-5000
info@jbpub.com
www.jbpub.com

Jones and Bartlett Publishers
Canada
6339 Ormindale Way
Mississauga, Ontario
L5V 1J2

Jones and Bartlett Publishers
International
Barb House, Barb Mews
London W6 7PA
UK

Jones and Bartlett's books and products are available through most bookstores and online booksellers. To contact Jones and Bartlett Publishers directly, call 800-832-0034, fax 978-443-8000, or visit our website www.jbpub.com.

Substantial discounts on bulk quantities of Jones and Bartlett's publications are available to corporations, professional associations, and other qualified organizations. For details and specific discount information, contact the special sales department at Jones and Bartlett via the above contact information or send an email to specialsales@jbpub.com.

ISBN-13: 978-0-7637-2748-2
ISBN-10: 0-7637-2748-2

Library of Congress Cataloging-in-Publication Data
Nash, David B.
      The quality solution: the stakeholder's guide to improving health care
/ by David B. Nash, Neil I. Goldfarb.
         p. ; cm.
      Includes bibliographical references.
      ISBN 0-7637-2748-2
      1. Medical care--United States--Quality control.   2. Medical care
--Standards--United States.   3. Health care reform--United States.
      I. Goldfarb, Neil I.   II. Title.
      [DNLM: 1. Quality of Health Care--standards.   2. Health Care Evaluation Mechanisms.   3. Health Care Reform.   4. Quality Assurance,
Health Care--methods.   W 84.1 N248q 2006]
      RA399.A3N13 2006
      362.1'0425--dc22

                                                                        2005008278

Production Credits

Executive Editor: David Cella
Editorial Assistant: Lisa Gordon
Production Director: Amy Rose
Production Assistant: Rachel Rossi
Marketing Manager: Emily Ekle
Associate Marketing Manager: Laura Kavigian
Manufacturing Buyer: Therese Connell

Composition: Shepherd, Inc.
Cover Design: Timothy Dziewit
Cover Image: © Mike Tolstoy/Ukranian Photobank/
      ShutterStock, Inc., © AbleStock
Printing and Binding: Malloy, Inc.
Cover Printing: Malloy, Inc.

6048

Printed in the United States of America
10 09 08 07 06   10 9 8 7 6 5 4 3 2

To our fellow travelers on the road to improve quality,
To our families who accompany us on the journey,
To our mentors who helped uncover the trail, and
To our students who follow it into the future.

Contents

"It was the best of times, it was the worst of times, it was the age of wisdom, it was the age of foolishness." Almost one hundred and fifty years ago, Charles Dickens began his classic *A Tale of Two Cities* with these famous lines that still resonate with readers today. But like most great literature, the quote speaks to us not only about our own personal experiences, but also about our society's journey. Many find these sentiments accurate descriptors as we struggle to make sense out of the perplexing way in which our society can reach seemingly superhuman heights of accomplishment while simultaneously tolerating conditions of almost inhuman depravity.

It may not be an overstatement to suggest that these lines also describe the current state of health care in America. At the dawn of the 21st century, our healthcare system, building upon the robust tools provided by science and technology over the past century, provides us with the means to lead remarkably productive and protected lives, even compared with our ancestors of only two or three generations ago. At the same time, the healthcare delivery systems that sustain this achievement have become comparably complex, and the interplay of all the stakeholders in the drama has become proportionately intricate.

A few measures of the problem: despite having some of the most sophisticated diagnostic and treatment technologies in the world, among the developed countries we rank extremely low in infant mortality. Some patrons can obtain treatment on-call 24/7 in "boutique medicine" operations; millions of others are uninsured, with emergency rooms serving as their only access to health care. Finally, regardless of socioeconomic status, many Americans simply fail to receive timely and effective treatments for a wide variety of reasons.

If one seriously hopes to contribute toward an improvement in the delivery of health care and the operation of the healthcare system in America, a first step on that path is to be educated about its dimensions. David Nash, a leader in this field for many years, and his colleagues are to be commended for this well-organized and clear volume written by experts in the field. It comprehensively develops the ways in which quality of healthcare delivery has come to be increasingly appreciated; the metrics that help to quantitatively define the distance between the ideal situation, as we presently understand it, and the practical experience that patients undergo; the major players in the healthcare delivery system and their perspectives; and what we can look forward to as efforts to reduce the quality chasm move forward.

The intended audience for this book will be as diverse as the field of public health itself. It will encompass those on the frontlines of healthcare delivery as well as those responsible for its administration, planning, and management. Even laboratory scientists conducting disease- and patient-oriented research, who wish to understand how their efforts will ultimately be translated into the public good, will find this volume of interest, as will those with only a financial stake in the operation of the system. It will certainly be invaluable to educators and researchers in the field. In this context, it will undoubtedly become central to our curriculum in Public Health at Thomas Jefferson University and can be expected to contribute to many around the country as well.

At some point in our journeys, we are all destined to be touched by the quality of health care. Naturally, there will always be disparities of the kind that Dickens so pithily described, but that will not preclude us from striving toward quality solutions. This volume is an important and effective step in that direction.

James H. Keen, PhD
Dean of the College of Graduate Studies
Vice President for International Affairs
Thomas Jefferson University
Philadelphia, PA

Preface

The central theme of this book is unambiguous—improving the quality of health care in our nation is a public health emergency. The status quo regarding healthcare quality is untenable. *The Quality Solution* provides the reader with a deeper understanding of the extent of this public health emergency and a set of skills to affect change. By focusing on the health of the public as it relates to quality, this book breaks new ground as a text for courses in public health, health administration, medical care, and related fields. Its message is broad in scope and comprehensive in its reach.

The Quality Solution is also indicative of the natural evolution of the field; that is, the timing for our work is appropriate. Students in many disciplines and in many graduate programs have expressed a deep interest in learning how to close the quality chasm. We believe our book will help. The tools described have gained widespread acceptance and are ready for implementation in different sectors. In short, the science of quality measurement and improvement has reached a critical juncture for those who recognize that the status quo is indeed untenable. *The Quality Solution* will enlighten, inform, and challenge you to participate in the transformation of the system for the future.

Our intended audience is learners across the spectrum of professional schools including public health, medicine, health administration, and health law. Professionals in each field will also resonate with the key message of the text. Practitioners and leaders in the emerging field of quality improvement will be attracted to the "one-stop shopping" that the book delivers. Policy makers will appreciate the insights from many of our prominent contributors, while organizational leaders will benefit from the succinct nature of many of the key chapters.

How is the book organized? The book is structured with four sections including an Introduction to Quality in Health Care; The Measures and Tools of Quality Improvement; Stakeholders in Quality Improvement, and Looking Toward the Future of Quality Improvement. Each section comprises component chapters that are organized in a consistent fashion. Each chapter is followed by a representative case study and examples of study questions for further classroom reflection. The book pulls no punches, and the editors recognize that sacred cows often make the best hamburger! Some readers will be delighted by our approach. Others will be vexed by the provocative nature of some of the content. Everyone will learn something new and useful.

Of course, any multi-authored, edited text has inherent limitations. Different authors and different editors utilize different styles and bring differing prejudices to bear. We strive to smooth out these rough edges and deliver a text that is tightly woven into a fabric that is succinct, logical, and compelling.

The editors are indebted to many individuals and organizations for the success of *The Quality Solution*. We thank three key internal leaders at Thomas Jefferson University (TJU) including Thomas J. Nasca, MD, the dean of Jefferson Medical College, Thomas J. Lewis, the chief executive officer of Thomas Jefferson University Hospital; and James H. Keen, PhD, the dean of the College of Graduate Studies at TJU. They have provided us with unwavering support and have evidenced a very public commitment to *The Quality Solution* at Jefferson and beyond. We also thank the many members of the Department of Health Policy who lent their insights and critical eye to the process of creating a multi-authored, edited volume of this size and scope. We also wish to acknowledge the many learners across the educational continuum, such as our medical students and house officers, who questioned us every step of the way and provided us with an opportunity to hone our thinking and simplify the take-home messages.

As editors, we take full responsibility for any error of commission or omission in the final version of the text. Our sincere hope is that *The Quality Solution* will help many readers to recognize the extent of the public health emergency we face, and will stimulate those same readers to participate in the public discourse regarding change. We hope our readers will ultimately close the quality chasm and thereby greatly improve the health of the public. This is, in part, the legacy we seek.

Contributors

Anne-Marie J. Audet, MD, MPH
Assistant Vice President
The Commonwealth Fund
New York, NY

Alon Y. Avidan, MD, MPH
Clinical Assistant Professor
Director, Sleep Disorders Clinic
Department of Neurology
Michael S. Aldrich Sleep Disorders Laboratory
University of Michigan Health Systems
University Hospital
Ann Arbor, MI

Kevin L. Bowman
Medical Student
Jefferson Medical College
Philadelphia, PA

Clair M. Callan, MD, MBA, FACPE, CPE
Vice President
American Medical Association
Science, Quality, and Public Health
Chicago, IL

Darrell A. Campbell, Jr., MD
Chief of Staff of University Hospital
Professor of Surgery
University of Michigan Health System
Ann Arbor, MI

Donald E. Casey, MD, MPH, MBA
Chief Medical Officer
Catholic Healthcare Partners
Cincinnati, OH

Carolyn M. Clancy, MD
Director
Agency for Healthcare Research and Quality
Rockville, MD

Karen Davis, PhD
President
The Commonwealth Fund
New York, NY

Jan De La Mare, MPAff
Research Associate
Center for Delivery, Organization, and Markets
Agency for Healthcare Research and Quality
Rockville, MD

Walter H. Ettinger, Jr., MD, MBA
President
UMass Memorial Medical Center
Worcester, MA

Adam S. Evans
Medical Student Fellow
Department of Health Policy
Jefferson Medical College
Philadelphia, PA

Irene Fraser, PhD
Director
Center for Delivery, Organization, and Markets
Agency for Healthcare Research and Quality
Rockville, MD

Neil I. Goldfarb
Program Director for Research
Department of Health Policy
Jefferson Medical College
Philadelphia, PA

Jonathan E. Gottlieb, MD
Senior Vice President for Clinical Affairs
Thomas Jefferson University
Philadelphia, PA

John R. Griffith, MBA, FACHE
Professor of Health Management and Policy
University of Michigan
Ann Arbor, MI

Stuart Guterman
Senior Program Director, Medicare's Future
The Commonwealth Fund
Washington, DC

Christine W. Hartmann, MSS, PhD
Assistant Professor
Department of Health Policy
Jefferson Medical College
Philadelphia, PA

James H. Keen, PhD
Dean, College of Graduate Studies
Vice President for International Affairs
Thomas Jefferson University
Philadelphia, PA

Karen S. Kmetik, PhD
Program Director, Clinical Quality Improvement
American Medical Association
Chicago, IL

Stephen T. Lawless, MD, MBA
Chief Knowledge Officer
Associate Professor of Nemours Pediatrics
Jefferson Medical College
Philadelphia, PA

Vittorio Maio, PharmD, MS
Research Assistant Professor
Department of Health Policy
Jefferson Medical College
Philadelphia, PA

Gregg S. Meyer, MD, MSc.
Medical Director
Massachusetts General Physicians Organization
Partners Healthcare System
Boston, MA

Michael L. Millenson
The Mervin Shalowitz, MD Visiting Scholar
Health Industry Management Program
Kellogg School of Management
Northwestern University
Evanston, IL

David B. Nash, MD, MBA
The Dr. Raymond C. and Doris N. Grandon Professor of Health Policy
Chairman, Department of Health Policy
Jefferson Medical College
Philadelphia, PA

Rachel Nelson, MHA
Special Projects Task Leader, Quality Improvement Group
Office of Clinical Standards and Quality
Baltimore, MD

Erin T. O'Brien, MPH
Policy Analyst
American Medical Association
Chicago, IL

Judith Owens, MD, MPH
Division of Pediatrics
Rhode Island Hospital
Providence, RI

Michael D. Parkinson, MD, MPH
Executive Vice President, CMO, and CHO
Lumenos
Alexandria, VA

Roy Proujansky, MD
Chief Executive of the Practice
Nemours Children's Clinic
Robert L. Brent Professor and Chair
Department of Pediatrics
Jefferson Medical College
Philadelphia, PA

Elizabeth R. Ransom, MD
Vice Chair, Board of Governors
Residency Director
Otolaryngology/Head and Neck Surgery
Henry Ford Health System
Detroit, MI

Scott B. Ransom, DO, MBA, MPH
Director, Program for Healthcare
    Improvement & Leadership Development
Associate Professor of Obstetrics,
    Gynecology, Health Management, and Policy
University of Michigan
Ann Arbor, MI

William C. Rollow, MD, MPH
Director, Quality Improvement Group
Office of Clinical Standards and Quality
Centers for Medicare and Medicaid Services
Baltimore, MD

Sheila H. Roman, MD, MPH
Senior Medical Officer, Quality Measurement and Health Assessment
Centers for Medicare and Medicaid Services
Baltimore, MD

Thomas N. Ricciardi, PhD
Manager, Medical Quality Improvement Consortium
GE Healthcare
Clinical Assistant Professor
Oregon Health and Science University
Hillsboro, OR

Stephen C. Schoenbaum, MD, MPH
Senior Vice President
The Commonwealth Fund
New York, NY

Vincenza T. Snow, MD
Senior Medical Associate (DEL Research)
Department of Scientific Policy
American College of Physicians
Philadelphia, PA

Kevin Tabb, MD
Chief Quality and Medical Information Officer
Stanford University Medical Center
Stanford, CA

Margaret C. Toepp, PhD
Director, Clinical Quality Improvement
American Medical Association
Chicago, IL

Introduction to Quality in Health Care

Chapter 1

An Overview of Quality in the Healthcare System

David B. Nash
Adam S. Evans
Kevin L. Bowman

EXECUTIVE SUMMARY

If there is one idea that you should take away from reading this book it should be this: Improving the quality of health care is a public health emergency. In the late 1990s, the Institute of Medicine produced two landmark national reports, *To Err is Human* and *Crossing the Quality Chasm,* which exposed the inadequacies that plague the US healthcare system and the need for major reform. Despite these red flags, there has been marginal improvement since then. A quintessential report published as recently as 2003 by McGlynn and colleagues points out that these inadequacies still exist in the healthcare system, revealing that 50 percent of all adults are still not receiving care that corresponds with basic prevention and treatment guidelines.[1] After decades of research and numerous press reports indicating just how poor the quality of health care is in the United States, how can we continue denying that improving the quality of care is one of the most, if not the most, pressing public health issue today? This book addresses these deficiencies in quality and the actions society can take to close the quality chasm.

LEARNING OBJECTIVES

1. To gain a better understanding of what the term public health means.
2. To identify the challenges facing the healthcare system today.
3. To understand how quality plays a role in public health.
4. To be aware of why improving quality is a public health emergency.

KEYWORDS

Institute of Medicine (IOM)
Quality Improvement
Public Health

Introduction

As the United States moves forward in the early twenty-first century, healthcare consumers are increasingly exposed to new challenges and opportunities in healthcare delivery, relating Internet information, the sequencing of the human genome, proliferation of pharmaceuticals, and other technologic advances. At the same time, there still exists many of the public health problems that were faced in the twentieth century, such as increased numbers of individuals with chronic diseases, limited access to care for the poor and uninsured, and rising healthcare costs.

As these forces collide, even more problems will arise if action is not taken now. The best way to address this is by focusing attention on the quality of healthcare delivery, which is currently both inadequate and costly. Simply put, this is a public health emergency that must be addressed. This chapter sets the framework to understand the problem, its magnitude, and steps that can be taken to remedy the current situation.

What Is Public Health?

Before we address quality as a public health emergency, we must first discuss what public health means. For some, it conjures up ideas about reducing the spread of epidemics such as AIDS and SARS, for others it is about improving life expectancy, and for others it deals with improving the overall health of communities.

Why does the term public health evoke so many different meanings, and what is the right one to use? The answer is that as a society we have faced numerous and diverse health issues over the past few centuries, and this has led people to arrive at different notions for the definition of public health itself.

Tracing the Roots of Public Health

Before 1850, public health was characterized by epidemics of infectious disease such as cholera, smallpox, tuberculosis, typhoid, and yellow fever. Because science had not yet proven the existence of microorganisms as the cause of these diseases, society's approach to dealing with epidemics involved evacuating people from areas where epidemics were located and quarantining the infected individuals.[2]

After 1850, social forces such as the industrial revolution and key findings by individuals such as Edward Jenner, John Snow, and Lemuel Shattuck helped to lead the way public health was viewed and dealt with. Efforts then focused on reforming the unsanitary conditions—such as crowded living conditions and inadequate sewage infrastructure—that were believed to bolster these outbreaks. Local and state health departments were established to prevent the outbreak of epidemics by improving waste disposal, street and swamp drainage, and any other measure that would provide a more sanitary environment.[3]

These sanitation reforms along with better nutrition, a rising standard of living, and other health practices such as increased pasteurization and sterilization, resulted in large decreases in mortality due to infectious diseases. At the same time, the scope and view of public health began to broaden during the early part of the twentieth century. Advances in modern medicine—such as the creation of antibiotics, childhood immunization programs to prevent polio, legislation targeting the quality of food and drugs, and regulations to prevent injuries in the workplace—have contributed to the growing agenda of public health.[4]

As a result of these improvements, people have started to live longer and chronic conditions such as cardiovascular disease and certain cancers have become more prevalent than the acute infectious diseases that affected previous generations. By 1950 chronic diseases had become the major cause of death in the United States and efforts since then have focused on elucidating the causes of chronic diseases in order to prevent them.[5]

It has become apparent that the list of important issues affecting the health of the public has become more extensive over the years. With the aging population, mapping of the human genome, and the increased use of technology it can be expected that the scope of public health will only continue to expand.

In light of the expanding agenda of public health, in 1994 The United States Public Health Service sought to define public health in a statement titled "Public Health in America."[2] The following roles of public health were outlined:

- Preventing epidemics and the spread of disease
- Protecting against environmental hazards
- Preventing injuries
- Promoting and encouraging healthy behaviors
- Responding to disasters and assisting communities in recovery
- Assuring the quality and accessibility of health services

As mentioned previously, society has devoted significant resources to the first five bulleted points. However, efforts to improve the quality of healthcare in America are still lagging significantly. The remainder of the chapter will focus on understanding quality and the emergent need to improve it.

Defining Quality and Its Relationship to Public Health

In *Crossing the Quality Chasm* the IOM defined quality as "the degree to which health services for individuals and populations increase the likelihood of desired health outcomes and [the degree to which they] are consistent with current professional knowledge."[6] But what exactly does this mean and how does it apply to the health of the public? In general, the IOM interprets quality along six domains:

1. Safety
2. Effectiveness
3. Patient-centeredness
4. Timeliness
5. Efficiency
6. Equity

The first domain, safety, refers to "avoiding injuries to patients from the care that is intended to help them."[6] Problems that fit into this category occur all too often in health care. Examples of safety errors include administering the wrong drug or wrong dosage of medicine, incorrect diagnoses, or injuries from patient falls. Deaths due to preventable medical errors are more common than deaths due to breast cancer, motor vehicle accidents, or AIDS.[7]

Effectiveness refers to "providing services based on scientific knowledge to all who could benefit and refraining from providing services to those not likely to benefit."[6] This means utilizing proper and effective services when they are warranted, and avoiding both overuse and underuse.

The third domain is patient-centeredness, which involves providing care for patients that takes into account their preferences, their values, and their needs.[6] Specifically, to adequately address a patient's healthcare needs, his or her values must be respected; care should be coordinated so information between the different healthcare providers is seamless; patients should be well informed about their condition and any treatments available; they deserve to live without unnecessary and avoidable pain; they need an adequate support system; and their family and friends need to be involved in the healing process.

The fourth domain is timeliness—how long it takes to deliver care to patients.[6] For example, it refers to how long a patient must wait to receive a biopsy once a breast mass is detected, or to receive any follow-up care that might be needed. Waiting times should be reduced to allay the patient's fears and to increase the efficacy of treatments.

Efficiency has to do with resources slated for patient care being administered in a way that minimizes waste.[6] For example, it might involve reducing unnecessary duplication of tests, achieving more a streamlined approach to ordering prescription drugs, or having fewer layers of administrative control.

The final domain has to do with delivering care that is equitable. That is, all individuals should receive the same level of care regardless of "gender, ethnicity, geographic location, and socioeconomic status."[6]

The Quality of Health Care in the United States

Now that we have a working definition of quality, the next step is to look at the current state of quality in the American healthcare system. Significant research shows that the quality of care delivered in the United States is substantially lower than what it should be.[8]

In October 2000, an article in the *Journal of the American Medical Association* (*JAMA*) found wide variations in the care that Medicare beneficiaries received. For example, only 11 percent of beneficiaries who needed pneumococcal immunization screening prior to discharge actually received it; 95 percent nifedipine was used with acute stroke patients. The report goes on to add that had these services been provided hundreds to thousands of lives could have been saved each year.[9] A subsequent report in January 2003 dealing with Medicare beneficiaries confirmed that though care had improved from 2000 to 2001, there still remained large areas for improvement.[10]

In June 2003, a prominent article in the *New England Journal of Medicine* that examined 439 quality-of-care indicators reported that individuals were receiving about 55 percent of recommended care, regardless if it was preventative care, acute care, or care for chronic conditions. For example, when considering coronary artery disease, only 68 percent of patients received the recommended care. This includes individuals not receiving medications such as aspirin and beta-blockers, which are proven to reduce the risk of cardiac complications. Similar gaps in quality were also found in other high prevalence diseases such as diabetes and hypertension.[1]

These studies are consistent with the results of the first *National Healthcare Quality Report* released in late 2003 by the Agency for Healthcare Research and Quality. While the report states that some areas where quality is measured—such as diabetic hospital admissions and childhood vaccinations—have improved, it concluded that overall there remains significant areas for improvement.[11] The report found that:

> More than 57,000 Americans die needlessly each year because they do not receive appropriate health care. The majority, almost 50,000, die because known conditions—high blood pressure or elevated cholesterol—are not adequately monitored and controlled. Others die or are at increased risk of death because they have not received the right preventative or follow-up care. [This is because] people with high blood pressure do not have it controlled, . . . people who have suffered a heart

attack do not have their cholesterol levels monitored . . . [and] smokers receive no advice to quit. Put simply, the healthcare system regularly fails to deliver care we know to be appropriate.[11]

It might be assumed that this lack of quality only occurs in inner cities or rural areas: It is in fact pervasive. Two prominent studies in the *Annals of Internal Medicine* published in 2003 found that residents in the highest-spending regions received approximately 60 percent more care than those in the lowest-spending regions. However, this did not translate into better care. For example, patients being given cardiac care in the highest-spending regions were less likely to receive aspirin after acute MI and were no more likely to receive acute reperfusion, compared to those regions that spent less on healthcare. Therefore, inadequate care is being delivered regardless of the amount of money being spent on it.[12,13]

Indeed this is a significant problem, but there are other issues undermining the quality of health care—such as deaths due to medical errors. Consider this: 44,000 to 98,000 preventable deaths occur each year due to medical errors. This is greater than the number of deaths from AIDS, motor vehicle accidents, and breast cancer in any given year.[7] How can this be? How can the quality of care delivered to patients be so inadequate for a country that prides itself so much on having the best health care in the world?

Reasons for Inadequate Quality

The quality of health care in the United States continues to be inadequate for a variety of reasons. First, the growing complexities of science and technology have made it difficult, if not impossible, for one physician to possess all the necessary information to practice evidence-based medicine. And to complicate matters further, the rate of new information being made available through various sources does not seem to be slowing down. The problem is that all of these new and exciting treatments, procedures, devices, and pharmaceuticals are making their way to the market much quicker than healthcare providers are able to safely, effectively, and efficiently utilize them.[6]

Second, individuals today are living longer than previous generations. The US Census Bureau has projected life expectancy to increase from 74.1 and 79.8 years for males and females, respectively in 1999, to 77.6 and 83.6 years for males and females in 2025.[14] Probably more impressive is the recent growth in the proportion of Americans living to old age. In 1940, a 65-year-old had a 7 percent chance that he/she would live to be at least 90 years old. But by 2000, that same 65-year-old had a 26 percent chance of living to 90.[15] As a result of people living longer, the prevalence of chronic conditions in the population is increasing. The problem is that the systems in place today to care for people are generally geared toward individuals with acute disease and not chronic disease. For better or worse, the US healthcare system does not have a model in place to care for individuals with chronic disease.[6] And this mismatch in how healthcare resources are delivered and how they need to be or should be delivered, given the ailments that afflict society today, are merely furthering the poor quality of care being provided.

Third, the healthcare delivery system is poorly organized. To many, the existing model for healthcare delivery is not easy to navigate, but rather a confusing web that is characterized by numerous unnecessary handoffs from one provider to another.[6] This complex arrangement has a tendency to decrease safety, waste precious resources, and lose patient information.

Finally, health care has not invested adequately in information technology (IT). Information technology is laden with opportunity yet health care, an industry that could benefit immensely from IT, has fallen far short in exploiting the many benefits it has to offer.[6] In 2000, only 17 percent of US general practitioners were connected to their patient's electronic medical records. In the same year, connectivity to a patient's digitized records in Sweden was at 90 percent; the Netherlands had 88 percent; Denmark had 62 percent; the United Kingdom had 58 percent; Finland had 56 percent; and Germany had 48 percent.[16] This is especially disturbing considering the United States claims to have the best healthcare system in the world, if not at least the best resources to pool from. Clearly, the United States must step up its efforts to integrate IT into health care.

Potential Problems if the Status Quo Persists

Regardless of why the quality of health care in America is deficient or how it came to be, the delivery of health care in the United States is so expensive and so flawed that the country faces imminent threats if the status quo persists. First of all, if health care continues to be funded in the current manner, the Medicare Trust Fund will go bankrupt in the future. According to Medicare's government trustees the program is already alleged to go bankrupt seven years earlier than originally projected because of rising healthcare costs.[17]

As a result of the skyrocketing costs of health care, it is predicted that fewer people will have access to it in the future. In 2003, two thirds of companies with 200 or more employees responded to increasing healthcare costs by shifting a greater burden of the costs onto their employees, in addition to eliminating coverage for some services. Also, smaller companies, which make up the majority of the US economy, are finding themselves unable to afford healthcare insurance altogether. This is a real concern considering employee-sponsored insurance is the primary source of coverage for most Americans under age 65. This means more working families will have less access to the healthcare insurance they need as more employers drop healthcare benefits, and health insurance overall becomes less affordable.[4]

But this is not only a problem for spouses and dependents of employees. It is also a major concern for retirees who face more health problems as they age. Consider the seven-year period from 1993 to 2001. During this period, the percentage of companies with 500 or more employees offering some type of retiree health benefit declined by 17 percent—from 46 percent to 29 percent.[4] It is very unusual to find a retiree whose employer still covers a large portion of their medical expenses. More often people find themselves responsible for covering their own medical expenses, which can be daunting given the rising costs of health care and the increased need for these services in a person's old age.

Equally as dangerous as an inefficient healthcare system on the verge of financial ruin is a system that is beset by lapses in safety. The organization of the current health-care system renders it prone to a host of medical errors, and more will occur if the system is not changed. Take for example the case of one medical center in California. Physicians were putting patients directly in harm's way by performing inappropriate and unnecessary procedures even though the hospital staff were well aware of such unacceptable behavior.[18] How long will these occurrences continue to be tolerated?

To understand how a delivery system can contribute to the poor quality of health, look only as far as the culture under which that system operates. The culture of the healthcare system, comprising many organizations and professionals, is one steeped in secrecy, deference to authority, defensiveness, and protectionism. And despite what people want to believe about dedication to patient interests, all too often these interests are subordinated to the needs of the organizations and the professionals themselves.[18] This illustrates a lack of accountability in the system of healthcare delivery and the inherent, sometimes dangerous implications.

Solutions for Improving Quality

Given the many problems facing the US healthcare system, what can be done to fix it? The only way the quality of health care in the United States will be improved is if all stakeholders take greater responsibility. This includes consumers, employers, insurers, providers, and the government.

First, greater efforts need to be made to get patients more involved in the care they receive. To truly realize the notion of consumer-driven health care it is not enough to simply put more of the financial burden on consumers. They also need to be provided with more information about the health care that they should receive so that they can fully embrace the idea of being responsible for their own health and health-care needs. To be successful though, "that information needs to be authoritative, easily accessible, easy to understand and to act on, and personalized."[8]

In order to have consumer-driven health care, information technology must also be utilized more in the healthcare system. It is believed that the Internet will radically change the way health care is delivered. Information technology has the potential to provide physicians and patients with greater access to medical knowledge, reduce medical errors, enable greater patient-provider communication, and enable more information to be captured in the clinical visit.[8] Until the gains of IT are captured, the healthcare system will continue to be characterized by inadequate quality.

Third, greater transparency and accountability among healthcare organizations and providers need to be put in place. Patients should have information that allows them to make informed decisions when selecting between health plans, healthcare providers, and hospitals. This means that the quality of healthcare provided by hospitals and physicians must be measurable and reported to purchasers and consumers. The metrics should be based on guidelines and standards for care and performance that are devised from general consensus and are widely accepted. Devising guidelines and standards of care will necessitate the cooperation of many parties; ideally, the federal government will take a leading role because it is the only entity that can effectively influence all interested parties.[8,18]

This notion of greater accountability and public reporting is changing the culture of medicine. A more frank discussion of medical errors with patients and among healthcare providers is needed. This will provide a fulfilling environment that not only allows lessons to be learned from mistakes but also sets the stage for appropriate steps to be taken to decrease their occurrence. In addition, an upfront and more frank discussion of errors with patients will foster greater confidence in the healthcare system and will enable the patient to be included in improving patient safety.

Fourth, financial incentives from purchasers and payers must be better aligned to actually encourage, rather than discourage, quality improvements in health care. Health plans that provide pay-for-performance opportunities bring into alignment the needs of providers and purchasers. These plans have the potential to improve efficiency and generate cost-savings that can then be passed on to purchasers in the form of reduced premiums while at the same time demonstrating to purchasers that they are getting more value for their dollar. From a provider standpoint, these economic incentives will further promote the use of evidence-based medicine.[18,19]

Finally, more physicians need to become involved in leadership positions. Of all healthcare providers, a physician's actions are known to influence the largest percentage of healthcare outcomes. Therefore, having physicians in leadership positions, which is more likely to elicit physician "buy-in," will lead to changes in practice patterns and, subsequently, improve quality. Additionally, physicians with skills in both medicine and business can bridge the gap between the administrative and clinical sides of medicine, which will further lead to improvements in the quality of healthcare delivered. However, care improvement ultimately needs to involve *all* system stakeholders, be they nurses, caregivers, hospital administrators, public health program administrators, among others. Only then, can a start be made in addressing and correcting the current system's deficiencies.

Organization of This Book

What follows is a brief description of the sections in this book. In their entirety, these sections illustrate the need for society to take serious steps toward closing the quality chasm through a comprehensive strategy that involves purchasers, providers, employers, and the government.

The first section of the book, *Introduction to Quality in Health Care,* builds a framework for thinking about quality in the context of public health. In this chapter, we defined what we mean by public health and quality, and the relationship between the two. Chapter 2, *Duty Versus Interest,* reviews the literature on how quality issues began in America and how they have reached their state of importance in society today. The various stakeholders within the meshwork of health care and their relationship to quality are analyzed. Chapter 3, *Public Health Implications of Quality Improvement,* reveals how different populations of individuals in America may be affected by the quality chasm. The chapter describes how without proper attempts to define quality, public health concerns for specific members of the health community will be neglected.

Section Two, *The Measures and Tools of Quality Improvement,* provides the framework to understand what quality is, how it can be measured, and how it can be improved. Chapter 4, *Conceptualizing and Improving Quality* establishes a definition of quality and how various stakeholders have examined quality over time. The lack of a clear definition of the concept of quality has provided major obstacles to improving quality. Chapter 5, *Analyzing Quality Data,* discusses traditional challenges of analysis and how newer methods of data collection can help to ease the analytic confusion. Chapter 6, *Fundamentals of Outcomes Measurement* explains the relationship between outcomes measures and quality management. It discusses how an institution dedicated to outcomes management can improve quality. Chapter 7, *Basic Tools for Quality Improvement,* discusses how tools such as evidence-based measures, clinical practice guidelines, report cards, and financial incentives can contribute to improving quality.

Section Three, *Stakeholders in Quality Improvement* provides the framework to understand how the actions of providers, employers, patients, payers, and government can be leveraged to improve quality. Chapters 8, *The Provider's Role in Quality Improvement,* addresses the relevance of physicians to the quality chasm and how they are going to be held more accountable for their actions in the future. Chapter 9, *Employers Focus on Quality,* emphasizes the role of employers in today's healthcare system and how they can encourage greater transparency and accountability. Chapter 10, *A Patient-Centered Approach to Care,* discusses how empowering patients and newer technology will improve quality. Chapter 11, *The Payer's Perspective,* examines the various payment methods that payers have used to improve quality. Chapter 12, *The Government's Perspective,* details the effects of the new Medicare legislation in improving quality in health care and various quality-demonstration projects that are either underway or in planning.

Section Four, *The Future Road to Quality* provides the framework to understand what will keep the quality agenda moving forward. Chapter 13, *Role of Information Technology in Measuring and Improving Quality,* defines information technology and its relationship to improving quality for the major stakeholders in the healthcare industry. Chapter 14, *The Research Agenda for the Future of Health Care,* discusses priorities for future research in quality that will continue to bolster this quality-driven healthcare approach. Chapter 15, *Medical Education for Safety* emphasizes the importance of addressing patient safety for physicians in training, and its influence on the culture of healthcare. Finally, Chapter 16, *Visions of the Future*, addresses the many challenges health care faces in the upcoming years and the need for increased emphasis and understanding of quality improvement.

Study/Discussion Questions

1. Why is quality improvement a public health challenge?
2. What are the six aims proposed by the Institute of Medicine (IOM) for improving quality?
3. What are some potential crises facing the healthcare system if the status quo persists?
4. What are some of the recommended solutions for improving quality?

Suggested Readings/Web Sites

Joint Commission on Accreditation of Healthcare Organizations (www.jcaho.com).
National Committee for Quality Assurance (www.ncqa.org).
National Quality Forum (www.qualityforum.org).
Institute for Healthcare Improvement (www.ihi.org).
Agency for Healthcare Research and Quality (www.ahrq.gov).
Agency for Healthcare Research and Quality. WebM&M (www.webmm.ahrq.gov).
Kohn LT, Corrigan JM, Donaldson MS, eds. *To Err Is Human: Building a Safer Health System.* Washington, DC: National Academy Press; 1999.
Institute of Medicine. *Committee on Quality of Health Care in America. Crossing the Quality Chasm: A New Health System for the Twenty-first Century.* Washington, DC: National Academy Press; 2001.
Gibson R, Singh JP, *Wall of Silence.* Washington, DC: Lifeline Press; 2003.
Wachter RM, Shojania KG. *Internal Bleeding.* New York City, NY: Rugged Land; 2004.

References

1. Institute of Medicine, Committee on Quality of Health Care in America. *Crossing the Quality Chasm: A New Health System for the 21st Century.* Washington, DC: National Academy Press; 2001.
2. Kohn LT, Corrigan JM, Donaldson MS, eds. *To Err Is Human: Building a Safer Health System.* Washington, DC: National Academy Press; 1999.
3. Raffel MW, Raffel NK. *The U.S. Health System: Origins and Functions.* 4th ed. NY: Delmar Publishers, Inc., Albany, 1994.
4. Clinton HR. Now can we talk about health care? *The New York Times Magazine.* April 18, 2004;26–56.

5. Grob GN. *The Deadly Truth: A History of Disease in America.* Cambridge, Mass: Harvard University Press; 2002.

6. McGlynn EA, Asch SM, Adams J, et al. The quality of health care delivered to adults in the United States. *N Engl J Med.* 2003 Jun 26; 348(26): 2635–45.

7. Turnock BJ. *Public Health: What It Is and How It Works.* 2nd ed. Gaithersberg, MD: Aspen Publishers, Inc.; 2001.

8. Steinberg EP. Improving the quality of care—can we practice what we preach? *NEJM.* 2003 Jun 26; 348(26):2681–83.

9. Jencks SF, Cuerdon T, Burwen DR, et al. Quality of medical care delivered to medicare beneficiaries: A profile at state and national levels. *JAMA.* 2000; 284(13):1670–76.

10. Jencks SF, Huff ED, Cuerdon T, et al. Change in the quality of care delivered to medicare beneficiaries, 1998–1999 to 2000–2001. *JAMA.* 2003; 289(3):305-12.

11. National Committee for Quality Assurance. The State of Health Care Quality: 2003. Available at: www.ncqa.org. Accessed on June 15, 2004.

12. Fisher ES, Wennberg, DE, Stukel TA, Gottlieb DJ, Lucas FL, Pinder EL. The implications of regional variations in medicare spending. Part 1: The content, quality, and accessibility of care. *Annals of Internal Medicine.* 2003 Feb 18; 138(4):273–87.

13. Fisher ES, Wennberg, DE, Stukel TA, Gottlieb DJ, Lucas FL, Pinder EL. The implications of regional variations in Medicare spending. Part 2: Health outcomes and satisfaction with care. *Annals of Internal Medicine.* 2003 Feb 18; 138(4):288–98.

14. Leppel K. Racial/ethnic projections of the U.S. retired population. Available at: http://www. iaes.org/conferences/past/philadelphia_52/prelim_program/j15-1/leppel.htm. Accessed on June 1, 2004.

15. Cutler NE. *Advising Mature Clients: The New Science of Wealth Span Planning.* New York: John Wiley & Sons, Inc.; 2002.

16. Reinhardt UE. Does the aging of the population really drive the demand for health care? *Health Affairs.* 2003; 22(6):27–39.

17. Despeignes P. Report: Medicare could go broke by 2019. Available at: www.usatoday.com March 23, 2004. Accessed on May 15, 2004.

18. Walshe K, Shortell S. When things go wrong: How health care organizations deal with major failures. *Health Affairs.* 2004; 23(3): 103–11.

19. Strunk BC, Hurley RE. Paying for quality: Health plans try carrots instead of sticks. Center for Studying Health System Change. Available at http://www.hschange.com/CONTENT/675/. Accessed on June 1, 2004.

Chapter 2

Duty versus Interest

The History of Quality in Health Care

Michael L. Millenson

EXECUTIVE SUMMARY

Like the civil rights movement, the quality improvement movement cast doubts on deeply held traditional beliefs; in this case, those of the individual physician. While it might have been the individual doctor's "duty" to pursue process improvement and outcomes measurement, it was not in his "interest," given traditional financial incentives. As a result, the history of the quality of care movement has been largely invisible—until now. That history can be divided into four eras: Good Doctors Practice Good Medicine, 1847–1948; Good Doctors, Left Alone, Practice Expensive Medicine, 1949–1971; Medicine Encounters Accountability, 1972–1994; and In Search of Safe and Effective Medicine, 1995 to the present.

LEARNING OBJECTIVES/QUESTIONS

1. To identify phases of the quality improvement movement.
2. To recognize early practices in quality measurement and their present-day effects.
3. To understand the history of quality measurement in health care.

KEYWORDS

Outcomes Measurement

End Results

Process Improvement

Purchasers

Accountability

Empowerment

Consumer-Driven Health care

Duty

Interest

Incentives

Safety

Efficiency

There is nothing more difficult to plan, more doubtful of success, nor more dangerous to manage than the creation of a new order of things.

Niccolò Machiavelli, *The Prince* (c. 1513)

Introduction

Years before the Institute of Medicine's call to "cross the quality chasm" between the care patients do receive and the care they should receive, quality-of-care activists were silently clawing their way up from another type of chasm. Those who sought to improve American medicine were largely invisible, the evidence of their efforts pushed deep into an Orwellian memory hole.

Times change. Ernest Amory Codman, the Boston surgeon who pioneered medical outcomes in the second decade of the twentieth century, died impoverished and forgotten. Today, the Joint Commission on Accreditation of Healthcare Organizations (JCAHO) reprints his writings and awards a prestigious annual prize in his name. In the mid-1950s Vergil Slee began using (yes) computers to analyze hospital outcomes. Slee's contributions were largely overlooked for decades. Today, a chair at the School of Public Health of the University of North Carolina is named in his honor.

One of the key instigators of the IOM's quality activities, Donald Berwick today moves easily in the top tiers of American medicine. But Berwick was long a prophet without honor in his own country, leaving his job as a health plan vice president in the late 1980s when fellow physicians paid little heed to his proposals for systemic quality improvement.

Codman would have understood. Toward the close of his life, Codman concluded he failed because doctors and hospitals believed they gained nothing tangible from changing the old ways. He wrote:

> There is a difference between interest and [professional] duty. You do your duty if the work comes to you, but you do not go out of your way to get the work unless it is for your interest.[1]

Much the same duty-versus-interest dichotomy was explored in a different context in biographer Robert Caro's multi-volume examination of the life and times of Lyndon Baines Johnson. When he was in Congress, Johnson owed his Senate Majority Leader post to the support of Southern Democrat segregationists. Nonetheless, he pushed through the first major civil rights legislation since the end of the

Civil War. Was it duty—a quiet sense of moral outrage fueled by his own childhood spent in poverty—that motivated Johnson to maneuver the Civil Rights Act of 1957 into law? Or was it calculated interest—courting crucial Northern support for a presidential bid? The answer goes to the core of Johnson's character, and Caro spends some one thousand pages of his book *Master of the Senate* showing why Johnson's behavior involved both "pragmatism . . . and something higher."[2]

The character of American medicine has been similarly tested by the quality improvement movement. The response has included pragmatism—resisting when possible, giving way when advantageous—and at other, far fewer times, something higher. Like the civil rights movement, the quality improvement movement cast doubts on deeply held traditional beliefs; in this case, those of the individual physician. The quality movement looks at individual care within an epidemiologic context. By contrast, the traditional clinical model, as sociologist Elliot Freidson put it:

> . . . encourage[s] individual deviation from codified knowledge on the basis of personal, firsthand observation of concrete cases. This deviation is called "judgment" or even "wisdom.". . . Since it is intimately bound up with the personal life of the knower . . . it is no wonder it has a dogmatic edge to it, resisting contradiction by embarrassing facts and contorting itself to reconcile contradictions.[3]

Author and philosopher George Santayana wrote, "Those who fail to understand history are doomed to repeat it." Accordingly, the history of past successes and failures to transform American medicine must first be thoroughly understood for the effort to complete that transformation to succeed.

In real life, historical eras usually do not divide neatly. But for purposes of this article, the history of the quality of care movement is grouped into four periods.

Good Doctors Practice Good Medicine: 1847–1948

From the formation of the American Medical Association in 1847, with its public code of ethics, until the publication in 1948 in the *British Medical Journal* of the first randomized controlled clinical trial, medicine struggled to be, and to appear to be, scientific. Absent many reliable quantitative measures, the central measure of scientific rigor became the minimum standards agreed to by professional consensus. These standards offered the opportunity to do well (interest) while also doing good (duty). For example, the Flexner Report in 1910 led to minimum standards for medical education, a good thing that also had the happy economic side effect of allowing scientific physicians to "do well" against competitors.

In 1913 the American College of Surgeons (ACS) was organized to promote professional standards in surgery; other specialties soon followed suit. The ACS also tried to establish minimum quality standards for hospitals. However in 1919, after the first hospital survey results were tallied, they were taken to the basement furnace of a New York hotel where the ACS was meeting and burned; only eighty-nine of 692 hospitals with at least a hundred beds passed the minimum quality standards.[4] Hospitals, though, were unfazed by failure. National Hospital Day was established in 1921 as hospitals began to promote low-cost access to their services by, for example, offering free lines of credit to surgical patients. By the 1930s, only about half of the hospitals met ACS standards, but hospital care had still grown to become one of the largest industries in the nation.[5]

Indeed, Frederick W. Taylor's breakthrough time-and-motion studies and Frank Gilbreth's scientific management research—both aimed at improving business efficiency—found a receptive audience in American medicine and helped create the atmosphere for Flexner's work and for the equally ambitious proposals of Ernest Codman.

Codman sought to improve the "product" of the hospital—cured patients. To increase "efficiency," he said, "every hospital should follow *every* patient it treats long enough to determine whether or not the treatment has been successful, and then to inquire, 'if not, why not?' with a view to preventing similar failures in the future." His End Result Idea employed a standardized "end result card" containing each patient's symptoms, original diagnosis, treatment plan, complications, diagnosis at discharge, and the results of care a year later—what is called longitudinal data. Codman even published five years of end results at a small hospital he started.[6]

The ACS—of which Codman was a founder—unanimously endorsed the End Result Idea in 1913, the same year Henry Ford set up the first moving assembly line for large-scale manufacturing. Yet widespread implementation never occurred—interest versus duty, Codman concluded. He added:

> I am called eccentric for saying in public: that hospitals, if they wish to be sure of improvement, must find out what their results are, must analyze their results, to find their strong and weak points, must compare their results with those of other hospitals [and] must care for what cases they can care for well, and avoid attempting to care for cases [that] they are not qualified to care for well . . . must welcome publicity not only for their successes, but for their errors. . . Such opinions will not be eccentric a few years hence.[7]

Codman's optimism was misplaced. Still, there were hopeful signs. In 1924, Walter Shewhart of Bell Labs invented the control chart, a statistics tool allowing managers to move from inspecting for defects to process redesign. A 1928 article by T. R. Ponton proposed standard comparative statistics to improve hospital efficiency. And in 1934, a study in New York City public schools of how doctors decided on the need for a tonsillectomy came to the startling conclusion that, "variation is not so much due to the differences in the conditions of the children as it is to differences in the viewpoint and standards of the [medical] examiners."[8]

In 1946, with World War II over, Congress wanted to ensure access by all citizens to the scientific miracles, such as penicillin, promised by American medicine. That meant building more and better hospitals, and the Hill-Burton Act passed that year eventually provided hundreds of millions of dollars to do exactly that. Soon, though, the nation started to learn that more care is not always better care.

Good Doctors, Left Alone, Practice Expensive Medicine: 1949–1971

Surgeon Robert T. Morris warned colleagues back in 1908 against "surgical art for art's sake." By the late 1940s, there was an unprecedented outbreak of surgical artistry.

The medical literature documented a virtual plague of unnecessary hysterectomies (many on young women with only a vague preoperative diagnosis), tonsillectomies, and other dubious procedures. Popular magazines in the mid-1950s warned of commercial surgeons, while comedians joked about the wallet biopsy performed in the hospital emergency room before treatment was given.[9]

The "inspecting-in" quality approach epitomized by minimum standards was starting to be challenged in the wider business world. Joseph M. Juran, a colleague of Shewhart's at Bell Labs, published his *Quality Control Handbook*. The savings from reducing "quality waste," he said, amounted to "gold in the mine." W. Edwards Deming's statistical process control methods so impressed the Japanese—Deming was largely ignored in his own country—that they established the Deming Prize to reward companies that excelled using these methods. General Electric's Armand V. Feigenbaum called for "total quality control," asserting that quality was everyone's job. Meanwhile, the ACS gave up trying to inspect-in hospital quality—that is, gave up trying to do it alone, not the approach itself. The surgeons formed a coalition with other medical and hospital organizations that was chartered in 1952 as the Joint Commission on the Accreditation of Hospitals. (The name changed in 1987 to include Healthcare Organizations.)

It was in this atmosphere that Paul Lembcke of the New York State Health Department introduced the medical audit. The phrase was a deliberate tribute to Codman, who had urged hospital trustees to audit clinical results as thoroughly as they would a hospital's financial results.

Lembcke's standardized audit arranged hospital information into disease classifications, verified statements in the clinical record, and independently established the accuracy of test results. The audit also compared performance to outside standards, such as appropriate surgical indicators. The final step compared the audited hospital with a group of hospitals "of acknowledged merit"—an early form of benchmarking.

In 1952 Lembcke reported on appendectomies in twenty-three hospital service areas. The result: "considerably more operations . . . done than are necessary."[10] In the same article Lembcke articulated a standard for appraising quality of care that was far ahead of its time. He wrote: "The best measure of quality is not how well or how frequently a medical service is given, but how closely the result approaches the fundamental objectives of prolonging life, relieving distress, restoring function, and preventing disability."

Lembcke died of a brain tumor in 1964 at age 56. The W. K. Kellogg Foundation—which in 2001 helped lead the Institute of Medicine committee that issued the *Crossing the Quality Chasm* report—recommended Lembcke's audit methodology to a physician-researcher in Michigan using a new tool few people really understood: the computer.

Slee's computerized Professional Activity Study (PAS) system gave hospitals a standardized way to examine their care and compare it to that of other institutions. The medical staff could also use the system to examine individual physician performance, making possible Codman's goal of sending each patient to the best qualified doctor. Still, the PAS involved tedious hand-coding of procedures and transferring those codes to computer punched cards. More to the point, participation was much more a duty than an interest. A pilot study, for example, found that about a third of surgeons who performed ten or more appendectomies a year were consistently wrong in their diagnosis. And the range of hospitalized diabetics who never even had their blood sugar tested ranged from 5 percent to 55 percent.[11]

Things were not much better outside the hospital. Family physicians in North Carolina whose education and training resembled national norms were observed in their offices by internists. Even with observers present, a stunning 45 percent of the family doctors failed to meet such minimal standards as putting the stethoscope directly on the patient's bare chest rather than on clothing.[12]

Yet countervailing forces were slowly building. In 1955, the *Journal of the American Medical Association* (*JAMA*) addressed misuse with the first major article on medical errors, "Hazards of Modern Diagnosis and Therapy—The Price We Pay." The *New England Journal of Medicine* followed the next year with a study on "Diseases of Medical Progress." The list of iatrogenic diseases stretched for pages.[13]

Medicaid for the poor took effect on January 1, 1966, and Medicare for the elderly on July 1, suddenly making the federal government the most powerful payer for health care. By June 1967, the federal government was convening its first national conference on out-of-control Medicare costs.

In 1969 *Marcus Welby, MD* debuted on television, Congress held its first hearings on Medicare fraud by real-life general practitioners; and Richard Nixon became the first US president to declare the existence of a healthcare crisis. "We face a massive crisis in this area . . . in the next two or three years unless something is done about it immediately," proclaimed Nixon in July. As it turned out, it was easier to land a man on the moon than to solve the problems of American medicine.

During the late 1960s and early 1970s, researchers such as Benjamin Barnes, Robert Brook, John Bunker, C. Wesley Eisele, Alan Gittelsohn, Lincoln Moses, Lawrence Mosteller, Duncan Neuhauser, Osler Peterson, Heather Palmer, Beverly Payne, Milton Roemer, Paul Sanazaro, Sam Shapiro, Lawrence Weed, John Wennberg, John Williamson, and others began to publish articles on institutional differences in risk-adjusted death rates, missed diagnoses, practice variation, doctor-induced medical demand, and end-result measurement. Avedis Donabedian's "structure, process, and outcome" construct for evaluating quality of care became the accepted template.[14] Growing evidence documented a dangerous, even fatal, gap between the care patients should receive and the (often costly) care they did receive.

The postwar belief that more is better and the doctor knows best crumbled as it became clear that individual physicians' decisions as to the necessity of "more" too often yielded only a marginal amount of "better"—or even made things worse. For the first time, society began to insist that provider autonomy be balanced with provider accountability.

Medicine Encounters Accountability: 1972–1994

The best-known provision of the Social Security Act Amendments of 1972 expanded Medicare to cover the disabled. The most profound impact, though, might well have been the establishment of Professional Standards Review Organizations (PSROs). These would later be renamed Peer Review Organizations (PROs) and then, later still, Quality Improvement Organizations (QIOs).

The original Medicare legislation read: "Nothing in this title shall be construed to authorize any federal officer or employee to exercise any control over the practice of medicine or the manner in which medical services are provided." Just seven years later, the 1972 amendments authorized Medicare to disallow "any costs unnecessary to the *efficient* [emphasis added] provision of care," an authority that was automatically extended to Medicaid. Put differently, a powerful third-party payer was given the right to second-guess a doctor's decisions about an individual patient—albeit a payer relying on the advice of other doctors—because the scientific validity of those decisions could not be accepted at face value.

The PSRO provisions prompted the formation of a special IOM committee. Its long-forgotten 1974 report, *Advancing the Quality of Health Care*, presciently declared:

> The United States has begun an experiment, unique to world experience,
> that attempts to assure quality in medical care. Many nations have sought
> to assure access to care, but none has established a national system of
> quality assurance.[15]

The report goes on to discuss "bettering the health status and satisfaction of a population," within available societal resources and moving beyond structure and process measures "toward the measurement of the outcomes of care." The committee also calls for communitywide data systems and for informing "consumers [their word] of the relative effectiveness of various health providers . . . so they can make their choices accordingly."

Talk of accountability was in the air. In 1972, the Joint Commission unveiled a new survey system "based primarily on optimal outcomes." British epidemiologist Archie Cochrane published *Effectiveness and Efficiency*, which later became the basis for the evidence-based medicine movement. In Salt Lake City, Latter-Day Saints (later LDS) Hospital installed computerized medication monitoring to prevent adverse drug events. NASA physician Carmault B. (Jack) Jackson, Jr. concluded that if computers could help astronauts land on the moon they could help doctors provide more efficient medical care—so he quit his job to form a company to do exactly that. Again, it was easier to land a man on the moon than to persuade physicians to use computers.

Fending off a Democratic push for national health insurance, President Nixon borrowed Minneapolis pediatric surgeon Paul Ellwood's plan to unleash market forces in the form of health maintenance organizations. In December 1973 Nixon signed the Health Maintenance Organization Act, thereby turning what had been called "prepaid group practices" (long denounced as socialized medicine) into a capitalistic tool for competition based on cost and quality. At the time, about 98 percent of the total insured population was in unmanaged indemnity insurance. Thirty years later, about 2 percent of the privately insured population remained in unmanaged indemnity plans.

Although Ellwood's idea for a national commission for quality assessment was not adopted, other accountability mechanisms outside professional control grew rapidly during the 1970s and have been important ever since. Activist Ralph Nader turned his attention from unsafe automobiles to unsafe medical care and formed a consumer watchdog called the Public Interest Health Research Group. Congress stopped Hill-Burton funding of new hospitals and began its own watchdog hearings on unnecessary surgery, starting with tonsillectomies. The Employee Retirement Income Security Act of 1974 did not mention health care, but its provisions allowed employers to self-insure and avoid state regulation. That, in turn, led to large corporations banding together in coalitions to share knowledge and control healthcare costs. (Employers were paying twice as much for employee healthcare in 1980 as in 1975.) Victor Fuchs's *Who Shall Live?* sparked a national conversation about medical rationing—by hospitals and doctors. Concern about rationing by health plans was not even a blip on the health policy horizon. A Supreme Court decision of 1975, meanwhile, opened the way for professionals to advertise and even compete on price—a key ingredient of a functioning market.

In 1977, the Health Care Financing Administration (HCFA) was formed to oversee Medicare and Medicaid. In 2001, HCFA was renamed the Centers for Medicare & Medicaid Services (the use of the ampersand in its name allowed it to be legally known as CMS rather than CMMS). The national Blue Cross and Blue Shield Association flexed its muscles by listing surgical and medical procedures it considered obsolete and inappropriate, but use of the list by local Blues plans was voluntary. Also voluntary was the "consensus development" program begun by the National Institutes of Health. As were hospital cost controls, mandatory controls proposed by the Carter Administration were defeated in Congress in 1979.

Voluntarism unaccompanied by incentives proved ineffective, and so-called appropriate care began increasingly to be defined by outsiders. Insurers began to adopt mandatory second opinions and utilization review. On October 1, 1983, in a radical break with past policy, Medicare began changing hospital payment from a cost-plus method to a prospective payment method that set prices based on the average cost of treating a particular diagnosis (also known as Diagnosis Related Groups, or DRGs). Economic efficiency—a steep drop in the use of hospital inpatient services—did not affect the quality of care, although it did lead to an increase in outpatient procedures and the cost of those procedures. In 1988, physician payment was changed from a straight-fee basis to one involving a resource-based relative value scale (RB-RVS).

In the mid-1980s Congress discovered Wennberg's work on small-area practice variations, and used it to ask the politically attractive question: "How much money could we save if the lowest rate was the norm?" *The Painful Prescription* by Henry J. Aaron and William Schwartz of the Brookings Institution, became a bestseller when it raised the possibility of medical rationing.

Media coverage of healthcare began to probe deeper. In 1973, *Newsday* reporter David Zinman revealed that Nassau County Medical Center had nearly triple the death rate for bypass surgery as the second-worst Long Island hospital, and nine times the rate of the best one.

In 1986, a Freedom of Information Act request from Joel Brinkley of *The New York Times* forced HCFA to release hospital mortality data, a practice it then regularized until early in the Clinton Administration. That same year Congress passed the Health Care Quality Improvement Act, aimed primarily at "bad" doctors and hospitals (i.e., those guilty of malpractice or of turning away the uninsured), while Berwick—turned on by colleague Paul Batalden to the potential of applying Deming's teachings to medicine—started a national demonstration project on continuous quality improvement in healthcare.

The triumph of accountability in medicine seemed inevitable in the late 1980s and early 1990s. The Joint Commission announced an outcomes-based Agenda for Change. The journal *Inquiry* devoted its spring 1988 issue to "the challenge of quality," including a detailed examination of the work of Codman. And the editor of the *New England Journal of Medicine* proclaimed the arrival of "Era of Assessment and Accountability."[16]

Congress set up the Agency for Health Care Policy and Research in 1989, and the American Medical Association (AMA) endorsed "practice parameters" (eschewing the word, guidelines) the next year. Meanwhile, a 1990 IOM report provided a definition of quality to supplant the "I know it when I see it" hegemony of individual practitioner judgment. Wrote the IOM: "Quality consists of the degree to which health services for individuals and populations increase the likelihood of desired health outcomes consistent with current professional knowledge and patient expectations."[17] In 1991, the Harvard Medical Practice Study caused a blip of interest in medical errors, as had a somewhat less comprehensive national study, with similar results, in 1975.[18] Both studies, by their own admission, were motivated in signifi-cant part by physician concern over high malpractice premiums.

An AMA poll in 1993 found that 70 percent of respondents were beginning to lose faith in their doctors, with 69 percent thinking doctors were too interested in making money. Managed care membership rose steadily. Riding a wave of popular support for healthcare reform, newly elected president Bill Clinton introduced an ambitious Health Security Act designed to simultaneously address access, cost, and quality problems. It drew on the "managed competition" approach of Ellwood, Alain Enthoven, and Lynn Etheridge.

By the fall of 1994, however, the Clinton health plan was dead—pilloried as tak-ing control away from doctors and giving it to bureaucrats and health plans—and Republicans, with an interest in privatization, had taken control of both houses of Congress. Managed care organizations—HMOs and variations on the theme—that were supposed to manage costs while ensuring high-quality care found themselves accused of rationing care to ensure low costs. The presence of new organizations such as the National Committee for Quality Assurance, whose mission was to intro-duce standardized quality measures into managed care, did nothing to stem the tide of public distrust. The subsequent managed care backlash left HMOs at the same level of public esteem as car salesmen and tobacco companies.

The economy was booming, while healthcare inflation—thanks to managed care economic clout and the political threat of reforming high-cost providers—was low. The pressure to pursue the duty of accountability weakened. A renewed push had to wait for renewed public concern over the cost and quality of care.

In Search of Safe and Effective Medicine: 1995–Present

On March 23, 1995, a page one article in the *Boston Globe* related the tragic tale of a 39-year-old mother with breast cancer who died after a hospital administered a massive overdose of a powerful anti-cancer drug. A tragic irony was the fact the patient, Betsy Lehman, was the medical columnist for the *Globe*. A further incon-gruity: The hospital was the nationally renowned Dana-Farber Cancer Institute. "If this can happen at a place like Dana-Farber," one anguished expert asked, "what is happening in other places?"[19]

What, indeed? In Grand Rapids, a surgeon performing a mastectomy on a 69-year-old woman removed the wrong breast. A New York woman died when a doctor mistook her dialysis catheter for a feeding tube and pumped food into her abdomen. At Tampa's University Community Hospital, a 51-year-old diabetic had the wrong foot amputated; a 77-year-old retired electrician died when a therapist mistakenly disconnected his ventilator; and a female patient got arthroscopic surgery on the wrong knee.[20]

None of these incidents, of course, had anything to do with managed care. Shaken, the leaders of American medicine began to reassess the lessons of the Harvard Medical Practice study and the subsequent work of study co-author Lucian Leape. The news media, meanwhile, began to shine a spotlight on medical safety problems. The IOM report *To Err Is Human,* issued in late 1999, showed the influence of converging trends. The report combined tragic stories of real people (taken from the news media); the "don't blame individuals, change the systems" approach of continuous quality improvement doctrine; a compelling summary of health services research; and a savvy penchant for sound bites.[21]

Phrases like "44,000 to 98,000 preventable deaths in hospitals each year"; "more deaths than from motor vehicle accidents, breast cancer, or AIDS"; and "the equivalent of two 747s crashing every three days" caught the eye of the public and politicians. State and federal legislation targeting error reporting (the federal database relied on voluntary reporting) followed, as did renewed attention by doctor and hospital groups.

In 1998 the generalized warnings about widespread and serious care problems by a presidential commission and an IOM quality committee had drawn little attention. The notable exception was the "Patient's Bill of Rights," adopted by the US Advisory Commission on Consumer Protection and Quality in the Healthcare Industry. Now, the pendulum began to swing back from a focus on access to a more balanced consideration of what the access was *to.* Every layperson could understand that bad care cost money and lives. The "overuse, underuse, and misuse" denounced by the 1998 IOM committee report found new resonance in the 2001 *Chasm* report when linked to potential savings of as much as 30 percent of national healthcare expenditures—thereby echoing the "quality is free" mantra of industrial quality improvement.[22]

Value purchasing—looking at quality as well as cost—became the purchaser's battle cry, if not always a behavior.[23] Evidence-based medicine evolved from oddity into accepted wisdom. In November 2000 a coalition of Fortune 500 employers called The Leapfrog Group launched an initiative whose centerpiece was pushing hospitals to undertake a series of evidence-based safety and quality steps. Ninety years after Codman's "eccentric" proposals, "pay for performance" started to become a routine purchasing tool, even for Medicare. Monetary incentives melded "duty" and "interest," and of course purchasers now needed some sort of medical audit to ensure the reliability of results.

By 2001 the economy was no longer booming, and the nation was at war. At a time of federal and state budget deficits and intense cost pressures on US businesses, the impact of rising healthcare expenditures took on a strategic national significance. Providers, payers, and plans alike worried about potential government regulation and the cost of overlapping and duplicative private efforts (interest)—as well as the ability to provide the best possible care (duty). So they joined together in a voluntary National Quality Forum to develop a consensus on safety and quality standards. In this they were aided by the Agency for Healthcare Research and Quality, as AHCPR had been renamed. The "national system of quality assurance" referred to by the IOM in 1974 took a step closer to reality with the issuance in 2003 by AHRQ of the first National Healthcare Quality Report.

Technology emerged as a powerful force to destabilize tradition. In the Internet Age, professional knowledge is far more difficult to protect; the amount of sophisticated health information easily available to patients has exploded. Meanwhile, the benchmarking of providers that was the goal of Slee's Professional Activity Study, already available through risk-adjusted Medicare claims data, was now encouraged on a more sophisticated basis by the spread of electronic medical records (EMRs). The potential of EMRs for improving health system efficiency was so clear that implementation drew widespread political and business community support.

By 2004, disease management firms hired by health plans and employers routinely used telephone call centers and Web-enabled guidelines to bring evidence-based care to patients with chronic ills. Nurses called patients and physicians directly to try to influence them to follow best evidence—and, of course, save money in the process.

The social power of consumerism, the pressures of cost, and the widespread availability of digitized information combined to make patients the kind of partners in their own health care as was envisioned by the quality movement's pioneers. While hope and hype still exceeded reality, interest by employers and policymakers alike in consumer-driven health care promised to accelerate the process, particularly at a time when the presidency and both houses of Congress were controlled by a political party that championed the use of market forces. Indeed, the roots of consumer-driven health care derive from the work of political conservatives who championed the power of market-driven purchasing behavior.[24] It was an idea employers and consultants found particularly attractive after managed care plans lost much of their clout. And financial motives notwithstanding, consumer-driven healthcare offered the promise of patient empowerment in a clinical sense, as well. Costs can be controlled by giving consumers a greater financial incentive to spend health insurance funds wisely while—and this is crucial—providing information on healthcare quality to allow consumers to accomplish that goal.

Implementation issues were key to this goal. Early research released in mid-2004 found that little reliable information was available to consumers on cost or quality of care, and there remained significant concerns as to whether this model of care could actually enhance overall system performance.[25] Nonetheless, enrollment in the plans was expected to increase exponentially from a modest base of about one million in 2004. The search for safe and effective medicine was not near completion as 2004 came to an end; rather, the momentum promised only to accelerate in the years ahead.

The Lessons of History

The success of the civil rights movement in the 1960s grew out of social, economic, and technologic changes that swept through post-World War II America—changes that were exploited by an inspired leadership. The problems were not new; the response to them was. Similarly, little of today's knowledge about quality-of-care problems is new. What has changed are the social, economic, and technologic forces that affect the healthcare system and, perhaps, the leadership exerted by those who make their living within that system. Genuine transformation, however, will be slow.

The physicist Max Planck wrote: "A new scientific truth does not triumph by convincing its opponents and making them see the light, but rather because its opponents eventually die, and a new generation grows up that is familiar with it." Perhaps, then, someday all doctors will use information technology as a matter of course to practice safe and evidence-based care in partnership with patients—perhaps those doctors have just been born.

Case Study

The Professional Activity Study (PAS) was one of the first efforts to measure quality in a healthcare setting. While working as a county health officer and hospital administrator, Vergil Slee, MD, found it difficult to measure the health and well-being of people in his community and whether or not their healthcare needs were being met. Information was garnered by going to each hospital, looking through individual patient records, and then manually recording the desired data.

In 1954, Dr. Slee initiated a pilot program to systematically collect statistical information from patient records as a means to analyze individual hospital clinical care and comparatively study thirteen area hospitals. This program became PAS.

PAS has been criticized for a lack of uniform definitions and calculations. In addition, some believe the program collected too much data that was unusable. Nevertheless, Dr. Slee laid the groundwork for future measurement tools.

Study/Discussions Questions

1. What is the distinction between interest and duty?
2. What are the factors that have contributed to the historical resistance to the quality improvement movement and how might these barriers be overcome in the future?
3. What role did the federal government play in bringing the issue of quality measurement in health care to the forefront?

Suggested Readings/Web Sites

Aaron HJ, Schwartz WB. *The Painful Prescription: Rationing Hospital Care.* Washington, D.C.: Brookings Institution; 1984.

Mallon WJ. *Ernest Amory Codman: The End Result of a Life in Medicine.* Philadelphia, PA: Saunders; 2000.

Millenson ML. *Demanding Medical Excellence: Doctors and Accountability in the Information Age.* Chicago: University of Chicago Press; 1997 hardback and 1999 paperback with updated afterword.

Rosenberg C. *The Care of Strangers.* New York: Basic; 1987.

Starr P. *The Social Transformation of American Medicine.* New York: Basic; 1982.

Stevens R. *American Medicine and the Public Interest.* New Haven: Yale University Press; 1971.

Stevens R. *In Sickness and In Wealth.* New York: Basic; 1989/

Quality and Safety in Health Care (journal) (http://qhc.bmjjournals.com/).

References

1. Codman EA. The product of a hospital. *Surg Gynecol Obste.* Apr 1914; 18:491–96.

2. Caro RA. *The Years of Lyndon Johnson: Master of the Senate.* New York: Alfred A. Knopf; 2002.

3. Freidson E. *Profession of Medicine: A Study of the Sociology of Applied Knowledge.* New York: Dodd, Mead; 1970.

4. Roberts JS, Coale JG, Redman RR. A history of the Joint Commission on Accreditation of Hospitals. *JAMA.* 1987 Aug 21; 258(7):936–40.

5. Stevens R. *In Sickness and in Wealth: American Hospitals in the Twentieth Century.* New York: Basic; 1989.

6. Millenson ML. *Demanding Medical Excellence: Doctors and Accountability in the Information Age.* Chicago: University of Chicago; 1997.

7. Codman EA. *A Study in Hospital Efficiency.* Oakbrook Terrace, Illinois: Joint Commission on Accreditation of Healthcare Organizations; 1996. Reprint of 1917 text with extra commentary material.

8. *American Child Health Association. Physical Defects: The Pathway to Correction.* American Child Health Association; 1934.

9. Millenson. 149–50.

10. Lembcke PA. Measuring the quality of medical care through vital statistics based on hospital service areas: 1. Comparative study of appendectomy rates. *Am J Public Health.* 1952; 42(3):276–86.

11. Millenson. 153–56.

12. Peterson OL, et al. An analytical study of North Carolina general practice. *J Med Educ.* 1956; 31(2):1–65.

13. Moser RH. Diseases of medical progress. *NEJM.* 1956 Sept 27; 255(13):606–14.

14. Donabedian A. Evaluating the quality of medical care. *Milbank Memorial Fund Quarterly.* 1966; 44(2):166–203.

15. Institute of Medicine. *Advancing the Quality of Healthcare: Key Issues and Fundamental Principles.* A policy statement by a committee of the Institute of Medicine. Washington, DC: National Academy of Sciences. August; 1974.

16. Relman AS. Assessment and accountability: The third revolution in medical care. *NEJM.* 1988; 319(18):1220–22.

17. Lohr KN, ed. *Medicare: A Strategy for Quality Assurance.* Washington, DC: National Academy Press; 1990.

18. Mills DH. Medical insurance feasibility study—a technical summary. *West J Med.* 1978; 128(4):360–65. Brennan TA, Leape LL, Laird NM, et al. The incidence of adverse events and negligence in hospitalized patients: Results of the Harvard Medical Practice Study, I. *NEJM.* 1991; 324(6):370–76.

19. Knox RA. Doctor's orders killed cancer patient. *Boston Globe.* March 23, 1995:A1.

20. Millenson. 53.

21. Institute of Medicine, Committee on Quality of Health Care in America. *To Err Is Human: Building a Safer Health System.* Washington, DC: National Academy Press; 1999.

22. Institute of Medicine, Committee on Quality of Health Care in America. *Crossing the Quality Chasm: A New Health System for the 21st Century.* Washington, DC: National Academy Press; 2001.

23. Maio V, Goldfarb NI, Carter C, Nash DB. Value-based purchasing: A review of the literature. The Commonwealth Fund, Report No. 636, May 2003. Available at: http://www.cmwf .org/programs/quality/maio_valuebased_636.pdf. Accessed on August 1, 2004.

24. Goodman JC, Musgrave GL. *Patient Power: The Free-Enterprise Alternative to Clinton's Health Plan.* Washington, DC: Cato Institute; 1994.

25. Davis K. Consumer-directed health care. Will it improve health system performance? *HSR.* 2004; 39(4):1219–33.

Public Health Implications of Quality Improvement

How to Implement National Quality Goals at the Local Level

Clair M. Callan
Erin T. O'Brien
Karen S. Kmetik
Margaret C. Toepp

EXECUTIVE SUMMARY

Everyone is affected by the public's health, not just those who are ill. A healthy nation and a sound public health infrastructure have the potential to lower health-care costs, reduce the number of school and work days missed, and increase the quality and years of life.

Historical interventions to improve public health have mirrored historical epidemics: containment of communicable diseases, public education campaigns, and government-mandated vaccinations. These interventions were effective for acute illnesses and outbreaks of infections. In contrast, today's epidemics are largely chronic illnesses; therefore, today's public health interventions must be designed to address long-term diseases. Quality improvement represents the nation's best approach to reducing the burden of chronic illness.

The United States stands poised to address the health of the entire public, especially vulnerable populations who are disproportionately burdened by chronic illness. Now more than ever, national quality reports are beginning to identify where the gaps in care occur. From these gaps, national goals are established to improve health care. Quality improvement tools to be used at the individual patient level currently exist to help meet these national goals by treating all Americans with high quality, evidence-based care. Tools such as clinical performance measures and information technology can be the link between local efforts and national initiatives.

The medical profession has an obligation to embrace today's information and quality revolutions to ensure that all patients receive consistent, safe, and effective health care.

LEARNING OBJECTIVES

1. To be aware of national gaps in care, using the application of cardiovascular care as an example.
2. To recognize that racial/ethnic minority populations are disproportionately affected by gaps in care.
3. To understand how current national quality initiatives involving performance measurement and information technology (IT) are implemented at the local level.
4. To envision how local data can be aggregated to inform national goals.

KEYWORDS

Disparities

Vulnerable populations

Performance measures

Introduction

It has been said that all politics is local. Environmental issues are proclaimed on bumper stickers as "Think globally, Act locally." In health care it can be argued that all quality improvement is local. The term public health refers to global, population-based health care. Improving public health, however, requires local information and action, in the physician's office, at the point of care.

In July 2004, the US National Coordinator for Health Information Technology, David Brailer, MD, PhD, described a new vision for healthcare made possible through the use of information technology (IT).[1] Of the three specific strategies he outlined for improving population health, the following highlights the view that quality improvement stems from local activity:

> Strategy 2: Many different state and local organizations collect subsets of data for specific purposes and use it in different ways. A streamlined quality-monitoring infrastructure that will allow for a complete look at quality and other issues in real-time and at the point of care is needed.

This strategy is within grasp. The potential to dramatically improve the availability of individual and population health data and in turn to act on that data is tremendous.

Tools and standards currently exist to collect valid, reliable data on the quality of care delivered; however, they have not yet been uniformly applied. Moreover, to be effective these quality measurement initiatives must be applied consistently and equally to all practice locations. Dr. Brailer's vision for the role IT will play in improving the quality and efficiency of the nation's health care must not exclude the thousands of health centers caring for vulnerable populations. Safety nets in the United States cannot be left behind in this IT revolution. To do so would perpetuate vulnerable populations' susceptibility to substandard care and poor health outcomes.

This chapter is organized in four major sections. First, cardiovascular disease (CVD) is used as a focus condition for this chapter. Next, the national picture for population health is discussed: quality gaps in CVD care, particularly for vulnerable populations; national health care goals for CVD; and national quality initiatives involving performance measures and IT. Third, local quality efforts are explored as they relate to the larger national picture. Finally, the circle is completed by offering a pathway by which local quality initiatives can be used to influence regional health care, and eventually national healthcare. Using the cardiovascular objectives set forth in Healthy People 2010 as national goals, it will be demonstrated how public health can be impacted by local measurement and quality improvement.

National Measurement Supports National Goals: Tangible Application at the Local Level

To think globally and act locally in public health using a quality improvement framework requires a clear statement of purpose for the healthcare system, national goals to support that purpose, and translation of these goals into local action.[2] Just as the assessment of the nation's health care shapes national healthcare goals, so too should an assessment of the local health care picture shape local goals.

Over the last several decades, the healthcare needs of Americans have shifted from primarily acute, episodic care to long-term care for chronic conditions. Chronic illnesses are now the leading causes of death and disability in the United States, and 40 percent of patients with a chronic condition have more than one.[3]

Identification of a Health Condition

By way of example, consider why cardiovascular disease (CVD) has been identified as a target condition for national health goals.

Among all chronic conditions, CVD is the leading cause of morbidity and mortality, and accounts for the majority of the nation's healthcare costs. Cardiovascular disease was responsible for 38.5 percent of all deaths in 2001. Diseases of the heart and strokes are also the leading causes of death among males and females who are

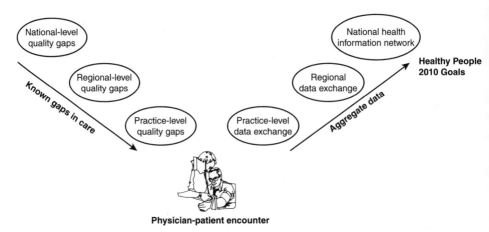

Figure 3–1 *Clinical Performance Measurement Impacts Patient Care and Influences Population Health*

Caucasian, African American, Hispanic, Asian American, Pacific Islander, American Indian, or Alaska Native.[4] In terms of prevalence, more than 64 million Americans, 40 percent of whom are over age 65, have one or more types of CVD. By 2010, an estimated 40 million Americans will be over age 65 years. The three most prevalent types of CVD are:[5]

- Hypertension (HTN)—50 million men and women
- Coronary Artery Disease (CAD)—13.2 million men and women
- Heart Failure (HF)—5 million men and women

Racial and ethnic minority populations are disproportionately affected by CVD. Compared to 6 percent of whites with CAD, the prevalence among African Americans and Mexican Americans is 8 percent and 7 percent respectively. African Americans have a 43 percent prevalence of HTN, compared to 31 percent in the white population and 32 percent of Mexican Americans.[6]

National Picture of CVD: A Target for Quality Improvement

Before specific national quality improvement strategies for CVD are developed, a baseline assessment of the nation's current quality of care for this condition is an important first step.

Data on Gaps in Care for CVD

A baseline assessment of the nation's current quality of care for CVD shows significant gaps that, if addressed, could improve care (see Figure 3-1). Despite conclusive evidence for the use of medications and therapies, patients with CVD are not being optimally managed for their disease, and prevention efforts are similarly disappointing. For example:

- Rates for blood pressure screening are 90 percent. However, only 25 percent of people with HTN have it under control.[7]
- Approximately 11 percent of patients with known HTN are not receiving pharmacotherapy.
- Although the cholesterol screening rate for patients age 45 or older is 80 percent, the rate for patients under age 45 is only 53 percent.[7]
- Both aspirin and beta-blocker therapy are underused in the management of patients with CAD, despite conclusive evidence of distinct long-term benefits. Approximately 21 percent of Medicare patients hospitalized for an acute myocardial infarction were not prescribed a beta-blocker on discharge.[8]
- In 2002, only about 44 percent of patients with CAD who did not have a contraindication to aspirin were using aspirin prophylactically.[9] Two thirds of patients with elevated cholesterol levels were not receiving lipid-lowering medication.[10]
- While studies show a gradual increase in the use of ACE inhibitors in the 1990s, current utilization remains less than optimal for patients with HF.[9]

McGlynn and colleagues telephoned a random sample of adults to ask them about specific healthcare encounters, then reviewed their medical charts.[11] They discovered that participants received 55 percent of recommended care. In general, care requiring an encounter or other intervention (e.g., the annual visit recommended for patients with HTN) had the highest rates of adherence (73 percent), and processes involving counseling or education (e.g., advising smokers with chronic obstructive pulmonary disease to quit smoking) had the lowest rates of adherence (18 percent). For CAD specifically, McGlynn et al. reported adherence to the guidelines occurred about 68 percent of the time.

Data also shows gaps in care for vulnerable populations. By definition, vulnerable populations, such as underserved patients, are at some form of disadvantage in the healthcare system.[12] The addition of substandard care and healthcare disparities puts these patients in a double jeopardy situation. Underserved populations become ill more often because of lack of access to primary care and preventive services; poor quality care only serves to keep them ill longer. In this way, inconsistent and substandard care increases the vulnerability of patients already at risk for poor outcomes.

The Institute of Medicine (IOM) report *Unequal Treatment: What Healthcare Providers Need to Know about Racial and Ethnic Disparities in Healthcare* received a great deal of attention both for its comprehensive examination of variations in care and for the actual data, which lent validity to the observations. The IOM defines health disparities as, "racial or ethnic differences in the quality of health care that are not due to access-related factors or clinical needs, preferences, and appropriateness of intervention."[13] Racial and ethnic disparities in health care constitute significant barriers to ongoing quality improvement activities, because they signify a systematic bias that the provider must overcome. Minority race/ethnicity has been linked to a lower likelihood of having a regular source of care, fewer physician visits, less intensive hospital visits, and lower total healthcare expenditures.[13]

Literature reviewed by the IOM study committee found minority race or ethnicity to be linked to disparities in receipt of appropriate cancer diagnostic tests and treatment; screening, diagnostic, and therapeutic interventions for heart disease and stroke; diabetes care; clinical procedures for cerebrovascular disease; HIV care; renal transplantation; asthma care; and a range of other preventive and specialty health services. Most studies have examined disparities in healthcare only among adult populations. However, racial and ethnic minority children and adolescents are also at considerable disadvantage, with minority status associated with a lower likelihood of: a usual source of care,[14] treatment for common but significant health problems, access to selected preventive services,[15] and medications.[16]

The following statistics reflect the current disparities in cardiovascular care, suggesting there is much work to be done to reach the Healthy People 2010 objective for CVD:[13]

- Thrombolytics

  Caucasian patients were 50 percent more likely to receive thrombolytics than African American patients, after controlling for patients' gender, education, and age.

- Cardiac procedures

  African-American and Hispanic patients are less likely to receive angioplasty; African Americans were less likely to receive CABG, after controlling for patients' gender, education, and age.

- Medications

  Mexican Americans received 38 percent fewer medications than whites, after controlling for patients' gender, education, and age.

There is growing consensus regarding the need to integrate efforts to eliminate disparities in health care with clinical quality improvement strategies.[17,18] While the pathways through which socioeconomic position and race/ethnicity affect health care are complex, quality is a natural lever for advancing the dialogue on the issue of disparities among physicians, nurses, healthcare organizations, insurance agencies, government, accreditation agencies, and consumers.[17] The use of standardized clinical performance measures to identify and address disparities in healthcare enables clinicians to track individual patient care over time and pinpoint areas that require improvement (e.g., whether or not patient received at least one lipid profile each year). Currently, there is no consensus regarding the value of assessing quality by race or ethnicity.[18]

National Goals for CVD Care

Given the statistics on gaps in care for CVD and disparities in care, national goals for this condition have been established in Healthy People 2010. Healthy People 2010, a comprehensive set of objectives for the nation to achieve in the first decade of this century, represents a high-level initiative to streamline national efforts to attain good quality care for all populations. The two overarching goals are to 1) increase quality and years of healthy life, and 2) eliminate health disparities. The Healthy People 2010 objective for cardiovascular health is:[19]

> Improve cardiovascular health and quality of life through the prevention, detection, and treatment of risk factors; early identification and treatment of heart attacks and strokes; and prevention of recurring cardiovascular events.

National Clinical Performance Measures and Tools for CVD

Nationally accepted, evidence-based performance measures are an integral step toward reaching the objectives set forth by Healthy People 2010. A clinical performance measure is a mechanism that enables the user to quantify the quality of a selected aspect of care by comparing it to a criterion.[13] Measures facilitate the delivery of clinical services that are appropriate for the patient in the optimal time period. Evidence-based measures developed by the medical profession for CAD, HTN, and HF currently exist.

The AMA convenes the Physician Consortium for Performance Improvement (called the Consortium) in an effort to fulfill the medical profession's responsibility to deliver high quality health care to all Americans. The Consortium is a national, physician-led initiative comprising clinical experts representing more than sixty national medical specialty societies, medical state associations, methodology experts, the Agency for Healthcare Research and Quality (AHRQ), and the Centers for Medicare & Medicaid Services (CMS). The Consortium is dedicated to the development and implementation of standardized, evidence-based performance measures and tools to give the provider quality improvement activities. For medical providers, the measurement tools also promote improved patient care by providing them with comprehensive feedback reports that aid in managing their patients' conditions.

Consortium Measurements for CVD Gain National Attention

In response to the known gaps and goals for CVD, the Consortium began collaborating on the development of performance measures with the nation's leading guideline developers for CVD: the American College of Cardiology (ACC) and the American Heart Association (AHA). The ACC is a professional society of more than 25,000 cardiovascular physicians and scientists committed to providing optimal cardiovascular care. The AHA is a national voluntary health organization with more than 30,000 scientist and physician volunteers dedicated to reducing disability and death from CVD and stroke. Together these groups have joined with the Consortium to ensure that the cardiovascular community speaks with one voice on clinical performance measurement.

The ACC/AHA clinical guidelines were the basis for the physician-level performance measures. Table 3-1 illustrates the performance measure for beta-blocker therapy from the CAD measurement set. The ACC/AHA/AMA Consortium measures are designed with the flexibility to accommodate physician and patient judgment for all measures related to prescribed medications. This flexibility results in a clinically realistic assessment of performance without adverse consequences from performance scores.

These CVD measures are gaining national attention. The National Quality Forum (NQF), a private, not-for-profit membership organization created to develop and implement a national strategy for healthcare quality measurement and reporting, is conducting an expedited review process for the CVD and other measures to identify a clinical measurement set for NQF's Ambulatory Care Project. The initial measurement set to be reviewed by NQF is a collection of process measures developed by three leading organizations: the AMA/Consortium, CMS, and the National Committee for Quality Assurance (NCQA). The mission of the NQF is to improve American health care through endorsement of consensus-based national standards for measurement and public reporting of healthcare performance data that provide meaningful information about whether care is safe, timely, beneficial, patient-centered, equitable, and efficient.

Table 3-1 *Performance Measure for Beta-Blocker Therapy*[20]

Clinical Recommendation	Performance Measure
Beta-blocker therapy is recommended for all patients with prior MI in the absence of contraindications (Class I Recommendation, Level A Evidence)	**Per Patient:** Whether or not patient with prior MI was prescribed beta-blocker therapy **Per Patient Population:** Percentage of patients with prior MI who were prescribed beta-blocker therapy
	Denominator Inclusion: Prior MI Denominator Exclusion: Documentation that beta-blocker was not indicated; documentation of medical reason(s) (e.g., contraindication, allergy) for not prescribing a beta-blocker; documentation of a patient reason(s) (e.g., economic, religious) for not prescribing a beta-blocker

Source: The ACC/AHA/AMA Consortium

In addition, to facilitate measurement standardization across all populations, the AMA is working with the Bureau of Primary Health Care (BPHC) to align data elements from Consortium performance measures with data elements from the BPHC's Health Disparities Collaboratives performance measures. The BPHC is the federal bureau within the Health Resources and Services Administration responsible for funding the Community Health Center (CHC) program. This program is a federal grant program funded under Section 330 of the Public Health Service Act to provide for primary and preventive healthcare services in medically underserved areas throughout the United States and its territories. The cooperative venture between the BPHC and the AMA will enable health centers to collect standardized data that satisfy multiple national initiatives. The Health Disparities Collaboratives represent a systematic approach to transforming the way health care is delivered, starting with the collection of performance measures across all participating sites.[21] Health centers that join the Collaboratives submit data on process measures to a Web-based registry. Aggregate data is then returned to the centers to guide their quality improvement efforts.

Measuring Race, Ethnicity, and Primary Language to Understand Disparities

In addition to the collection of clinical data via performance measures, the IOM report on unequal treatment calls for the collection of racial, ethnic, and primary language data as well. Collection of these statistics as part of a quality improvement strategy will increase awareness and support the potential elimination of health disparities.

To ensure that race, ethnicity, and language data is collected in a uniform manner, the Health Research and Education Trust (HRET), the research arm of the American Hospital Association, has been working on a project since 2003 to develop a framework for collecting race, ethnicity, and primary language data in hospitals and clinics. This framework was conceived as a first step in addressing disparities in health care and lays the foundation for long-term efforts to improve quality of care and reduce disparities for vulnerable populations. Clinics can select a set of clinical conditions and a core set of measures—stratified by race, ethnicity, and primary language—to track over time and examine the care process. They can then develop targeted interventions to improve quality of care. The HRET developed this framework for collecting data on patient race, ethnicity, and primary language by utilizing the Office of Management and Budget Standards for Classification of Federal Data on Race and Ethnicity.[22]

To date, this framework has been tested solely in the hospital setting. The AMA has begun collaborating with HRET to pilot test the framework in the outpatient environment, namely at urban community health centers. The goal is to marry data collected via the uniform framework with clinical data collect via the uniform performance measures developed by the AMA/Consortium. In this way, performance measures can be stratified by demographic variables, allowing for in-depth analysis of where the gaps exist, followed by targeted interventions.

National Goals for Information Technology

Performance measures alone are not sufficient to improve health care. According to Donald Berwick, a national champion for performance measurement and improvement, "[I]n the pursuit of healthcare quality improvement, measurement is necessary but is no more sufficient than measuring a golf score makes for better golf."[2]

Following Berwick's analogy, performance measures provide a snapshot, or baseline assessment of current care being delivered at a specific point in time. Knowing that 40 percent of patients in a practice receive recommended medication therapy for a given instance is a necessary starting point, but does not in itself improve that rate. However, if more data is captured about these patients at the time they were in the physician's office—such as recent laboratory results, allergies, whether or not the patient received the medication from another physician, and patient preference—improvement could occur.

National leaders have identified IT as a vehicle to facilitate the availability of data at the point of care, and to support evidence-based measures. With IT, physicians can quickly access a patient's medical history, radiography or laboratory results, and treatment preferences to make care more patient-centered. In April 2004, President Bush called for widespread adoption of interoperable electronic health record system (EHRS) within ten years. To reach this objective, Dr. Brailer has formulated a strategic framework to incrementally advance our nation's use of IT in health care. The four national goals highlighted in David Brailer's report are:[1]

- *Goal 1—Inform Clinical Practice:* Bringing information tools to the point of care, especially by investing in EHRS in physician offices and hospitals.
- *Goal 2—Interconnect Clinicians:* Building an interoperable health information infrastructure, so that records follow the patient and clinicians have access to critical healthcare information when treatment decisions are being made.
- *Goal 3—Personalize Care:* Using health information technology to give consumers more access and involvement in health decisions.
- *Goal 4—Improve Population Health:* Expanding capacity for public health monitoring, quality of care measurement, and bringing research advances more quickly into medical practice.

With the momentum from President Bush and Dr. Brailer's initiatives, efforts are under way to guide the uniform integration of performance measures into EHRS. To this end, the AMA has been collaborating with CMS to develop technical specifications to facilitate the integration of performance measures, including those for CVD, into any EHRS.

The BPHC has sponsored several IT initiatives over the past several years. Holding to its goal, "moving toward 100 percent access and zero health disparities," the BPHC has created multiple grants to promote EHRS integration among the nation's health centers.[23] In preparation for EHRS integration, the BPHC encouraged the formation of community health center networks with its Integrated Services Development Initiative (ISDI). This evolutionary process began with the funding of Integrated Service Networks in 1994. In 1997, the emphasis of the ISDI shifted toward integrated delivery systems that were designed to increase the efficiency and effectiveness of health centers through the sharing of specific functions. Building on these grants, the BPHC funded several new grants in 2003, such as the Integrated Information Communications Technology to support EHRS integration into networks of health centers. These BPHC-led initiatives represent a commitment to ensure that its safety net health centers are not left behind in the national quality measurement and IT movements.

Local Implementation of National Goals

With the national priorities in place to improve quality care (goals, measures, IT specifications) physicians, nurses, and other health professionals can apply them from "the bottom up."

Individual Assessment

Local enactment of national goals begins with assessment. Given the well-documented national gaps in CVD care, assessment of an individual practice using standardized measures establishes a baseline evaluation of care that can guide change. With the use of standardized measures, individual practices can benchmark their performance with that of the nation's. In addition, practices can assess where variations in care exist across the different populations they serve.

Regional Collaborations

Once practices are able to reliably collect data using national measures, joining a regional collaboration permits health information exchange to determine through aggregate data where a community or region's opportunities for improvement lie.

Quality improvement collaboratives, largely popularized by the Institute for Healthcare Improvement's Breakthrough Series collaborative program, will likely provide the greatest response to quality and safety gaps.[24] The collaborative model emphasizes learning, knowledge sharing of best practices, and dissemination. Information sharing via networks of physician practices and health centers symbolizes the profession's shift away from the current culture of blame and information suppression to a culture of informed, interconnected health systems. Collaborations acknowledge that everyone is striving toward the same high quality care, everyone experiences successes and shortcomings in their practices, and everyone can learn from others' experiences.

An example of a successful regional collaboration is the Northern New England Cardiovascular Disease Study Group. Since the late 1980s, cardiothoracic surgeons, invasive cardiologists, nurses, and other providers from six medical centers have compared and contrasted their knowledge, theories, and practice through pooling of CVD outcomes (e.g., coronary artery bypass graft surgery) data and the study of process. Data is collected using a single-page form that is transmitted either electronically or via registered mail. During the first post-intervention period (1991–1992), the Group realized a 24 percent reduction in coronary artery bypass graft mortality rates.[25] The Group has met at least three times each year since its inception.

While many state or regional collaboratives are currently functional as information exchange networks, there is no consistency across collaboratives as to exactly what data is collected, nor to what system changes occurred based on these findings. Though they are increasing in number, regional collaboratives are often poorly funded and lack sustainability.[1] In addition, many initiatives are focused on outcomes in the surgical or inpatient setting and do not fully utilize EHRS.

Ideally, enhanced quality of care will grow from the individual physician's office outward, a goal Dr. Brailer calls bringing about "quality improvement in healthcare from the inside out." Eventually, IT-centered quality improvement can lead to national interoperability to form a national health information infrastructure. Protected by coordinated, secure pathways, data from standardized clinical performance measures could feed into a national health network that would inform policy makers and highlight where gaps still exist and where quality enhancement is needed. Furthermore, public health monitoring, research, and bioterrorism surveillance would also benefit from access to national data.[1]

Completing the Circle

Quality improvement has recently been described in a push/pull paradigm. The pull often refers to external forces—such as payers, the government, and consumers, who are trying to improve the quality of health care through use of incentives and regulation. The push is generated by the profession and by science. The medical profession has the capacity to improve care from the inside out by creating a culture of quality. Physician leaders who encourage the adoption of evidence-based performance measures and quality improvement strategies into their practices can push the nation's healthcare toward national goals.

The physician-patient relationship is at the heart of health care. Data collected during a single clinical encounter are building blocks that, once aggregated with data from other patients, practices, and regions, can present a concrete picture to the nation of where real opportunities for improvement lie. Current national quality reports are based on several sources including national telephone surveys, national surveillance data, and claims data. While these reports represent an important first look at the quality of care in America, they are not based on uniform data collected using standardized, evidence-based measurement tools.

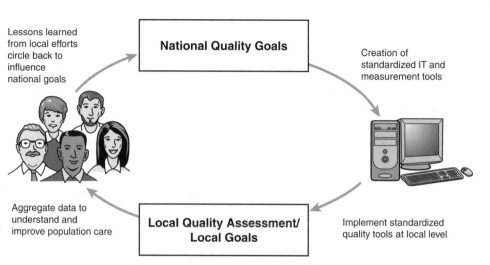

Figure 3–2 *Quality Improvement Information Cycle: Data from Standardized Clinical Performance Measures, Used at the Point of Care, Can Be Aggregated to Inform New National Quality Goals*

Therefore, widespread use of standardized quality measures for CVD not only has the potential to move the nation toward the cardiovascular goals in Healthy People 2010 but also has the potential for using locally collected data to shape the goals for Healthy People 2020. In this way, the quality circle is completed (see Figure 3-2); national goals inspire use of performance measurement by individual physicians, and data from performance measures inspires new national goals.

Case Study

The promise of individual assessment, regional collaboration, and national information sharing anchored in nationally recognized, evidence-based quality improvement tools is already being made a reality. The following case study demonstrates how a current initiative can influence CVD care.

Midwest Heart Specialists, a fifty-physician cardiology practice near Chicago, Illinois, has been fully using an EHRS for six years to treat patients with CVD. In 2002, this large cardiology practice successfully integrated all CVD data elements into their EHRS.[26] Led by Dr. Michael O'Toole, the practice electronically mapped each data element for all of the nationally recognized CVD measures. Once the mapping was complete and the data elements were validated, the EHRS was modified to generate point-of-care reminders to support the measures. Eventually, Midwest Heart Specialists was able to use queries and feedback reports to provide practicing physicians with clinically relevant data. This model practice is now using aggregate data to monitor one patient over time, or assess the entire practice.

To disseminate the quality improvement culture at Midwest Heart Specialists to other practices, regionally or nationwide, would be a crucial step in working toward the CVD goals set forth by Healthy People 2010. For example, if several practices also integrated the ACC/AHA/AMA/Consortium CVD performance measures into their EHRS offices, de-identified data could be shared using a data warehouse to assess the quality of CVD care in a region, or in different parts of the country. Aggregate data on standardized CVD measures could identify opportunities for care improvement, as well as influence new national health goals. The type of EHRS a practice has, or where it is located geographically is irrelevant as long as the data elements are identical and allow for meaningful comparison.

Although vulnerable populations are not specifically targeted in this case study, use of standardized performance measures reduces variations in care, eliminates physician uncertainty, and accounts for patient preference, thereby improving the health of *all* patients. This regional collaborative represents a shift in the nature of public health interventions to mirror today's public health challenge of chronic illness. Cardiovascular disease is one of the most prevalent chronic illnesses in the United States, and CVD is disproportionately prevalent among vulnerable populations. Having multiple practices collect, share, and act on data from standardized evidence-based performance measures demonstrates how quality improvement initiatives can positively impact the public's health.

Study/Discussion Questions

1. How are vulnerable populations defined and what are the effects of poor quality care on underserved communities?
2. What is a clinical performance measure?
3. What is the potential impact of integrating IT into healthcare?

Suggested Readings/Web Sites

American Medical Association, Clinical Quality Improvement (http://www.ama-assn.org/go/quality).
Healthy People 2010 (http://www.healthypeople.gov/).
IOM Report: Unequal Treatment (http://www.iom.edu/report.asp?id=4475).
American Hospital Association (http://www.aha.org).
Health Research and Education Trust (http://www.hret.org).

References

1. US Department of Health and Human Services. *The Decade of Health Information Technology: Delivering Consumer-centric and Information-rich Health Care. Framework for Strategic Action.* Washington, DC; 2004.
2. Berwick DM, James B, Coye MJ. Connections between quality measurement and improvement. *Medical Care.* 2003;41(1):I-30-I38.

3. Institute of Medicine, Committee on Quality of Health Care in America. *Crossing the Quality Chasm: A New Health System for the 21st Century*. Washington, DC: National Academy Press; 2001.

4. Centers for Disease Control and Prevention National Center for Health Statistics. Mortality Data. Available at: http://www.cdc.gov/nchs/about/major/dvs/mortdata.htm. Accessed on April 16, 2004.

5. Centers for Disease Control and Prevention. National Center for Health Statistics. The Third National Health and Nutrition Examination Survey (NHANES III, 1988–1994) Reference Manuals and Reports October 1996. Available at: http://www.cdc.gov/nchs/about/major/nhanes/NHANESIII_Reference_Manuals.htm. Accessed July 2004.

6. American Heart Association, American Stroke Association. *Heart Disease and Stroke Statistics—2004 Update*. Dallas, Texas: American Heart Association; 2003.

7. Agency for Healthcare Research and Quality. US Department of Health and Human Services. *National Healthcare Quality Report*. Rockville, MD; December 2003.

8. Jencks SF, Huff ED, Cuerdon T. Change in the quality of care delivered to Medicare beneficiaries, 1998–1999 to 2000–2001. *JAMA*. 2003;289:305–12.

9. Stafford RS, Radley DC. The underutilization of cardiac medications of proven benefit, 1990 to 2000. *J Am Coll Cardio*. 2003;41(1):56–61.

10. Miller M, Byington R, Hunninghake D, Pitt B, Furberg CD. Sex bias and underutilization of lipid-lowering therapy in patients with coronary artery disease at academic medical centers in the United States and Canada. *Arch Intern Med*. 2000;160:343–47.

11. McGlynn EA, Steven MA, Adams J, et al. The quality of health care delivered to adults in the United States. *NEJM*. 2003;348(26):2635–45.

12. Shi L. The convergence of vulnerable characteristics and health insurance in the United States. *Soc Sci Med*. 2001;53(4):519–29.

13. Institute of Medicine. *Unequal Treatment: What Healthcare Providers Need to Know About Racial and Ethnic Disparities in Healthcare*. Washington, DC: The National Academies Press; 2002. Available at: http://www.iom.edu. Accessed July 2004.

14. *Key Facts: Race, Ethnicity & Medical Care*. Menlo Park, Calif: The Henry J. Kaiser Family Foundation; 1999.

15. Stevens GD, Shi L. Racial and ethnic disparities in the quality of primary care for children. *J Fam Pract*. 2002;51:573.

16. Wilson KM, Klein JD. Adolescents who use the emergency department as their usual source of care. *Arch Pediatr Adolesc Med*. 2000;154:361–65.

17. Fiscella K, Franks P, Gold M, et al. Inequality in quality: Addressing socioeconomic, racial, and ethnic disparities in healthcare. *JAMA*. 2000;283(19):2579–84.

18. Aaron KF, Clancey CM. Improving quality and reducing disparities: Toward a common pathway. *JAMA*. 2003;289(8):1033–34.

19. US Department of Health and Human Services. *Healthy People 2010: Understanding and Improving Health*. 2nd ed. Washington, DC: US Government Printing Office; November 2000.

20. American College of Cardiology, American Heart Association, Physician Consortium for Performance Improvement. *Clinical Performance Measures, Chronic Stable Coronary Artery Disease*. American Medical Association; 2003.

21. The Health Disparities Collaboratives: A national effort to improve health outcomes for all medically underserved people with chronic diseases. Available at: http://www.healthdispar ities.net/. Accessed July 2004.

22. Office of Management and the Budget. Recommendations from the Interagency Committee for the Review of the Racial and Ethnic Standards to the Office of Management and Budget Concerning Changes to the Standards for the Classification of Federal Data on Race and Ethnicity; July 1997. Available at: http://www.whitehouse.gov/omb/fedreg/directive_15.html Accessed July 2004.

23. Bureau of Primary Health Care. Key Program Areas: Community Health Centers. Available at: http://bphc.hrsa.gov/chc/. Accessed July 2004.

24. Mittman BS. Creating the evidence base for quality improvement collaboratives. *Annals Int Med.* 2004;140(11):897–901.

25. Malenka DJ, O'Connor GT. The Northern New England cardiovascular disease study group: A regional collaborative effort for continuous quality improvement in cardiovascular disease. *J Qual Improvement.* 1998;24(10):594–600.

26. O'Toole MF, Kmetik K, Schwaumberger P, Kostos T. Embedding clinical performance measures into an electronic medical record. Abstract presented at the American Heart Association annual meeting. May 2004.

The Measures and Tools of Quality Improvement

Chapter 4

Conceptualizing and Improving Quality: An Overview

Scott B. Ransom
John R. Griffith
Darrell A. Campbell, Jr.
Elizabeth R. Ransom

EXECUTIVE SUMMARY

While it is convenient to discuss the concept of quality from the patient's or provider's perspective, the US healthcare delivery system involves many constituents that have different perceptions of healthcare quality. The various healthcare constituents include: patients, families, physicians, nurses, hospitals, health plans, employers, government, Centers for Medicare & Medicaid Services, the Joint Commission on Accreditation of Healthcare Organization, the Veterans Administration, long-term care facilities, pharmaceutical manufacturers, device companies, and others. Each of these constituents has their own needs and desired outcomes that are frequently in conflict with each other. As patients seek luxurious amenities and more personalized care, the payers present continued pressure to lower, or at least limit, the costs for care. The lay public demands the most state-of-the-art and personalized care with an expectation of only paying, at most, a small fraction of the actual cost of care. Entrepreneurs and businesses attempt to earn their fortune through new products and services that can expand the 15 percent Gross National Product that currently goes toward health care. Simultaneously, employers are screaming that healthcare is already too expensive and making their businesses less competitive on the world stage. All said, American health care remains a cottage industry, where providers are preoccupied with financial survival and challenged by regulation and litigation. They are driven by highly individualized value needs, not by an abstract or common desire to improve health care.[1] How can the healthcare delivery system develop new technologies and pharmaceuticals, have top-knotch amenities and personalized services, and lower costs for employers and government? These questions set up an inherent conflict in defining quality.

LEARNING OBJECTIVES

1. To gain an appreciation of the various healthcare stakeholders and their individual perspectives on a definition of quality.
2. To understand the techniques used in improving healthcare quality.
3. To be able to describe the quality triad, the Institute of Medicine goals for quality health care, and methods to improve performance.

KEYWORDS

Quality Triad
Total Quality Management
Six Sigma
Disney Institute
IOM Report
The Leapfrog Group
Clinical Quality
Service Quality
Financial Quality
Baldrige Award
Institute for Healthcare Improvement
National Quality Forum
Performance Improvement

Introduction

Many reports suggest that the US healthcare delivery system is in crisis. The economy has experienced double-digit healthcare inflation that now approaches $2 trillion and absorbs over 14 percent of the Gross National Product. Malpractice premiums are exploding, with several areas experiencing 50 percent inflation last year alone and annual premiums as high as $211,000 for obstetricians.[2] A recent study showed that 31 percent of healthcare costs go to healthcare administration.[3] Other studies have shown that as much as 8 percent of hospital revenues go to malpractice and other tort expenses. And for this incredible cost, several studies have shown that the public is frequently mistreated by the healthcare delivery system.[4] McGlynn et al.[5] showed that over 50 percent of patients are not optimally treated. While the nation has a complicated healthcare delivery model, there is no coordinator that is dedicated to efficiently improving the health of American citizens.

The past several years have highlighted several deficiencies in the healthcare delivery system. Countless reports of patients being harmed by medication errors, wrong site surgery, and being over-treated, under-treated, and miss-treated exist in the media. Three major reports have highlighted substantial evidence of quality problems in the US healthcare system, including:

1. The Institute of Medicine's (IOM) National Roundtable on Health Care Quality report *The Urgent Need to Improve Health Care Quality*[6]
2. The IOM's *To Err Is Human* report[7]
3. The IOM's *Crossing the Quality Chasm* report[8]

These reports present several problems with quality but still fall short of defining quality. The Institute of Medicine[9] suggested, "Quality of care is the degree to which health services for individuals and populations increase the likelihood of desired heath outcomes and are consistent with current professional knowledge. . . . How care is provided should reflect appropriate use of the most current knowledge about scientific, clinical, technical, interpersonal, manual, cognitive, and organization and management elements of health care." And then in 2001, the IOM suggested that health care should be safe, effective, efficient, timely, patient centered, and equitable. As Stephen Shortell highlights:

> The US healthcare system can be likened to a shoddily constructed building located in the pathway of an impending disaster. The system has been constructed by thousands of different architects, engineers, masons, and carpenters working from wildly different blueprints. For the most part, it has been built to the codes of the nineteenth century.[2]

Another perspective is that the healthcare delivery system is perfectly designed to get the results it gets.[10] Stockholders demand profits and an increasing share price in pharmaceutical companies; patients want instant cures; providers want more money; and citizens "want fries with that." There is no simple fix. The system must be rebuilt, even redesigned, and in the process most constituents must change the way they think about getting, giving, and paying for health care.

The Quality Triad

Healthcare providers and patients tend to look at quality from different perspectives. Physicians, nurses, pharmacists, and technologists have spent countless years learning the technical dimensions of clinical practice. They tend to judge quality on these dimensions; surgeons for example, assess quality by counting complications. When an adverse event occurs, it is often attributed to an unavoidable mishap. Conversely, patients assume technical quality and expect their providers to deliver excellence. The knowledge gap between providers and patients is generally very large, reinforcing the patient's trust in the provider's intellectual and technical skill. Patients and families tend to evaluate quality based on areas they have experience with—service and amenities. The patient's subjective experience is often based on the ease of access to care, the friendliness and responsiveness of the providers, the décor of the treatment facility, the taste of the food, the temperature of the room, and the physical comfort while going through an examination. The patient's perception of quality is placed center stage as discussed in "Through the Patient's Eyes" (Gerteis et al. 1993).

Quality in health care has at least two major dimensions. Technical excellence is the skill and competence of health professionals and the ability of the diagnostic or therapeutic equipment, procedures, and systems to accomplish what they are meant to accomplish reliably and effectively. The experiential dimension of quality is the heart of what patients want in health care—enhancement of their sense of well-being and relief from suffering. Any healthcare system, however it is financed or structured, must address both aspects of quality to achieve legitimacy in the eyes of those it serves.

Donabedian's conceptualization of quality goes well beyond this dichotomy. He suggests that quality includes access as well as satisfaction on the experiential dimension, and continuity, comprehensiveness, prevention, and compliance, as well as accurate diagnosis and effective treatment, on the technical dimension.[11] Important as these concepts are, they still exclude any direct reference to cost and efficiency. Most of Donabedian's elements indirectly promote efficiency. Effective, comprehensive treatment, including prevention and continuity is almost certainly cheaper in the long run—as well as better.

A basic view of quality health care can be summarized in reviewing the quality triad: clinical quality, service quality, and financial performance (see Figure 4–1). This conceptual model differs from Donabedian's classic quality triad of structure (the "bricks and mortar" of care delivery), process (the way care is delivered), and outcome (the result of care). Practitioners, trained to expertly diagnose and treat patient modalities, tend to focus on "doing the right thing" and "doing the right thing right." That is to say, surgeons work to make an appropriate diagnosis of appendicitis, and then perform a complication-free appendectomy. The surgeon assumes excellent patient quality when both the appropriate diagnosis and treatment have been completed.

Patients tend to focus on their own subjective experiences. They evaluate quality based on staff courtesy, immediate access to the provider, "whether my doctor listens to me," office décor and cleanliness, ease of parking, and quality of food. They prefer the physician's office that provides these services, even in situations where healthcare professionals see poor clinical quality. Recognition of the importance of service has led many hospitals to measure patient, employee, and physician satisfaction through formal surveys and focus groups. Leading healthcare organizations have built on this tendency to establish "service excellence," a deliberate program

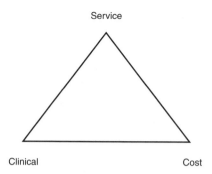

Figure 4–1 *The Quality Triad*

of collaboration with caregivers to meet both technical and service needs.[12] The Disney Institute has taken the tradition of service excellence from its theme park and has assisted hospitals in developing a polished customer orientation. While many providers initially look on service excellence as a commercialization of care, the program's focus on their needs as well as the patients' soon changes their minds. Hospitals that pursue service excellence have some of the best records of recruiting and retaining caregivers. It is also true that patient attitude is sometimes important in technical quality, and is central in compliance, prevention, and continuity.

Lastly, cost and financial performance often define quality for the individuals and groups that pay for healthcare services. Negotiated payments are a fixture of twenty-first century healthcare, and the federal government and large employers drive hard bargains. This necessitates efficient practice, limiting length of stay, regulating ancillary costs, and striving to reduce waste. As a private and frequently "mission-centric" business, the hospital must have adequate financial performance to exist. Financial crisis can be attributed to poor payer mix, high malpractice premiums, increasing cost of employee wages, and ever increasing pharmaceutical costs. Despite the daunting challenge, effective management teams must maintain financial viability for their organization.

In the past few years, buyers have begun to think in more holistic terms. Buyers have promoted the public disclosure of clinical quality data through the federal Centers for Medicare & Medicaid Services (CMS) Voluntary Hospital Quality Program; commercial sources such as Solucient and Health Grades; and voluntary initiatives such as the National Committee for Quality Assurance, the Joint Commission on Accreditation of Healthcare Organizations, and the National Quality Forum. While quality information is becoming more transparent, the dissemination nationally is only beginning. The CMS is moving to "pay for performance" with both quality and satisfaction measures. The Leapfrog Group, a consortium of large employers, has moved to both "pay for performance" and support of electronic medical records. Although many aspects of the payment programs are still not properly aligned with either clinical or service excellence, providing cost-effective and financially prudent healthcare services is an integral part of the quality triad.

The "Quality Triad" provides a useful, albeit basic, view to healthcare quality. The conflicting views of quality from the perspective of the provider, patient, and financial officer provide a challenge and important dynamic in health care. The organization that thrives pursues all three perspectives and balances them, whether it is a solo primary care practice or a large health system. The organization that over-emphasizes one portion of the triad places its existence in jeopardy. While it would be wonderful to offer providers state-of-the-art equipment and one-on-one nursing care for patients, the cost is often prohibitively high—ultimately resulting in bankruptcy. Similarly, patients that have beautiful and lavish suites, personalized amenities, and absolutely pain-free care, are not necessarily receiving the highest level of clinical care, let alone financially prudent care. Lastly, financial stability is essential if equipment is to be updated and nursing wages maintained at a competitive level. The healthcare leader must carefully balance the quality triad to provide high quality services for the long run.

Understanding Conflicting Quality Perspectives

Quality in health care is something that is commonly discussed, yet rarely clarified. Each healthcare constituent has their own definition of quality that often changes as life events are unveiled. As a start, this chapter seeks to identify the different ways to look at the decisions that support quality. To illustrate the many faces of quality, the chapter will present eight real-life perspectives.

Eight Perspectives: A Theoretical Case Study

1. Doctor Mary is a well-trained, 30-year-old, obstetrician and gynecologist in private practice. She wanted to be a physician for as long as memory serves and worked hard to achieve her goal. She graduated from residency three months ago with an $180,000 student loan, $100,000 bank loan to start her small town private practice, and hopes to purchase her first home later this year. While patients are beginning to make appointments, her schedule is mostly open and she fears that she will require another bank loan to keep her private practice financially viable. A 42-year-old patient presents to Doctor Mary with a four-month history of dysfunctional uterine bleeding that might be related to a two-centimeter uterine fibroid detected by her office ultrasound. The patient has a normal blood count and her hormone levels are all normal. Doctor Mary privately believes the patient has four options, including: close observation with a follow-up visit in six months, a trial of birth control pills to regulate the patient's bleeding, a hysteroscopy and laparoscopy to assess uterine pathology, or a hysterectomy. Doctor Mary wants to do what is best for the patient; however, she does a quick calcula-

tion and finds that she will earn $60 from a follow-up office visit, nothing for prescribing birth control pills, $1,000 for completing a hysteroscopy and laparoscopy, and $2,000 for completing a hysterectomy. All options have various benefits and risks; but, how does she explain the options to her patient?

2. Hospital Administrator Mary leads a 50-bed hospital in a small town and hopes to be promoted to a more prestigious post in the next two years. The hospital has shown a negative net income since her arrival. She recruited three new physicians to satisfy unmet patient demand and enhance revenues leading to a positive net income and her ticket to a better paying position at a larger facility. She is delighted that the new obstetrician and gynecologist is completing a large number of hysterectomies that has boosted hospital financial performance. The hospital pathologist, who chairs the Tissue Committee, has cited an unusual number of hysterectomy specimens without any pathologic evidence of disease. The hospital administrator has prioritized her goals to include a positive net income margin and good patient, staff, and physician satisfaction scores. Should the hospital administrator jeopardize the hospital net income and her new gynecologist's satisfaction by discussing the high number of inappropriate surgeries?

3. Medical Director Mary has been a physician for twenty-five years and recently assumed the medical director role at a 100,000-member managed care organization. She has a financial incentive to improve profitability for the organization's stockholders. A request was submitted to complete a hysterectomy on a 42-year-old patient with a four-month history of dysfunctional uterine bleeding and a small fibroid uterus. It appears that the patient has not attempted hormonal or other therapeutic options to resolve the problem. Medical Director Mary considers the $6,000 hospital payout and $2,000 physician payout for this procedure and wonders why the physician has recommended this aggressive therapy without attempts at cheaper and less risky options. Should Medical Director Mary approve the hysterectomy?

4. Employer Mary runs a small business with ten employees. She treats her employees well and earns government grants to support her farm. Despite the outrageous cost, she pays for health insurance for her employees. The health plan is a managed care organization that is the least expensive option for her business. An employee will be off work for eight weeks due to an upcoming hysterectomy. The employee has been an average worker and has required extensive time off for doctor appointments during her twelve-month employment. Employer Mary is concerned that the surgery will cause staffing problems during the main harvesting season for her tobacco farm. In addition, she is concerned that health insurance premiums might increase due to this employee's excessive use of the medical system. The business's health insurance premiums were discounted last year due to an

employee history of low utilization of medical services. The health insurance agent was very clear that the discount could be eliminated if the plan experienced increased costs. Should Employer Mary temporarily or permanently replace the employee? If the health insurance rates go up substantially, she might no longer be able to pay the premiums and her staff will be left to get insurance on their own.

5. Researcher Mary has studied variation in clinical practice for ten years. She specializes in medical practice variations for women with a particular personal interest in hysterectomy. Her research found a dramatic spike in the hysterectomy rate in a small town this past year. After performing a zip code evaluation, she finds the town and surrounding community seem to have a physician performing hysterectomies on women for apparently any reason at all. While the statewide average has been consistent for the past five years, this region seems to have a dramatic spike over the past twelve months. Researcher Mary's funding is highly dependent on insurance company contributions and this new finding can secure funding for the next three years and tenure at her university. How should Researcher Mary present her findings?

6. Attorney Mary was asked to review a possible case for medical legal action. The case involved a client who had a hysterectomy complicated by a damaged ureter that resulted in a damaged right kidney and a nephrectomy. Unfortunately, the patient has a partially developed left kidney and will require renal dialysis to survive. Attorney Mary reviewed the chart and wonders why the patient underwent a hysterectomy in the first place. She understands that the local hospital attempted to recruit an obstetrician for over five years to serve the community. The physician in this case is a new recruit that the community hopes will help attract a second obstetrician to the area. Attorney Mary worries that a lawsuit can damage the town's chances of recruiting new physicians; however, she believes the surgical injury was preventable and requires compensation for her client. In addition, she would enjoy earning one third of a judgment that could be as high as $1,000,000. Should Attorney Mary accept this case and file a malpractice action against her client's physician?

7. Pharmaceutical Representative Mary was hired by a startup pharmaceutical company with just one product. The new and innovative product is a hormone that regulates menses and reduces the size of fibroid uterus. The product is newly FDA approved and works about 60 percent of the time with 30 percent of patients experiencing reversible symptoms such as headaches, depression, and mood swings. Unfortunately, one company confidential report showed that 5 percent of patients using this drug experience a life-threatening stroke. Pharmaceutical Mary will get a big bonus if her target area physicians prescribe 500 doses of the product this year. The cost

of the product is $500 per dose and will require an average of three doses for cure. How should she explain the life-threatening side effects to her target physicians?

8. Patient Mary is looking for a gynecologist to complete a hysterectomy. She visited two big city gynecologists who refused to do the procedure because they believed she would be better served by hormone therapy for her mild dysfunctional uterine bleeding and small fibroid. She has read about the indications for a hysterectomy on the Internet and wants to convince a doctor that she is a good candidate. Privately she wants a tubal ligation but knows that her church believes this form of birth control is unacceptable. She sees hysterectomy as her way to permanent birth control while eliminating her monthly menses and the stigma of having a tubal ligation. Patient Mary has an appointment with the new gynecologist in town. What will Patient Mary do if the new gynecologist says no to her request for hysterectomy?

Each of the eight Marys is most likely to act in her own self-interest. Physician Mary is an independent business owner who must make a profit to support home ownership and prevent the risk of defaulting on loans. The hospital administrator hopes to lead the hospital to profitability so that she can secure a more prestigious position. The medical director hopes to earn a bonus and a good retirement through stock options. The employer hopes to earn a profit for her tobacco farm. The researcher strives to continue external funding to keep her laboratory functioning and earn tenure at the university. The attorney hopes to get a good judgment for her injured client while simultaneously earning a good living on fees. The pharmaceutical representative hopes to cash in on her investment and efforts in developing and distributing the new drug. And lastly, the patient will give her best effort to obtain the treatment she believes is of the highest quality and most convenient for her. The perspectives of the doctor, hospital administrator, medical director, employer, researcher, attorney, pharmaceutical representative, and patient are all important and valid. The healthcare system must consider each of the perspectives; however, the individual goals present obvious, and sometimes hidden, conflicts to the success of the healthcare delivery system. Perhaps quality should be defined as achieving the desired outcomes from the individual stakeholder's perspective. What happens to the perception of quality when the various outcome goals are in conflict?

Healthcare delivery in the United States can be organized in four levels.[13] The first level is that of the patient. The interventions and personal experiences with the healthcare delivery system must be focused on the patient to receive optimal care. The second level is the clinical microsystem that includes the providers who care for the patient. The small provider teams and care locations substantially influence the care received by the patient. The third level considers the organizational framework to deliver care. The organization includes several groups of the clinical microsystem that come together for the benefit of several, often diverse, patients. Lastly, the fourth level considers the external environment that influences the organizations, clinical

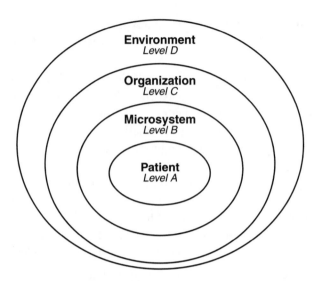

Figure 4–2A *Four Levels of Organizational Focus*

Reprinted with permission from Crossing the Quality Chasm: A New Health System for the 21st Century. © 2001 by the National Academy of Sciences, courtesy of the National Academies Press, Washington, DC.

microsystems, and patients. The environment includes community resources, reimbursement mechanisms, government regulations, and polices as well as natural resources such as food and water supply, air quality, street crimes, toxins, and weather. These four levels are integrated to influence the health of the individual as described in Figure 4–2A. As we rebuild our system, we will need to address all four levels.

Goals for Quality Health Care

The IOM established six aims for improvement.[9] These include:
1. **Safe:** avoiding patient injuries from the interventions and providers that are intended to improve health.
2. **Effective:** providing evidence-based services to all who could benefit and refraining from providing services not likely to benefit the patient.
3. **Patient centered:** providing care that focuses on individual patient preferences, needs, and values while being respectful of and responsive to the patient in all clinical decisions.
4. **Timely:** reducing wait times and delays for patients, families, providers, and staff.
5. **Efficient:** avoiding waste of patient and provider time, pharmaceuticals, equipment, supplies, ideas, and energy.

Current Approach	New Rule
1. Care is based primarily on visits.	1. Care is based on continuous healing relationships.
2. Professional autonomy drives variability.	
3. Professionals control care.	2. Care is customized according to patient needs and values.
4. Information is a record.	3. The patient is the source of control.
5. Decision-making is based on training and experience.	4. Knowledge is shared and information flows freely.
6. Do no harm is an individual responsibility.	5. Decision-making is evidence-based.
7. Secrecy is necessary.	6. Safety is a system property.
8. The system reacts to needs.	7. Transparency is necessary.
9. Cost reduction is sought.	8. Needs are anticipated.
10. Preference is given to professional roles over the system.	9. Waste is continuously decreased.
	10. Cooperation among clinicians is a priority.

Figure 4–2B *Simple Rules for the Twenty-first Century Health System*

Proposed by the Committee on Quality of Health Care in America. Institute of Medicine; 2001.

6. **Equitable:** providing care that does not vary in quality because of personal characteristics such as gender, ethnicity, geographic location, and socio-economic status.

They also proposed ten "Simple Rules for the Twenty-first Century Health System" (see Figure 4–2B) that emphasize Donabedian's concepts of continuity, comprehensiveness, prevention, and compliance. These goals have received wide support despite the challenge they represent. They probably are not enough. With an increasing aged population and a shrinking supply of caregivers, America simply must address prevention and health promotion as well.

Introducing Quality in Clinical Practice

Physicians practice medicine with a combination of art and science. While evidence-based medicine is a noble goal, only 20 percent of medicine has a scientific basis. This grim statistic reveals that at least 80 percent of healthcare services are provided as "best guesses." The sad truth is even worse. While 20 percent of medicine has a scientific basis, it takes over a decade to integrate new scientific findings to clinical practice.[14] The history of medical practice can often be viewed by observing different generations of physicians. Despite continuing medical education requirements, it is difficult for physicians to keep up-to-date and integrate new scientific findings into their clinical practice. As scientific discovery unfolds, the healthcare delivery system must consider ways to translate basic science research to clinical research to health services research to implementation in clinical practice.

While most physicians have an eye of providing high quality services to their patients, providers have a difficult time understanding their own compliance with even the most standard practices. While the standards of delivering a baby have become well established, even well-intentioned providers do not always follow evidence-based guidelines. Ransom et al. showed that 11.9 percent of obstetrical patients experienced care that diverged from a well-established clinical pathway without justification.[15] Similarly, McGlynn[5] showed the use of asprin and B-blockers for patients experiencing an acute myocardial infarction is sub-optimal. While providers believe they provide high quality care, the broader healthcare delivery system has a responsibility to insure that evidence-based services are provided. The Women's Health Initiative showed that hormone replacement therapy is associated with an increased risk of breast cancer, stroke, and heart disease in women. These contemporary stories show that even with the best intentions, providers deliver harmful care to their patients. This highlights the importance of optimizing the basic and clinical research enterprise in the United States. Better and balanced research that removes the inherent financial incentives and focuses on the best interests of the patient must be completed.

In an attempt to achieve the goals of the IOM report, research to better transition these findings must be introduced. Health services research to compare the cost-effectiveness of treatment options must be considered in contemporary medical practice. Choosing a more costly product where a cheaper alternative exists with similar or better quality cannot continue. As the IOM report suggests, care must be both effective and efficient. Health services research methodologies must be considered in developing the optimal organization and models of healthcare delivery services. Research on better implementation can help resurrect better delivery models to improve the ability to achieve the IOM goals.

Physicians with a passion for improving quality must encourage their colleagues to adopt evidence-based medicine. In addition, physicians must police their own profession and get rid of providers that are incompetent or unwilling to provide healthcare services. While bad providers are generally rare, physicians often develop problems with burnout, substance abuse, conflicts of interest, and disruptive behavior.[16] Medical leaders must be willing to challenge these potentially dangerous providers. Despite overwhelming evidence, it is the rare medical leader who is willing to tackle these very personal challenges. Given the current culture of medical practice, leaders have no incentive to perform these tasks and will often find themselves ostracized from the rest of the medical staff. Physicians must step up to the challenge and expect outstanding service and clinical quality at a reasonable cost. Balancing the quality triad is often a precarious challenge; however, it takes a physician's leadership to support a quality culture.

Basic science research is the traditional building block for medical practice. Some of the most innovative and exciting discoveries have changed the face of medicine forever, including: the germ theory, anesthesia for surgical procedures, organ transplantation, cardiac catheterization, and countless others. How does the community provider learn to adopt contemporary advances into practice as learned from the genome project, genetic engineering, proteomics, and stem cell research? Providers are confronted with an overwhelming daily influx of materials to read and understand. Pharmaceutical representatives, equipment vendors, professional societies, publishers, and now, e-alerts create a never-ending stream of information to the providers. Unfortunately, even well-meaning and energetic providers have a difficult time differentiating quality innovations from those that are harmful. Simultaneously, much of the marketing blitz experienced by providers are from individuals and organizations that seek profits but do not necessarily expect to improve the health of the individual patient. Still further, providers are reminded of the potential disasters of introducing innovations without proper scientific research. Even reputable companies sell products that are later found to be harmful, such as the research showing Cox-2 inhibitors, such as Vioxx and Bextra, increased the risk of heart disease of patients using the product.

Strengthening Quality in Provider Organizations

Hospitals, clinics, and group practices and other care-giving organizations succeed to the extent that they simultaneously meet the needs of patients, buyers, providers, and workers. There are many thousands of these organizations in the nation, despite recent trends toward integration and consolidation. Available data on overall performance indicates a startling range—the best hospitals are about half as good as the average, and twice as good as the bottom dwellers.[17] Furthermore, only a few institutions can document progress toward the IOM goals. However, the leading healthcare systems have developed a style of management that has now been implemented in over a hundred sites, across a broad range of American communities. The methods these leaders have used, detailed elsewhere, are similar.[18] The core strategy derives from the Continuous Quality Improvement philosophy of W. Edwards Deming. It emphasizes objective measurement, benchmarking (i.e., comparison to known best performance), and ongoing improvement of work processes, beginning at the smallest work units of the organization and aggregated upward to the whole. The leaders are also generous with rewards. Celebrations and cash recognize achievement of goals. People enjoy working in these organizations. The organizations also monitor physician and worker satisfaction. They have very low turnover, and many post awards for "Best Place to Work" alongside their "Top Hospital" placques.

These methods are teachable. The leading organizations have taught themselves, and they routinely and carefully teach newcomers. Measurable improvement occurs within a few years. Installing these methods requires profound shifts in organizational culture. Collaboration becomes the keyword at all levels. Evidence replaces authority as the criterion for decisions. Perspectives shift fundamentally—from inputs to outputs, from tradition to results, and from static to dynamic. Professional domains—the board's, the physician's, the nurse's—give way to dialogue about the cost and quality per case. Service lines, organized around patient need instead of clinical function, revise the accountability structure. Management becomes dually accountable—upward for results, downward for supporting and training associates and teams.

Strong governance is essential to achieve the change. Governance itself becomes pro-active rather than reactive. It turns to ongoing cooperation instead of negotiated settlements. Organizations cannot sustain these sorts of shifts without a firm, continuous mandate from their highest levels. That mandate is missing in too many institutions.[19] Unfortunately, too few governing boards understand the need or the opportunity. Many not-for-profit boards are appointed through a political process that is often more dependent on friendships and unwavering support than on talented representatives of the community interests. A counter-tradition called "the mushroom theory" (i.e., keep the board in the dark, covered with whatever you feed mushrooms) is all too popular among hospital administrators. Physicians serving on the board are too often focused on their practice rather than the needs of all caregivers. There is a tacit agreement: Don't rock the boat. Successful organizations have rocked their boats, and turned them in a new direction. The board must be moved to the center of the healthcare perfect storm. Until boards are engaged in creating high quality environments, the executive team and medical staff can do little except to struggle within their domains. That struggle is not likely to win, and it is a major source of the dissatisfaction heard from all sides.

The challenge of upgrading boards is daunting. Frequently, community leaders appoint friends to these posts, and successful business executives tend to populate the remainder of the board's membership. While these board members are generally smart and successful, many find health care intimidating. Being a successful retailer, educator, banker, or minister does not equip you to understand the complex issues involved in maintaining quality of cardiovascular care. Corporate financial officers can contribute to the Finance Committee and go home proud, while important clinical programs are neglected. The CEOs of first-class corporations can accept practices at the hospital that they would immediately change in their company, because they read the culture as accepting of those practices. Lacking data on quality or physician satisfaction, they accept the word of the doctors who rule the roost. The first task for doctors promoting quality is to reorient the board, moving from word-of-mouth reassurance to measured performance and evidence-based standards. This quality orientation is rarely in the established knowledge base for the new board member. Most boards must be upgraded through education and developing the right mix of talents to support the quality mission.

Historically, boards were too easily reassured about the quality of care. Today's boards must provide high-quality services for their communities. Particularly as decisions become more challenging, the weighing of financial performance must be tempered with measurable quality performance metrics. The board must drive the executive team and physicians to realize new levels of performance for the benefit of the community.

An effective board does the following things:

1. Routinely receives data on a balanced scorecard of performance that includes quality, safety, patient satisfaction, worker and physician satisfaction, efficiency, and financial stability.

2. Conducts an annual, in-depth, fact-based assessment of mission, achievement, needs, and opportunities. The assessment is used to establish strategies that meet community needs for care and prevention.

3. Uses a formal long-range financial plan to establish annual goals for cost and profit, and national benchmarks to establish goals for quality, efficiency, and satisfaction.

4. Acts deliberately but promptly on capital needs, physician privileges, compensation, and controversies that can impair overall success.

5. Reviews its own performance, individually and collectively, and makes changes as indicated.

Goal Setting and Incentives

Incentive compensation for executives is now widespread. In the best organizations, the bonus is based on quality, patient satisfaction, administrative and medical staff development, efficiency, and financial performance. The organizations set goals in each of these areas, with the expectation that the goal will be achieved and the bonus paid. The aggressiveness of the goals can be a difficult strategic judgment. At the highest level, the board identifies the desirable and the feasible, but as the process rolls out, every manager asks the question, "What should I do, and what can I do?" The incentive system encourages them to take the question seriously.

A key role for leadership, specifically including medical, executive, and board leadership, is pushing the organization toward more aggressive goals. The use of benchmarks—known best practice on a specific measure—is the starting point. These provide the evidence basis for what is possible. Some of the larger healthcare systems use inter-hospital communications groups to allow their lower performing members to identify how the best have achieved the benchmark. Organizations such as the Institute for Healthcare Improvement, the National Center for Healthcare Leadership, and VHA Incorporated provide similar learning opportunities for free-standing institutions.

Blame, punishment, and fear are counter-incentives, powerful de-motivators that are too prominent in most hospitals. People hide actions for which they can be punished; hiding makes it difficult to analyze and improve. The nature of an adversarial medical-legal system creates a culture of blame, and promotes hiding the truth.[20] Further, the medical-legal system supports a huge and expensive organization that includes both plaintiff and defense attorneys, physician expert witnesses, judges, juries, and administrators. Ransom et al. showed that only 12 percent of all the direct expenses of the medical-legal tort system actually go to the alleged victim. That is, 88 percent of the resources devoted to the system support the structure and all its constituents.[4]

While physicians often blame greedy plaintiff lawyers for these costs, it is the patient who goes to a lawyer to seek answers and often a financial settlement. This expensive system supports physician experts who often charge over $400 per hour for their opinions. While some experts provide balanced and reliable testimony, financial incentives often buy the opinion sought rather than a true and accurate statement. Further, the current medical-legal system tends to impede a quality culture by hiding mistakes and the processes that allow mistakes to occur. While the courts attempt to define quality, the jurors often do not have the intellectual capacity or understanding to reasonably pass judgment on the care provided. All too often, quality is defined through a process of lawyers presenting one well-spoken expert against another.

Leading institutions address the culture of blame frontally. They reward reporting "near misses." They analyze high-risk activities and redesign them to make them safer. They invest in safety training, safe environments, and safe processes. They offer immediate compensation for legitimate injury. Although the hard data is not yet available, many of the leaders are convinced that these steps pay off. In the end errors are reduced, costs are lower, and both patients and providers are happier.

Change by its nature is uncomfortable. Rewards are important, but protection is also important. Executives who push for a new quality paradigm without building the foundation to support it can find themselves in the unemployment lines. The good news is that well-planned, carefully developed improvement programs are their own reward. They are enormously satisfying to physicians and other workers. The "hassle factor" is gone. The frustration of knowing the patient might have survived, if only, is reduced. Unfortunately, some individuals will have trouble with the transition. A foreseeable problem is the physician who enhances his or her income with unnecessary care. Another are the older workers who suddenly discover they have been falling behind for years. Clearly, change must be implemented in a thoughtful way; training, encouragement, and peer support precede punitive steps. But sooner or later, a few individuals must be brought to face their inadequacies. Leadership at the governing board and on the senior management team addresses this inevitability. Until the board and the most senior executives demand high-quality services, there will continue to be overuse, underuse, and misuse of healthcare services. What is needed are committed and tenacious leaders to support the quality program.

Physicians are front and center in today's quality challenges. A common response among medical school applicants is that in their future careers they hope to help people. While most providers strive to help their patients, the many years in clinical training tend to make providers myopic. Professors and teachers are role models for providers. While many outstanding educators exist, faculties have built-in blinders that often steer them away from improving the actual health of patients. The variation in healthcare services at leading hospitals and universities highlight the quality challenge. As Wennberg and his team's Dartmouth Atlas have shown, patterns of care are highly variable and not consistent with evidence-based principles.[21] Despite the enormous progress with evidence-based care and the new core competencies of Accreditation Council for Graduate Medical Education (ACGME), "Do as I do" is still a common dogma at the leading medical schools. Students ultimately adopt the same blinders as their trainers. Physicians must continuously challenge themselves to a higher quality standard. Measuring performance is becoming more common among leading providers of healthcare services such as the Henry Ford Health System and Kaiser Permanente.

Process Improvement Tools

Effective process improvement in healthcare has about a twenty-five-year history. In the late 1970s Deming introduced the Plan-Do-Study-Act (PDSA) process (see Figure 4–3) as a cycle for learning and improvement.[22] Shortly after, Joseph Juran presented three interrelated processes that support improvement, including: quality planning, quality control, and quality improvement.[23] These early leaders supported a holistic approach to running an organization such that every facet earns the

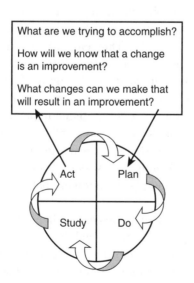

Figure 4–3 *Basic Model of Improvement*

Ransom SB, Pinsky WW, eds., Ward RE, Lafata JE. Clinical effectiveness: An emerging discipline. *Clinical Resource and Quality Management.* Tampa: American College of Physician Executives Press; 1999.

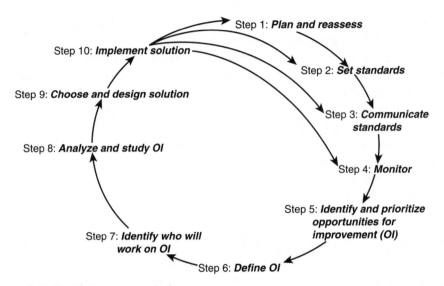

Figure 4–4 *Quality Improvement Cycle*

From the USAID Quality Assurance Project: http://www.qaproject.org/

description quality, and a basic model of identifying an opportunity and establishing a team to address it.[24] By the turn of the century, these approaches were widespread. Several specific programs implementing these concepts have been developed, including Six Sigma and Lean Manufacturing. These approaches, now available from a number of commercial sources, provide formal training in process improvement and programs for immediate results. They emphasize performance measurement as a basic foundation in supporting a quality culture. Data can be used to measure processes and outcomes. Measurement can determine if an organization is in control to better understand underlying processes to create adjustments leading to better quality (see Figure 4–4).[2] Systemic organizational improvements have begun to integrate the various quality tools for more substantial and long-lasting improvement. Developing the processes and systems necessary to treat every patient in an optimal fashion was highlighted by Deming, who wrote, "Transformation is required to move out of the present state, metamorphosis, not mere patchwork on the present state of management."

While the various tools and techniques can be helpful in improvement, the leader must establish clear and specific goals to lead the organization forward. Nolan[22] suggests answering three questions before beginning an improvement project, including: 1) What is your specific aim for improvement? 2) What can the organization do to achieve the specific aims? 3) How will the organization know it achieved its aims? While simple, a clear understanding of these questions will optimize the likelihood of achieving an improvement.

For example, a Women's Hospital learned that compliance with prophylactic antibiotics at the time of cesarean section was 35 percent. Despite an evidence-based guideline that required antibiotics after a cesarean section for eligible patients, the hospital was far from its goal. The Director of Quality established a clear and specific aim of achieving the goal of patients receiving antibiotics after cesarean at least 95 percent of the time. To construct possible strategies for improvement, the leader formed a team to better understand the process of actually providing the patient with the antibiotic. And finally, the leader developed a measurement system to assure that the goal had been reached.

The organization learned that the process to provide an antibiotic required twenty-two steps. A new process was developed that only required four steps to an antibiotic administration that ultimately reached a measurable outcome of 96 percent success. The reduction of these handoffs has the opportunity to dramatically reduce errors and improve quality.

Pharmaceutical companies have become very skilled at inducing change in healthcare providers. While Continuing Medical Education has shown at best minimal improvements, academic detailing has been wildly successful. Pharmaceutical representatives have been very successful at befriending physicians through personal relationships, gift giving, and offering product samples. These skilled professionals have mastered the challenge of modifying physician behavior through a personal connection. While academic detailing techniques have been developed by pharmaceutical companies, successful executives have used these approaches to further induce acceptance by physicians to change in hospitals. While a fairly simple and straightforward technique, personal relationships are very important for building a common vision for the future.

The Malcolm Baldridge National Quality Award strives to recognize this organizational transformation. While only four hospitals have won the National Award and achieved Baldridge status, more have used the approach without the label, or have won recognition at the state level. These leaders have set a course to challenge the rest of the healthcare delivery system. Take for example, Baptist Health Care in Pensacola, which received the 2003 Baldridge Award.[25] While only five years earlier the organization looked like many hospitals in the United States, the hospital executives, medical staff, and board led the hospital through a challenging transformation to achieve a new level of excellence. As highlighted by the organization's senior vice president for Medical Affairs, Craig Miller, MD, "the hospital achieved a new level of excellence by interrelating core values and concepts. Very early in the transformation, the organization looked to retain and recruit people with a shared vision while getting those not accepting the vision off our bus." This personnel issue helped disseminate the quality movement more efficiently throughout the organization by optimizing the acceptance of adopting change by organizations (see Figure 4–5).

The Baldridge is awarded to healthcare organizations that have visionary leadership and patient-focused excellence, encourage organizational and personal learning, value staff and partners, exhibit organizational agility, focus on the future, manage for innovation, manage by facts, maintain a focus on social responsibility and community health, focus on results and creating value, and maintain a broad

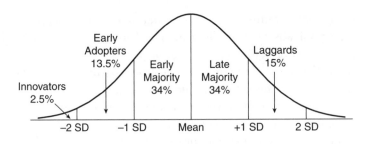

Time to Adoption (SD's from mean)

Figure 4–5 *Roger's Adopter Categories for Change*

Rogers EM. *Diffusions of Innovations.* 5th ed. New York: The Free Press, a Division of Simon & Schuster Adult Publishing Group; 2003.

systems perspective. Hospitals can take steps to achieve these transformational results; however, the challenge of leadership is highlighted by Gandhi, who said, "Change is possible if we have the desire and commitment to make it happen."

One of the obstacles to transformational change is related to an effective sharing and transmission of information. While the healthcare delivery system is a heavy user of information, it is the rare organization that uses information technology effectively to drive better performance. The Veteran's Administration (VA) has been an early leader in the use of information technology to lead change. The 1990s witnessed a true transformational change, led by the Ken Kizer, MD, MPH, at the VA.[26] The backbone of these incredible changes was related to the integrated information system that linked all outpatient and inpatient progress notes, laboratory and radiology information, problem lists, and active medication lists, among others. The system allowed the easy retrieval of information as the patient was cared for simultaneously by several physicians and consultants. Physicians could easily and immediately access all of the important information that allowed more effective and integrated care plans while reducing resource consumption by eliminating laboratory, radiology, and medication duplications. While the VA has long been a government establishment, it took the tenacity and will of its leaders to eliminate entrenched staff and physicians and look to a new future.

The use of these sophisticated information systems has the potential to drive change. Decision-support systems have been used to reduce medication errors and adverse medical events by establishing more standardized processes to reduce variation. Judy Gilliam, chief operating officer at Ohio State University Health System, highlighted one big benefit of the electronic medical record: the elimination of the need to decode poor penmanship by physicians and staff, which shows dramatic reductions in medication errors. In addition, online alerts and reminders have limited the use of drugs that the patient is known to be allergic to as well as reduce adverse medication interactions through these "smart systems." Finally, alerts and reminders can reduce the reliance on memory and underuse errors by highlighting medications that the patient requires.

These decision-support tools have been shown to improve compliance protocols for common disorders such as insuring use of aspirin and beta blockers for patients with an acute myocardial infarction. While Continuing Medical Education has not been shown to integrate new knowledge to clinical practice, decision tools have great potential in helping physicians understand and use state-of-the-art care. While physicians have been suspicious of cookbook medicine, the public reporting of physician-specific compliance data has highlighted the need to use every tool available to improve care.

Conclusion

While there are many perspectives of quality, the healthcare industry must look to a more comprehensive and integrated vision to improve the health and health care of all Americans. While many conflicts of interest exist in the present healthcare system, it is imperative to get beyond these conflicts and create a better vision for the future. The system must look to what is best for the individual patient in order to define quality.[27]

Similarly, while the pharmaceutical industry and device manufacturers provide an important and valuable service, providers must reconcile innovations with proven value of those innovations for patients. When a cheaper product exists that provides the same benefit, the system must aggressively encourage these less expensive options. Physicians must develop a focus on quality that appreciates the important contributions of other professionals such as nurses, pharmacists, laboratory technicians, clerks, and administrators. The administration of health care can become much more efficient and allow these nonpatient-focused resources to better care for the uninsured, develop new innovative products, and/or allow employers, individuals, and the government to invest their resources in other ways.

Systems need to be developed that support access to healthcare services for all Americans, rich and poor, at least to a minimum standard of care. A government-sponsored care model that supports a uniform level of care must be adopted to achieve the goals of quality care across the United States. A payment system supporting basic healthcare and public health services has the potential both to reduce costs for healthcare delivery and improve quality. In addition, a government-sponsored system would allow more effective negotiation for products that would, in turn, improve access to medications and devices; however, the current system is untenable. Admittedly, a quality-oriented system needs to allow for adequate profits and incentives to innovate. A model that provides access to physicians without the ability to pay for pharmaceuticals does not optimize health. The nation's healthcare system has a long way to go in realizing an exemplary quality vision.[28] This chapter is intended to help define quality in a holistic way. Other chapters in this book will delve deeper into areas that may help close the quality chasm.

Study/Discussion Questions

1. Describe the "quality triad" and how it can be used to improve healthcare delivery.

2. From your own personal experience, describe ways that your healthcare provider can close the chasm and achieve the six aims for improvement described in the IOM report.

3. Describe the importance of precisely defining what you mean by quality before undertaking an improvement project.

Suggested Readings/Web Sites

Institute of Medicine, Committee on Quality of Health Care in America. *Crossing the quality chasm: A new health system for the 21st century.* Washington, DC: National Academy Press; 2001.

Ransom SB, Joshi M, Nash D. *The Healthcare Quality Book.* Chicago: Health Administration Press; 2004.

Berwick DM. A users manual for the IOM's "quality chasm" report. *Health Affairs.* 2002;21(3):80–90.

University of Michigan Health System (www.med.umich.edu/obgyn/HealthServicesResearch/otherlinks.htm).

Institute for Healthcare Improvement (www.ihi.org).

The National Quality Forum (www.qualityforum.org).

Agency for Healthcare Research and Quality (www.ahrq.gov).

National Institute of Standards and Technology (www.quality.nist.gov).

Center for Studying Health System Change (www.hschange.com).

References

1. Kelley MA, Tucci JM. Bridging the quality chasm. *BMJ* 2001; 323:61–62.

2. Ransom SB, Joshi M, Nash D. *The Healthcare Quality Book.* Chicago: Health Administration Press; 2004.

3. Woolhandler S, Campbell T, Himmelstein DU. Costs of health care administration in the United States and Canada. *NEJM.* 2003;349:768–75.

4. Ransom SB, Dombrowski MP, Shephard R, Leonardi M. The economic cost of the medical-legal tort system. *Am J Obstet Gynecol.* 1996;174(6):1903–9.

5. McGlynn EA, Asch SM, Adams J, Keesey J, Hicks J, DeCrisofaro A, Kerr EA. The quality of healthcare delivered to adults in the United States. *NEJM.* 2003;348(26):2635–45.

6. Chassin MR, Galvin RH. The urgent need to improve health care quality. *JAMA.* 1998;280(11):1000–5.

7. Kohn LT, Corrigan JM, Donaldson MS. *To Err Is Human: Building a Safer Health System.* Washington, DC: National Academy Press; 1999.

8. Institute of Medicine, Committee on Quality of Health Care in America. *Crossing the Quality Chasm: A New Health System for the 21st Century.* Washington DC: National Academy Press; 2001.

9. Lohr KN. *Medicare: A Strategy for Quality Assurance.* Institute of Medicine. Washington, DC: National Academy Press; 1990.

10. Berwick DM. A user's manual for the IOM's "Quality Chasm" Report. *Health Affairs.* 2002;21(3):80–90.

11. Donabedian A. Explorations in quality assessment and monitoring. *The Definition of Quality and Approaches to its Assessment.* Vol. 1. Ann Arbor, Mich: Health Administration Press; 1980.

12. Griffith JR and White KR. Six strategies for highly successful organizations. In: *Thinking Forward.* Chicago; Health Administration Press; 2003. See also the Web site for Baptist Hospital, Pennsacola, Fla. The hospital has won the Baldrige Award for Quality, and several awards for service excellence. http://www.ebaptisthealthcare.org/

13. Fertlie E, Shortell SM. Improving the quality of healthcare in the United Kingdom and the United States: A framework for change. *The Milbank Quarterly.* 2001;79(2):281–316.

14. Ransom SB, Tropman J, Pinsky WW. *Enhancing Physician Performance.* Tampa: American College of Physician Executives Press; 2001.

15. Ransom SB, Dombrowski MP, Studdert D, Mello M, Brennan TA. Reduced medico-legal risk by compliance with obstetrical clinical pathways: A case-control study. *Obstet Gynecol.* 2003;101(4):751–55.

16. Campbell DA Jr, Sonnad SS, Eckhauser FE, Campbell KK, Greenfield LJ. Burnout among American surgeons. *Surgery.* 2001;130(4):696–702.

17. Griffith JR, Knutzen SR, Alexander JA. Structural versus outcomes measures in hospitals: A comparison of Joint Commission and Medicare outcomes scores in hospitals. *Qual Manag Health Care.* 2002;10(2):29–38.

18. Griffith JR, White KR. The revolution in healthcare management. *J Healthcare Manag.* In press.

19. Griffith JR, White KR. The revolution in healthcare management. *J Healthcare Manag.* In press.

20. Studdert DM, Mello MM, Brennan TA. Medical malpractice. *N Engl J Med.* 2004;350(3):283–391.

21. Wennberg JE. Unwarranted variations in healthcare delivery: Implications for academic medical centers. *BMJ.* 2002;325:961–64.

22. Nolan TW. System changes to improve patient safety. *BMJ.* 2000; 320:771–3.

23. Juran JM, Grya FM. *Juran's Quality Control Handbook.* New York: McGraw-Hill; 1951.

24. Grandzol JR. Which TQM practices really matter: An empirical investigation. *Qual Manag J.* 1997;4(4):43–59.

25. Griffith JR, White KR. The Revoluation in Hospital Management. In Preparation.

26. Ransom SB. *The Wisdom of Top Healthcare CEOs.* Tampa: ACPE Press; 2003.

27. Cleary PD, Edgman-Levitan S. Health care quality: Incorporating consumer perspectives. *JAMA.* 1997;278(19):1608–12.

28. Griffith JR, Alexander JA, Jelinek RC. Measuring comparative hospital performance. *J Healthcare Manag.* 2002;47(1):41–57.

29. Gerteis M, Edgman-Levitan S, Daley J, Delbanco T. (eds). *Through the Patient's Eyes: Understanding and Promoting Patient-Centered Care.* San Francisco, CA: Jossey-Bass; 1993.

Notes

Donabedian A, Bashur R. *An Introduction to Quality Assurance in Healthcare.* New York: Oxford University Press; 2003.

Leape LL, Berwick DM, Bates DW. What practices will most improve safety? Evidence-based medicine meets patient safety. *JAMA.* 2002;288(4):501–7.

Chapter 5

Analyzing Quality Data

Jonathan E. Gottlieb

EXECUTIVE SUMMARY

This chapter focuses on the challenges of collecting, organizing, and interpreting information about quality health care. Although these challenges are shared by other industries, the intricacies of health care pose unique problems in the analysis of quality. These intricacies include a rapidly and continually changing foundation of medical knowledge, a considerably individualized approach by clinicians, tremendous biological diversity among patients, and a highly complex system that can obfuscate accountability. This chapter will examine operational definitions of quality that facilitate measurement, discuss issues surrounding the quantification of quality, summarize techniques of measuring quality, explore pitfalls in comparing quality across settings, and discuss the challenges of interpreting information about quality. Physicians, nurses, and hospital administrators each see quality from their own perspective, which might or might not be similar to that of the patient. To minimize ambiguity, the patient's perspective will be assumed wherever possible in exploring issues of healthcare quality.

LEARNING OBJECTIVES

1. To learn about the challenges of collecting and analyzing quality data.
2. To understand the four components of quality.
3. To gain knowledge of quantitative measures of quality.

KEYWORDS

Outcomes Movement

Patient Satisfaction

Compliance

OSCE

Cost Sharing

Benchmarking

Case Mix

Risk Adjustment
Severity Score
Process Measures

Introduction

Operational Definition of Quality

The notion of quality in health care encompasses a broad array of concepts including safety, technology, compassion, skill, and thoroughness, among others. Both subjective aspects, in terms of the value placed on health care, and objective aspects, in terms of measurable results, are relevant to that value. It incorporates the sense of quality as described in *Zen and the Art of Motorcycle Maintenance*.[1] "Quality couldn't be independently related with either the subject or the object but could be found only in the relationship of the two with each other. It is the point at which subject and object meet".[1] This notion of quality emphasizes the result of interaction between a caring and competent individual and a process, analogous to that between a highly skilled and dedicated physician and a patient, or a carefully designed and managed clinic and its patient population. The value of such an interaction must be determined by patients or, collectively, by the society in which they live.

Patient Outcomes

Although healthcare quality must require the sort of interaction between healthcare professionals and patients envisioned in the preceding paragraph, progress in quality health care necessitates a deeper level of specificity. That quest for specificity has fueled in large part the "outcomes movement" in which intermediate health states at defined points in time (death defines all ultimate human outcomes) are quantified. Frequently measured outcomes include mortality, infection rate, remission rate, cure rate, survival and life expectancy, and complication rate, among others. Relatively simple methods have been developed to estimate life expectancy from summed disease-specific mortality.[2] Sources of outcomes information include administrative databases such as those maintained by the Centers for Medicare & Medicaid Services (CMS), clinical databases largely derived from provider institutions, payor data, and data from health-related quality-of-life initiatives. New developments in methodologic approaches to measuring and interpreting outcomes have been recently reviewed.[3] While there is little controversy about the importance of sophisticated value-adjusted outcomes, objections to using outcomes as the ultimate measure of quality include biologic diversity and patient heterogeneity, uncertainty in medicine, complexity of disease and the varied approaches to their diagnosis and treatment, and multiple uncontrolled and unrecognized confounders of outcome, among others. In other words, significant differences in outcomes can have a relationship to quality that is only approximate. Perhaps more important, the outcomes that can be so closely correlated with a specific care process by double-blind, prospective, placebo-controlled trials can be much more difficult to discern among the "noise" of real-world clinical medicine. For these reasons and others, Brook and co-authors opined, "the assessment of quality should depend much more on process data than on outcome data, especially when those systems are used to compare health plans or physicians."[4] Nevertheless, outcomes data has become increasingly available not only to healthcare professionals, but to the general public as well. For example, individual Pennsylvania hospital mortality "ratings" (higher, lower, or not different than expected) in infectious pneumonia can be viewed online at the Pennsylvania Health Care Cost Containment Council's Web site (www.phc4.org).

Patient Satisfaction

A second approach to defining quality emphasizes the perception of quality. Ultimately, it is the human value placed on outcomes, process, or experience that determines quality. At one extreme, quality is reduced to popularity or superficial allure, such as the physician with a great bedside manner but little skill or knowledge. Patients can flock to this "quality" physician despite his failure to follow evidence-based medicine and despite his being regarded with disdain by his colleagues. At the other is the emphasis on "hard data" and science to the exclusion of concern for or attention to the patient experience. Structured, explicit, and validated instruments that address patient satisfaction go a long way toward eliciting quantitative and reproducible patient preferences about specific aspects of care. Public reports of patient satisfaction are limited, but several initiatives have made individual hospital patient satisfaction data publicly available; Rhode Island reports on 10 dimensions of patient satisfaction (nursing care, physician care, treatment results, patient education, comfort/cleanliness, admitting, staff courtesy, food service, patient loyalty, and overall experience) at www.health.ri.gov/chic/performance/quality/quality10.pdf.

Compliance

To answer these objections, another approach to defining quality surrounds the compliance with a prescribed plan, emphasizing process in terms described by Donabedian.[5] If a robust plan is meticulously implemented, it provides the highest likelihood of achieving the best outcome, which should then be limited only by biologic diversity, inherent variation, and other complexities. This aspect of quality has been the cornerstone of accreditation by the Joint Commission on Accreditation of Healthcare Organizations (JCAHO) and similar organizations, emphasising adherence to standards, policies, or processes as a reflection of quality. A major limitation of this approach is that it is difficult to identify a consensus-driven evidence-based compilation of "right things" for most clinical conditions. Much is known about which "things" to do to achieve minimally appropriate outcomes (e.g., anticoagulation for atrial fibrillation to prevent stroke). But within a population of patients who receive appropriate anticoagulation for atrial fibrillation, there can be a broad range of outcomes that can be the result of patient diversity, comorbid conditions, and myriad other processes unrelated to the primary problem of atrial fibrillation, but which nevertheless impact the outcome from any one hospitalization (handwashing, intravenous catheter care, and so on). Moreover, unrecognized aspects of care can lead to better or worse outcomes than expected despite adherence to a circumscribed set of known standards. Another problem with this approach is that there is limited evidence for most of what healthcare professionals do, with the result that local practice, opinion leaders, economic pressure, and other factors can drive the details of medical care, which can show great variability from locale to locale. Finally, the process-oriented approach to quality clearly assumes the provider view and can be invisible to the patient except in its impact on outcome or as reflected by the satisfaction of the patient.

Compliance with the JCAHO standards by individual hospitals is readily available at www.jcaho.org/quality+check/index.htm. Compliance with general process standards is available at this Web site, as is information about compliance with disease-specific process measures. Similar hospital disease-specific process data is available through Medicare's website www.hospitalcompare.hhs.gov/hospital/home2.asp.

Efficiency

It is helpful to highlight a fourth domain of quality: efficiency of care. Efficiency in this context includes the provision of healthcare utilizing a minimum of resources, including time. Thus access to care, length of stay, waiting time, and turnaround time for test results can reflect quality through attention to efficiency. Here it is very important to maintain the patient perspective in assigning value to efficiency; what can be of high quality because of supreme efficiency to a healthcare chief financial officer can hold little value to the patient who is inconvenienced by the effort. In a broader sense the responsible steward of healthcare resources will have greater ability to direct healthcare resources effectively, resulting in potentially better outcomes, higher satisfaction, and increased compliance. Generally, cost of care is not publicly shared. Medicare cost reports are available for a fee at www.cms.hhs.gov/data/download.

In actual practice, each of these components (**O**utcomes, **S**atisfaction, **C**ompliance, and **E**fficiency, or **OSCE**) reflects a distinct but interrelated facet of quality, and attention to each is required to achieve a quality of healthcare that is comprehensive and durable (see Table 5–1).

In many industries, the interaction among caring, competent individuals and a well-structured and implemented process results in desirable outcomes, that is, a quality that can be depended on to occur repeatedly and predictably. The machining of a mechanical component or the delivery of a package, if well done, will result in high customer satisfaction, comply with necessary regulations, and minimize resource consumption—and will do so most every time. In addition, a "high quality" machine part or delivery service will excel when compared with competitors.

Table 5–1 *Outcomes, Satisfaction, Compliance, and Efficiency (OSCE)*

Quality Dimension	Definition	Comparator	Examples
Outcome	Intermediate patient health status	Severity-adjusted peer measure	Infection rate, survival from myocardial infarction
Satisfaction	Patient satisfaction measured by standard instrument	Local norms or within-institution over time	Satisfaction with nursing responsiveness
Compliance	Adherence to best practice, standards, or evidence-based care	JCAHO, state regulations, guidelines	Handwashing rate, timeliness of stroke treatment
Efficiency	Minimizing unnecessary patient or provider resources to deliver care	Marketing, group purchasing norms	Waiting time, cost of pharmaceuticals

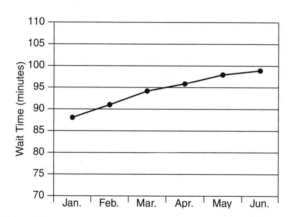

Figure 5–1 *Efficiency of Wait Time*

Thus, in addition to the OSCE quality dimensions, it is necessary to demonstrate reproducibility (or predictability) and excellence (or attainment of a benchmark). The operational definition of quality, then, is the interaction between a patient and a healthcare provider or system that consistently produces a favorable outcome, high patient satisfaction, compliance with best practice and efficient use of resources, and that compares favorably with others.

This quality measure of efficiency (e.g., as seen in Figure 5–1, the wait time in an emergency department) reflecting efficient use of patient time also overlaps with satisfaction, in that shorter waits are likely to result in greater satisfaction. To the extent that early evaluation and treatment can improve results, wait time can also impact outcome. In this example, wait time has been measured and plotted over six time periods, suggesting an increase in wait time has occurred.

Measurement of Quality

Patient Outcomes

In order to analyze quality, it needs to be measured. In order to measure it, healthcare quality has to be expressed in quantitative terms. Health outcomes lend themselves to quantification because when people think of quality in healthcare they tend to think of quantity of life (life expectancy, survival, mortality rates), at least for major health events (childbirth, surgery) and diseases (cancer, myocardial infarction). In-hospital mortality remains an important indicator that drives morbidity and mortality conferences, peer review, and other quality improvement processes. Cancer survival is perhaps the most commonly measured outcome of this disease, not because other intermediate outcomes are not important, but because the impact of cancer on survival eclipses most other considerations.

For global outcomes such as mortality, attribution becomes an important consideration. How can the contribution to life expectancy be measured from a single patient encounter with an endocrinologist, or a surgeon, or a midwife? Because numerous individual encounters with many healthcare professionals (as well as lifestyle, heredity, and myriad other factors) impact overall life expectancy and quality of life, these outcomes measures are most relevant in situations—such as cancer, major surgery, or stroke—that profoundly and imminently impact mortality. Although for any individual mortality is the nadir of all possible outcomes, its rare occurrence in, for example, appendectomy makes it a poor summary measure of outcome from that procedure. Definitions of survival and mortality can seem straightforward, but in fact there exists a wide variety of definitions. The Food and Drug Administration recognizes 28-day mortality as an endpoint in the testing of new drugs; CMS, JCAHO, and other organizations focus on mortality during a single hospitalization, whether one or one hundred days. Surgical mortality typically recognizes any death occurring within 30 days of the date of surgery as related to the procedure. Survival in cancer patients can be expressed in one-, three-, or five-year likelihood of survival, whereas survival from organ transplantation is reported by the United Network for Organ Sharing as three-month, one-year, or three-year survival.

In situations where mortality is not the major consideration, outcomes concerning symptom relief, improvement in functional status, achievement of target physiologic surrogate endpoints, and avoidance of complications can be the most meaningful factors. For example, favorable measurable outcomes from hip replacement include decreased pain assessed by a validated pain scale, ability to ambulate increased distances, and absence of wound infection. Favorable outcomes from treatment for hypertension include achievement of target blood pressure, absence of drug side effects, and avoidance of complications such as myocardial infarction or stroke. For individual patients, the impact of blood pressure control on stroke and heart disease occurs only over many years and only in a statistical sense; blood pressure control can make myocardial infarction and stroke less likely, but will not prevent their occurrence.

Despite a firm foundation in scientific evidence, measurement of outcomes has come late to contemporary medical care. Over the past decade CMS (formerly the Healthcare Financing Administration, or HCFA) has increasingly encouraged standard definitions of outcomes, alone or in partnership with other entities. For example, a recent initiative by CMS and Premier seeks to measure outcome and process quality indicators, compare healthcare institutions, and allocate reimbursement based on relative level of attainment of those quality targets (www.premierinc.com/all/informatics/qualitydemo). Professional, private, and government organizations have also independently developed repositories of outcomes-based data addressing issues such as hospital-acquired infections (the National Nosocomial Infection Surveillance System www.cdc.gov/ncidod/hip/SURVEILL/AboutNNIS.htm); mortality (University Healthsystem Consortium, CareScience); and outcome from organ transplantation (United Network for Organ Sharing, www.optn.org/latestData). These initiatives promise substantial progress in the ability to improve healthcare quality. For example the NNIS-defined catheter infection database provides an explicit definition of intravascular catheter-related infection, a standard denominator (device-days), and a standard procedure for capturing data. The challenges faced by healthcare institutions and the public is that unless other agencies employ the same definitions and procedures, comparisons about catheter-related infections would be problematic.

The sources of these outcomes data remain diverse and lack standardization, but are potentially readily available and inexpensive to obtain. For example, the universal billing form UB-92 includes data about outcome, is required by most regulatory agencies, and is readily available in many large databases. Use of the UB-92 to obtain outcome data requires little expense. However, the data present on the form reflects the accuracy and thoroughness of clinicians' documentation in the medical record, as well as the accuracy of coding by medical records personnel.

For other outcomes data, the situation is more complex. For example, the Pennsylvania Health Care Cost Containment Council, which reports publicly on outcomes at Pennsylvania hospitals, utilizes manual chart abstraction to enter clinical information into a database. In contrast, Premier and the University Healthsystem Consortium map out charge-level billing data into a standardized database to facilitate computerized transfer of information, in combination with chart abstraction. In general, the integrity of most of these outcomes data reporting methodologies (mortality being a notable exception) is highly vulnerable to variation in coding practices and clinician documentation.

Patient Satisfaction

Quantitative measurement of patient satisfaction depends on validated questionnaires; several are commercially available. Care must be taken in patient questionnaire construction to avoid bias, demonstrate face validity and stability, embody an appropriate reading level, and adhere to other standards of good questionnaire construction. Timing of the questionnaire must take into consideration such issues as accuracy of recalled events, fear of disapproval by physicians, and influence of family members. Satisfaction must be measured independent of outcome and disease severity. Recently, CMS has focused its Hospital-CAHPS program on the standardization of patient satisfaction across broad strata of the public, in order to make it easier to obtain reliable, uniform information about patient satisfaction; that project is slated for implementation in 2005 (www.ahrq.gov/qual/cahps).

The relationship between patient satisfaction and other quality measures remains complex. For example, in a study of more than 42,000 validated patient satisfaction questionnaires from 29 hospitals, hospital mortality varied inversely with satisfaction scores.[6] However, for some domains (physician care) there was no correlation, or the correlations were weak at best. More important, the interpretation of satisfaction data likely requires an underlying model far more complex than a simple linear approach. Some aspects of the patient care experience can have profoundly greater impact on overall satisfaction than others, although these aspects can be obscured in an overall score. Negative experiences in particular can affect overall satisfaction to a greater extent than positive experiences.[7] Satisfaction instruments that facilitate recall and recording of negative experiences can result in scores significantly lower than instruments that make negative experiences less accessible than positive experiences.

Compliance

Measurement of process indicators faces a different set of challenges because many of the target processes represent one intermediate step in the complex process of medical decision making. For example, most patients benefit from aspirin administration during the initial hours of an acute myocardial infarction. However, some patients will have already taken aspirin at home; others have aspirin sensitivity, a contraindication. Unless this information is documented and available to the abstractors, an accurate measurement of compliance with this evidence-based indicator will not be obtained. One approach is to set the target appropriately. If the incidence of aspirin sensitivity in the general population is 5 percent, and 10 percent of patients with chest pain take aspirin at home before presenting to an emergency room, then an 85 percent compliance with this indicator can be appropriate. However, levels above or below this target can reflect a different patient population rather than evidence of excellence or mediocrity, unless documentation is specific.

As in the case of outcomes measurement, measurement of compliance depends to a great degree on the accuracy and thoroughness of chart documentation. As more of the medical record becomes automated, the accuracy of measurement of compliance will improve. For example, rather than rely on a nurse to document the administration of aspirin and note the time correctly, automatic bar coding allows the patient, medication, and time of administration to be recorded accurately and automatically. Comprehensive ICD-9 based electronic problem lists that can include aspirin sensitivity (E93.5) can eliminate the need for costly manual chart abstraction.

Efficiency

Certain aspects of efficiency directly affect the patient experience, such as waiting time for a test result or appointment, hospital length of stay, and cost to the patient. As the trend toward cost-sharing with patients increases, patients will become increasingly sensitive to this aspect of quality. Purchasers in other industries have long been familiar with the relationship between quality and cost, or value. Assessment of value in medical care presents unique challenges not only because of the complexities in assessing quality, as previously discussed, but also because the cost to the patient will depend on a complicated interaction of provider efficiency, insurance coverage, and actual cost of care.

Other aspects of efficiency can be measured more readily. The time from request to first scheduled appointment, or the time from mammogram to result notification are measures of efficiency that are apparent to patients. The standardized collection and reporting of these measures, however, are far from routine. Increased pressure from patient groups will undoubtedly catalyze the collection and dissemination of this sort of information in the future.

Several measures can be combined into a composite quality measure of great richness and meaning. Utility theory provides both a framework and a methodology for adjusting a quantitative outcome, such as life expectancy, for qualitative patient preferences or values. For example, people (and patients) tend to value a year of life in the near term more than a year of life in the future, for many reasons. Health can be better and life more enjoyable now than in the distant future, or there is more certainty now than in the future. Utility theory helps to "discount" an outcome measure such as life expectancy for time, as well as for differences in perceptions about quality of life. Combining patient preferences or values with outcomes can result in a very patient-centered approach to quality, in contrast to efficiency and process measures, which are narrow surrogates for human values.

Variability of Quality Measures

All quality measures (outcomes, satisfaction, compliance, and efficiency) show variability over time. Random variation in biologic processes, inability to perfectly model innumerable variables, and true differences all contribute to the ups and downs of quality indicators. No two individuals have identical outcomes (no two individuals have identical genetic makeup, except for monozygotic twins), and no two patients demonstrate identical satisfaction. Efficiency of care can depend on patient variability, as well as the ability of the healthcare system to accommodate inconsistencies. However, it is not too much to expect a more uniform performance in measures of compliance, as long as they are sensibly defined.

Despite the caveats previously noted, high quality care includes a consistency in that level of quality. This consistency can be represented using tools of statistical process control—a detailed explanation of which is far beyond the scope of this chapter. Quantification of variability can be expressed in a variety of ways, several of which are briefly described as follows.

One of the most common ways of expressing variation among a series of measurements is in terms of the average (mean) and variance or standard deviation. Variance is calculated as the sum of the squared deviations of each measurement from the mean; the standard deviation is the square root of the variance, which has the advantage of being expressed in the same units as that which is being measured. The more "scatter" in the sample, that is, the further from the mean the individual measurements, the greater the variance and standard deviation. In the example of wait times, the average was 88.2 minutes; the variance was 434, and the standard deviation was 21. With the same mean, a smaller variance and standard deviation would reveal that more of the wait times were closer to the average wait time.

A more visual sense of variation among a sample is provided by a histogram (see Figure 5–2), which plots frequency on the vertical axis and magnitude on the horizontal axis. A combination of quantitative information and visual information is provided by the box-and-whiskers plot, which portrays the median (middle) value, the first and third quartiles, and the outer extreme values. From this plot, one can discern the symmetry of the distribution, the median value, how closely the middle values lie to the median, and how far away the outliers extend. In this histogram, wait times were between 90 and 100 minutes; 12 were between 80 and 90; and so on. The histogram provides a sense of how closely the times are grouped around a central tendency. Although most patients waited 90 to 100 minutes, some waited less than an hour, and several waited more than two hours. In addition to the sense of central tendency por-

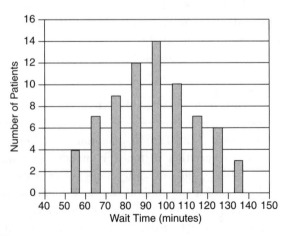

Figure 5–2 *The Histogram*

trayed in the histogram, the box plot (see Figure 5–3) shows the extreme ranges of values, the median, and the symmetry of the inner quartiles. The lower extreme measure is 50, and the upper extreme is 130. The second quartile of wait times lies between 70.75 and 92.5 minutes; the third quartile lies between 92.5 and 105.25 minutes. By definition, as many wait times fell below the median (92.5 minutes) as fell above it.

Measures and graphic representation of measures of central tendency can be useful in examining the reproducibility of a given measurement, such as wait time. A narrow histogram or a short box plot suggests a group of wait times characterized by a small standard deviation were consistent and reproducible. A better way to represent variability over time is to employ the control chart (see Figure 5–4). Under the assumption that the average value of a quality measurement (e.g., wait time) remains constant over time, fluctuations around that average should represent variation from "common causes" such as random busy times, emergencies that interrupt scheduling, and other factors. Should a pattern of measurements occur indicating that the wait times move consistently away from the average, or that significantly exceed the average the likelihood is that "special cause" variation systematically affected the wait time. This variation might include an influx of additional patients into the catchment

Lower Whisker	Lower Hinge	Median	Upper Hinge	Upper Hinge
50	71	93	105	130

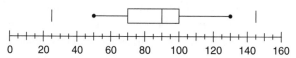

Figure 5–3 *The Box Plot*

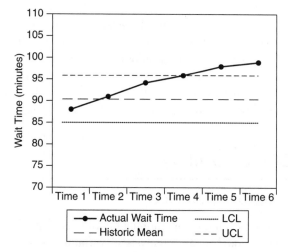

Figure 5–4 *Control Chart of Wait Time*

Table 5–2 *Data Characteristics of Special Cause Variation in a Control Chart*

Eight consecutive points above or below the mean
Any point above the upper control limit or below the lower control limit
Eight consecutive points that all change in the same direction
Non-random patterns including
Cycles
Trends
Clusters
Sawtooth
2 consecutive points beyond 2 sigma from the mean
4 consecutive points beyond 1 sigma from the mean

area, an inefficient clerk, a recently impaired physician, or other factors. The importance of identifying special cause variation lies in the ability to detect something going awry early on to enable efforts to address the problem. Although the average in the past had been 90 minutes, the control chart in Figure 5–4 suggests that there is special cause variation because there are multiple points all heading in the same direction, and because two points (Time 5 and Time 6) are associated with wait times that lie far from the expected average, beyond the upper control limit (UCL). Causes of increased wait time should be sought, such as increased patient volume, decreased staff productivity, increased patient complexity, and other factors. This pattern of variation is not consistent with random effects about a stable average wait time.

Control charts are useful tools to display such measures as mortality, infection rate, and patient satisfaction over time, not only because they accommodate the inherent variability of these biologic processes, but because they provide an indication of how much variation is "too much." They provide a statistical analysis that helps to differentiate random variation (common cause variation) from a true change (special cause variation). Commonly used criteria to identify special cause variation in control charts are shown in Table 5–2. If special cause variation is noted and is beneficial, it should be identified and promulgated. If it is detrimental, it should be identified and expunged.

Comparisons of Quality

Average or Expected Performance

This chapter has thus far examined operational definitions of quality, issues surrounding the measurement of quality, and analysis of variation as a reflection of quality.

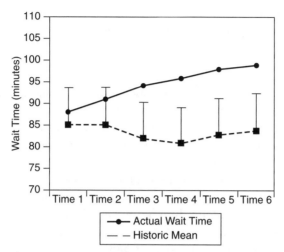

Figure 5–5 *Average Wait Time in the Emergency Room*

These considerations address quality in an absolute sense, whereas most people think of quality as something that distinguishes the better from the inferior. Whether the subject is diamonds, artwork, automobiles, or healthcare people expect a minimum level of quality to define quality that is merely acceptable and higher levels of quality to differentiate the superior. One way to set the expectation for acceptable healthcare quality is to see what everyone else is doing, to get a feel for the spectrum of performance. This requires that all parties divulge their performance, using standard definitions and employing similar methods of reporting; challenges in defining common measures and in reporting were described earlier in the chapter. Despite these challenges, substantial progress has been made in recent years by such states as New York and Pennsylvania, and by organizations such as the CMS; the JCAHO; and the AHRQ. These organizations have begun to promulgate explicitly defined quality measures, and have required timely and consistent reporting to permit comparison among healthcare organizations. The Agency for Healthcare Research and Quality provides an extensive list of well-researched and carefully defined quality indicators, including definitions of numerators and denominators for rate indicators, that have been gaining increasing acceptance by healthcare organizations and providers, as well as the public.

The hypothetical measure of wait time (e.g, an emergency department visit) could conceivably find its way into such a catalog of standard measures. The graph shown in Figure 5–5 can portray the average wait time. The dashed line represents the average wait time for a group of similar institutions during the same time period. The error bars reflect the 95 percent confidence interval of the group average. Because the wait times for Time 3 through Time 6 exceed the confidence interval, there is less than a 5 percent likelihood that the observed difference is due to chance alone. In other words, there is a 95 percent likelihood that these wait times are really longer than the average of the comparison group. The control limits and historic average from Figure 5–4 have been deleted for clarity.

Benchmarking

Beyond the concept of average lies the notion of the benchmark. This term refers to a level of achievement that defines superior. In the example of the emergency department, it can refer to the top few institutions that have achieved superior wait times. The comparator graph might look like Figure 5–6. The dashed line represents the benchmark wait time for the best performing group of similar institutions during the same time period. The error bars reflect the 95 percent confidence interval of the benchmark. There is less than a 5 percent likelihood that all wait times differ from the benchmark by chance alone. In other words, there is a 95 percent likelihood that the wait times are really longer than the benchmark.

Benchmarking is an important aspect of understanding and analyzing quality. It identifies a superior level of performance that is actually attainable and offers the opportunity to set an ambitious goal. By identifying specific institutions or processes associated with the benchmark, it also allows a deeper look into the potential factors that facilitated achievement of the benchmark performance. It might reveal, for example, a novel use of wireless technology, a pre-registration process, and the use of personnel as expeditors in the institutions with benchmark wait times.

The wait times in this example vary from under one to more then two hours, are increasing "out of control" over recent time periods, are significantly longer than comparator institutions, and are far from those of the best performing institutions. However, the defensive (and potentially appropriate) explanation might be: "You can't compare us to the other institutions fairly, because unlike them, our patients are more complex, and we have been experiencing a unique increase in volume over

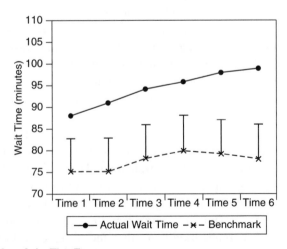

Figure 5–6 *Benchmark for Wait Times*

recent months." By focusing on the quality indicator of wait time, the implicit assumption is that longer wait times mean a lower performing institution. The preceding protest over unfair comparison emphasizes that non-institutional factors can be responsible for the special cause variation. What is needed is some method to compare wait times across institutions while adjusting for differences in severity of disease, volume of patients, and other non-institutional factors.

Risk Adjustment and Case Mix

The most common method of severity adjustment involves creating categories of risk or severity across all wait times and then comparing similar risk categories across institutions. A thorough discussion of this topic is beyond the scope of this chapter; the reader is referred to other sources for more detail.[8,9] In order to perform risk adjustment, an outcome variable must first be selected. Continuing with the example of wait time in an emergency department, the factors that are known or suspected to impact that variable can be considered, for example, frequency of patient arrivals, bed complement, and patient severity. Those variables that show a weak correlation with the outcome are discarded, until a model emerges that includes the most significant factors. Richardson cites four important characteristics of a good risk-adjustment model: parsimony (simplicity that is sufficient to describe the variability); goodness of fit (ability to account for a substantial proportion of the observed variability); theoretical consistency (the model must make sense); and predictive power (robustness using a new data set).

Having identified patient arrivals as an important factor, categories can be created for very low, low, medium, high, and very high arrival rate. Then comparisons can be made of wait times from institutions that demonstrate similar categories of arrival rates to "level the playing field." Or to go further by sub-categorizing each category of patient arrivals, an examination can be made of the ratio of bed complement to arrivals. In part, the specific adjustments really depend on the questions being asked.

Once the categories are defined for patient severity, arrival rate, and bed complement, the wait times associated with each combination of categories can be calculated. The characteristics of each institution can then be reconstructed in terms of severity, arrivals, and beds categories to calculate a wait time that is adjusted for those factors. Provided that the statistical assumptions are valid, the final result is a wait time that is expected given all of these factors. Wait times that are significantly different must be ascribed to other factors, which are more likely to reflect quality.

"Case mix" refers to the patient severity component of this adjustment. For example, in an emergency department that lies close to a major highway, the proportion of patients with major blunt trauma can be higher than that of a department in an inner city area away from major roadways. By calculating the average wait times associated with different types of trauma, the overall expected wait time can then be estimated by weighting the wait times by the particular mix of trauma types. As long as the patient severity factors have been worked into the equation, it can be confidently

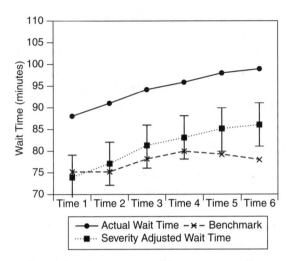

Figure 5–7 *Severity-Adjusted Wait Time*

shown that differences in observed wait time do not result from differences in patient severity. An example of severity-adjusted wait times is shown in Figure 5–7. When patient characteristics are taken into account, the wait times are not far from the benchmark. The interpretation is that the high patient severity is enough to explain the apparently long wait times; it need not be posited that there is a quality problem with the institution regarding wait time. Prior analysis demonstrated that the wait times are increasing due to a special cause—this remains true and should be investigated further. However, other causes that come into play can include increasing severity of patient illnesses or administrative factors, for example.

Risk adjustment must never be considered an infallible fix for potential differences in populations. Even the best risk adjustment methods seldom account for more than 30 percent of the observed variability in clinical outcomes.[10] In comparing several different major risk-adjustment methodologies across four conditions (acute myocardial infarction, stroke, pneumonia, and coronary artery bypass graft), it was found that the different methodologies frequently disagreed with predicted mortality by a factor of two.[10] Even accepting severity-adjusted differences in mortality, the relationship between "excess mortality" (as judged from the differences between actual and severity-adjusted predicted mortality) and other measures of quality (such as chart review of processes) is controversial. Some authors note a relationship between higher than severity-adjusted expected mortality and quality process problems, and others find no connection.

Unidentified factors not included in the risk adjustment can play an unanticipated role, so that attributing observed differences to differences in quality always entails some chance that not all of the important non-quality factors have been identified. There are practical limitations on risk adjustment as well, particularly when the number of strata are large and the population relatively small, leading to small numbers in any given cell and limitations in the ability to be confident about an important effect of a category on the overall outcome being measured.

Interpretation of Quality

In light of the foregoing discussion, it is time to ask: How can healthcare quality best be interpreted? The answer is both straightforward and complex. Just as no one would reasonably judge the quality of an automobile solely by the number of vehicle-specific accident deaths per 1,000 miles, the quality of a healthcare organization or practitioner cannot be judged by a severity-adjusted mortality statistic alone. Ultimately, quality health care is whatever it is perceived to be, so that patient satisfaction must figure prominently. Excellent compliance with processes that are known to produce good outcomes (e.g., aspirin for acute myocardial infarction) must be a prerequisite. Severity-adjusted outcomes that are in keeping with or that exceed average outcomes are desirable but serve better as a monitor than as a proof of quality. Finally—particularly from the provider perspective—highly efficient models of care mean that resources can be allocated to achieve superior satisfaction, compliance, or outcomes, and not to some extraneous task that detracts from the goal of high quality care.

The tools to analyze quality are largely quantitative and statistical. They help separate random events from real problems (e.g., the control chart); differentiate anecdotal from significant opinion trends (e.g., Likert scale); and make comparisons less subject to population-specific or external biases (risk adjustment).

Quality assessment of health care is far more complicated than quality assessments of manufacturing processes. A few measures such as frequency of repair record, fuel mileage, customer loyalty, and crash testing can be very helpful in assessing the quality of an automobile. In health care, each quality measure must be viewed in light of risk adjustment, common cause variation versus special cause variation, and benchmarks. Moreover, health care as an ongoing relationship among a group of professionals and patients must include the values and preferences of those patients. From a consumer perspective, individuals must weigh the entire spectrum of quality measures that can describe a single aspect of healthcare; no single statistical tool, number, or domain is sufficiently comprehensive to define healthcare quality. Like Phaedras in *Zen and the Art of Motorcycle Maintenance*, we must see quality as a series of interactions that combines the subjective with the objective and, in the end, make up our own minds.

Case Study

A 26-year-old woman developed gradual onset of shortness of breath over the past three days. She had no cough, fever, wheezing, or other symptoms. Because the sensation of shortness of breath increased in intensity, she went to her local hospital's emergency department (ED). At the ED, she waited in the busy reception area until her name was called to registration. After providing her general and insurance information, she was told to wait. Twenty minutes later, a triage nurse obtained a brief history and took vital signs. She returned to the waiting room, where she waited for two and a half hours. During this time, she witnessed a steady flow of patients with various degrees of injury and distress pass through the emergency area; most appeared much sicker than she was. She was eventually led to a stretcher, where another nurse took a detailed history. A physician entered the room, took a more detailed history, performed a physical examination, and ordered blood tests, a chest X-ray, lung scan, and electrocardiogram. Over the next three hours the tests were evaluated, after which time the physician told her that he thought that she might have asthma, but no serious disease. She was instructed to follow up with her primary physician and was given a prescription for an inhaled bronchodilator.

The afternoon previous to the patient's visit, a hospital administrator, the physician director of the emergency department, and the director of hospital performance improvement met to review several disturbing trends. Patient satisfaction with the emergency department was falling, the proportion of "elopements" (patients leaving the emergency department without being fully evaluated) was increasing, and there had been at least one instance of a patient falling in the crowded waiting room. The administrator wanted the physician director to organize the department more efficiently to address the fundamental problem of excess wait time; the physician director believed that the wait time was to be expected given the severity of illness of the patient population, and the existing resources. The performance improvement director suggested that the wait times first be measured and benchmarked before embarking on a performance improvement plan that focused on wait time.

Using the techniques described, with enthusiastic and substantive support from hospital administration and the medical staff, the emergency department embarked on a nine-month effort to measure, analyze, and improve the quality of care. They chose to focus on wait times; patient satisfaction with services delivered; timeliness of initiation of care for patients with time-sensitive diagnoses for cases such as stroke and chest pain; and return visits to the departments for the same complaint within 72 hours. Using tools from performance improvement organizations and ideas from staff within the hospital, they developed new policies and procedures, re-organized the functions of staff, hired additional staff, and instituted performance-based incentives. Some of the changes they initiated included:

- Hiring a "greeter" to establish contact with every patient from the time they entered the ED
- Moving triage out into the waiting area to better and more quickly identify seriously ill patients
- Completing registration in the examination areas, with the aid of wireless computers, to begin diagnosis and treatment more quickly
- Posting an electronic sign that reads, "Patients registering now may have an average wait time of . . . . "

In addition, the greeter, registration, nursing, and other staff were trained in the recognition of and appropriate action for time-sensitive conditions. Each person was then empowered to initiate an appropriate care process (e.g., the greeter knew to escort any patient complaining of chest pain to a wheelchair and then immediately to the triage nurse, bypassing registration). Other improvements were made to decrease wait times and improve the quality of care.

Study/Discussion Questions

1. What are some examples of challenges to collecting and analyzing quality data?
2. What are the limitations of some approaches to analyzing quality data?
3. What constitutes a catalyst for change to make health care more efficient?
4. How is variation measured?
5. What are control charts and why are they useful?
6. What are significant aspects of a good risk-adjustment model?

Suggested Readings/Web Sites

National Nosocomial Infection Surveillance (http://www.cdc.gov/ncidod/HIP/surveill/about_NNIS.htm).
University HealthSystem Consortium (http://www.uhc.edu/).
United Network for Organ Sharing (http://www.unos.org/).
Pennsylvania Health Care Cost Containment Council (www.phc4.org).

References

1. Pirsig RM. *Zen and the Art of Motorcycle Maintenance.* New York: William Morrow; 1974.
2. Beck JR, Pauker SG, Gottlieb JE, Klein K, Kassirer JP. A convenient approximation of life expectancy (the "DEALE"). II. Use in medical decision-making. *Am J Med.* 1982;73(6):889–97.
3. Lohr K. Health outcomes measurement symposium. *Med Care.* 2002;38:194–208.
4. Brook RH, McGylnn ME, Cleary PD. Measuring quality of care. *NE J Med.* 1996;335(13):966–70.
5. Donabedian A. *Explorations in Quality Assessment and Monitoring: The Definition of Quality and Approaches to Its Assessments.* Ann Arbor, Mich: Health Administration Press; 1980.
6. Jaipaul CK, Rosenthal GE. Do hospitals with lower mortality have higher patient satisfaction? A regional analysis of patients with medical diagnoses. *Am J Med Qual.* 2003;18(2):59–65.
7. Otani K, Harris LE, Tierney WM. A paradigm shift in patient satisfaction assessment. *Med Care Res Rev.* 2003;60(3):347–65.
8. Iezzoni L. An introduction to risk adjustment. *Am J Med Qual.* 1996;11(1):S8–11.
9. Richardson D, Tarnow-Mordi WO, Lee SK. Risk adjustment for quality improvement. *Pediatrics.* 1999;103:255–65.
10. Iezzoni L. The risks of risk adjustment. *JAMA.* 1997;278(19):1600–7.

Chapter 6

Fundamentals of Outcomes Measurement

Donald E. Casey

EXECUTIVE SUMMARY

This chapter will address a number of critical issues necessary to develop a fundamental understanding of the nature and complexities inherent in the field of Outcomes Measurement (OM). These issues range from the importance of one's time frame and frame of reference, measurement methods and sources of data, to barriers and opportunities of outcomes measurement.

LEARNING OBJECTIVES

1. To understand a simple taxonomy and basic conceptual framework for classifying OMs
2. To recognize and understand/appreciate the importance of specifying a frame of reference behind and related to OM
3. To identify sources and technical aspects of OM
4. To appreciate current challenges and future opportunities for OM

KEYWORDS

Outcomes Measurement
Scandinavian Simvastatin Survival Study
Indicator
Comparison
Assessment

Introduction

In the Affair of so much Importance to you, wherein you ask my Advice, I cannot for want of sufficient Premises, advise you what to determine, but if you please I will tell you how. When those difficult Cases occur, they are difficult, chiefly because while we have them under Consideration, all the Reasons pro and con are not present to the Mind at the same time; but sometimes one Set present themselves, and other times another, the first being out of Sight. Hence the various Purposes or Inclinations that alternatively prevail, and the Uncertainty that perplexes us.

Benjamin Franklin, London, September 19, 1772

The subject of Outcomes Measurement (OM) in health care is perhaps one of the most important and difficult issues to grasp. The purpose of this chapter is to introduce some basic technical concepts regarding OM. However, before the notion of "how" this is done, it is imperative to provide a conceptual framework around the process of approaching the "why" of OM.

When making a decision to measure outcomes, one must ask several fundamental questions:

1. What are the goals in attempting to measure outcomes? In other words, why bother?

2. What sort of OM expertise is available to assist with the measurement of outcomes? Outcomes Management is not for the amateur and requires specific prerequisite skills, knowledge, and experience.

3. What resources, especially computer software and hardware, are necessary and available to support the process of OM?

4. What are the costs and benefits of measuring outcomes?

5. Can other published or unpublished experiences be identified, consulted, and utilized that will assist in shortcutting the process of developing and measuring outcomes without sacrificing scientific accuracy? This includes identifying information that can be used in conjunction with or instead of that which might be generated by an expensive process.

6. What is the process for interpretation and identification of limitations of the OM that are generated?

Perhaps the biggest challenge is to measure outcomes for purposes of improving healthcare quality. In this case, it is absolutely imperative that evidence-based best practices can be identified that are directly linked to the outcomes that are measured. If so, then these specific processes can, for all practical purposes, be treated as outcomes. Some examples include:

- Time to reperfusion for Acute Myocardial Infarction—directly linked to the degree of myocardial necrosis, infarct size, and hence likelihood of death over the short-term (in hospital mortality and complications) and long-term (post-hospital survival and development of chronic heart failure).
- Glycosylated hemoglobin (Hb A1C), which is linked, over time, to the degree of glycemic control for patients with diabetes (both Type 1 and Type 2), which is, in turn, linked to the likelihood of complications such as diabetic nephropathy, retinopathy, and neuropathy.
- Early administration of appropriate antibiotics to elderly patients admitted to the hospital through the emergency department with community-acquired pneumonia (in- and post-hospital survival and disability).

As a result of this nuance, the use of the term "outcome" has varied meanings depending on the context of the discussion; the degree of sophistication of the researcher or quality improvement expert; and the transparency, reproducibility, and effectiveness of the measurement process. Another important decision to consider is whether previous use of a specific outcomes measure has been controversial and subject to disagreement and lack of consensus. On the other hand, given the flexibility and widespread appeal of OM, one must be on guard not to "overcook" one's intentions in measuring outcomes.

The United Way[1] has a particularly interesting and relevant online resource addressing many of the complexities related to outcomes and outcomes measurement:

> Outcomes are benefits or changes for individuals or populations during or after participating in specific health interventions. They are influenced by a program's outputs. Outcomes may relate to behavior, skills, knowledge, attitudes, values, condition, or other attributes. They are what participants know, think, or can do; or how they behave; or what their condition is, that is different following the program. Note: *Outcomes* sometimes are confused with outcome *indicators,* specific items of data that are tracked to measure how well a program is achieving an outcome, and with outcome *targets,* which are objectives for a program's level of achievement.

For the mathematically inclined, outcomes can typically be expressed as a (usually complex, rarely simple) function of intrinsic patient attributes and other factors, as described in more extensive detail by Iezzoni[2]:

> Outcomes = f (intrinsic patient risk factors, treatment effectiveness,
> quality of care, time frame, perspective, random chance)

Typically, data used for such methods is obtained from randomized, controlled experiments and clinical trials; prospective observational studies; and retrospective analytic methods, such as meta-analysis of several "like"—but not precisely methodologically concordant—published studies that focus on the same outcome endpoints.

Purpose/Aim of Outcomes Measurement

Before one begins to measure outcomes, several questions must be answered relative to the purpose/aim of OMs. The following represent several of the most typical reasons cited for measuring outcomes.

1. Measurement of health status, including mortality (either descriptive or defining risk of death); limitations of activity due to chronic health conditions; and patient characteristics (such as gender, ethnicity, race, income status, demographics, and other individual data).

2. For decision making relative to resource allocation, such as for health policymakers, either as a reaction to or in anticipation of private and public funding restrictions or opportunities within the care delivery system—for example an educational campaign designed to promote more widespread use of barrier methods (condoms) to prevent the spread of HIV/AIDS in African and Asian countries.

3. To determine effectiveness and safety of health improvement interventions, such as new pharmacologic or public health interventions, for example the Scandinavian Simvastatin Survival Study (4S)[3] trial to determine the effects of a cholesterol-lowering agent on a large population at risk for the development of ischemic heart disease, or a communitywide smoking cessation program to reduce the risk of ischemic heart disease (IHD), chronic lung disease, and cancer.

4. To assist government, healthcare insurance companies, and employers in defining and measuring quality of care among provider groups with the intent of improving care and stimulating competition on this basis.

Members of the European Research Group on Health Outcomes (ERGHO)[4] are from seven European countries and have formulated a set of critical questions and guidelines in choosing the best method of using health-related OMs:

What is your aim? Do you want to describe, to compare, or to evaluate health outcomes? The selection of your instruments is highly related to the endpoints of your project. What do you want to use it for? The psychometric qualities of the chosen instrument must be able to support your endpoints. There are three principal uses:

- *A health status measure can be used as an INDICATOR, measuring the situation at one point in time. The endpoint is descriptive. Besides validity, reproducibility and specificity, or the chosen condition are important.*

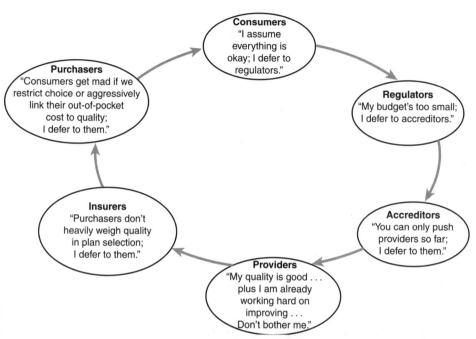

Figure 6–1 *Cycle of Unaccountability ©2000 Arnie Milstein, MD*

Galvin RS, McGlynn EA. Using performance measurement to drive improvement. A road map for Change. *Med Care*. 2003;41:I-48–I-60.

- *A health outcome measure can be used as a COMPARISON, relating differences at different points in time: before and after intervention. For this type of action sensitivity and responsiveness to change are important. That is, the measure must be able to register small changes in the health of patients over time.*
- *Health outcome ASSESSMENT implies, besides the measurement of outcome, an attempt to use the information through feedback to practitioners. In order to use that information some understanding of the process of care is required so that the project database must also include process data.*

Only after you have defined your aims and purposes and decided about the way to use the results, can you map these against a number of instruments and scales to decide on which most closely suits your purpose.

To get a better sense of specifics, let's turn to the *Closing the Quality Gap*[5] series from the Agency for Healthcare Research and Quality (AHRQ) that addresses many of the IOM-identified treatment priorities. It is AHRQ's hope that the series will stimulate ideas for further quality improvements across a broad range of users. For example:

- Policy makers can use the detailed evidence review to prioritize quality improvement strategies and choose how best to narrow the "quality gaps" in their organizations.

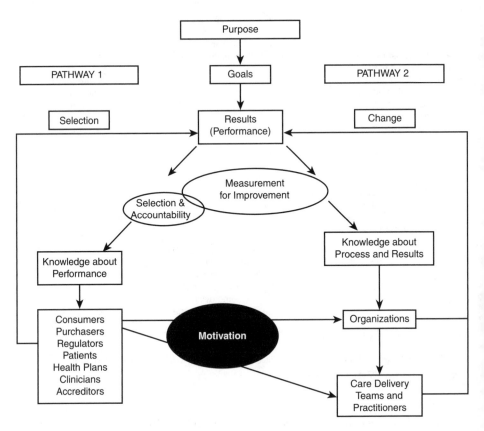

Figure 6–2 *Two Pathways to Quality Improvement*

- Researchers can find detailed information about well-studied areas of treatment, while learning of areas in need of greater exploration.
- Clinicians and trainees can see a broad spectrum of approaches to improving the quality of care. Some of these approaches fall within the control of individual practitioners, while others require major systemic changes at the local level or beyond.
- Patients can learn quality improvement strategies that they can help to promote, while gaining a deeper understanding of the nature and extent of quality gaps, as well as the systemic changes necessary to close them.
- Groups and individuals charged with funding research will be able to identify high-yield areas of concern that warrant future research support.

In defining one's purpose, it is important to specify whether one wishes to use OMs for the purpose of accountability or to improve care, or, perhaps both at once. According to

Galvin and McGlynn,[6] there are multiple reasons for wanting to do this. Six steps are recommended: (1) raise public awareness, (2) redesign measures and reports, (3) make the delivery of information timely, (4) require public reporting, (5) develop and implement systems to reward quality, and (6) actively court leaders. The recommended six steps are interconnected; action on all will be required to drive significant acceleration in rates of adoption of performance measurement and reporting. Leadership and coordination are necessary to ensure these steps are taken and that they work in concert with one another to avoid the "Cycle of Unaccountability" diagrammed in Figure 6–1.

According to Berwick,[7] clear purpose, focused goals, and valid and reliable performance metrics set the stage for the use of measurement to pursue changes that are improvements. But at this point, things become a little more complicated. The model in Figure 6–2 classifies approaches to the use of measurement in improvement into two different—although linked and potentially synergistic—agendas, or pathways. Pathway I relies primarily on the act of selection to improve quality and Pathway II relies primarily on process changes to improve quality. In a complete improvement strategy, both pathways are important. Both masters can be served in this regard, although it is critically important for those using OMs to continuously and clearly specify and separate these intentions (perhaps on a daily basis).

Types of Outcome Measurements

There are many types of OMs, some of the most common typologies of which are listed here with illustrative examples.

- **Clinical Status**, such as mortality, morbidity, patient characteristics (e.g., genetic predisposition for diabetes, chronic renal failure, all-cause mortality)
- **Functional Status** (e.g., ability to perform activities of daily living; exercise tolerance)
- **Patient Satisfaction/Perceptions** (e.g., satisfaction with providers; depressed mood; and other humanistic dimensions)
- **Financial/Economic Outcomes** (e.g., cost; cost-effectiveness)
- **Utilization Outcomes** (e.g., appropriateness of care; length of hospital stay)

One typology classifies outcomes as Economic, Clinical, or Humanistic Outcomes (the ECHO framework).

To show some of the complexities involved with using OMs an example is provided. The iSIM is a simulation model based on the Duke Stroke Prevention Policy Model, developed as part of the Duke Stroke Prevention Patient Outcomes Research Team (PORT).[8] In this study, the endpoint outcomes measured were death and disability from complex interactions due to co-morbid complications arising from an acute stroke or pre-existing conditions. The iSIM is designed to offer insight into the impact of acute stroke on a defined population and also to provide an estimate of the impact that an

Table 6–1 *Proximal, Intermediate, and Long Range OMs*

Proximal	Intermediate	Long Range
• Satisfaction with provider visit • Relief/control of symptoms (e.g., acute pain) • Physical status (self-care, ability to walk) • Prevention (cost to the patient and provider) • Appropriateness of care (appropriate clinical assessment and evaluation, e.g., the performance of dilated eye examination for a patient with diabetes)	• Affordability/access to healthcare • Cost (managed care contract) • Comorbidity development (e.g., neuropathy, renal function, AMI for patients with diabetes) • Delivery of appropriate services to a population (e.g., mammography)	• One-year mortality • Five-year mortality • Blindness, renal transplant, heart failure, other diseases/comorbidities (diabetes) • Cost (national health expenditures)

acute treatment unit might have on short- and long-term health and economic outcomes of stroke. By modifying the characteristics of the population of interest and the nature of the intervention, the user can examine how these factors influence the incidence and cost of stroke and the potential value of new treatment strategies. To make the use of the model more concrete, the iSIM includes a case study of a hospital medical director deciding whether to create an acute stroke service. A more detailed study of iSIM (outside the scope of this chapter) can be helpful for purpose of demonstrating the complexities that typically arise very rapidly in the course of developing and evaluating OMs.

Time Frame

Clear specification of time frame for which outcomes are to be measured is critical and should necessarily have a significant influence on which specific OMs are chosen or to be developed. Table 6–1 illustrates via example the conceptual differences between *proximal, intermediate,* and *long range OMs.*

A recurring and vexing issue in outcome measurement is deciding how far the outcome chain in a program should go in selecting its longest-term outcome. This decision requires a balance between two needs:

- *The longest-term outcome must be far enough out on the if-then chain to capture meaningful change for participants and reflect the full extent of the program's benefit for them.* As an example, participants knowing what constitutes good prenatal care is an important link in the if-then chain, but it is not meaningful as an end in itself and is not all the program aspires to achieve for participants. The program needs to go beyond that initial outcome in measuring its benefits.

- *On the other hand, the longest-term outcome should not be so far on the if-then chain that the program's influence is washed out by other factors.* It must be reasonable to believe that the program can influence the longest-term outcome in a nontrivial way, even though it cannot control it. In the prenatal program described, contact with the teen mothers ends when their infants are born. Extending the program logic chain from the outcome of healthy births to an even longer term outcome of "the children are developmentally on target at age two" is not sound in view of all the other factors that will influence mothers and babies in the intervening two years.[2]

Frame of Reference

Describing one's frame of reference is critical to the successful development and use of OMs. Table 6–2 developed by Radford[9] demonstrates this issue as it relates to the sincere and real differences that exist between physicians and health system administrators who use OMs to evaluate quality of care and practitioner performance. When different points of view are not acknowledged, dialogue can be easily (almost predictably) derailed into the abyss of arguing about the technical details of the measurement specifications, instead of serving as a pathway to improved care. Furthermore, when economic incentives are tied to such measurements, the ferocity of the debate can have serious and polarizing consequences that will subsequently quash meaningful conversations between parties (e.g., managed care plans and medical groups) for many years hence.

Up front and honest acknowledgment of these issues (in addition to making available in a transparent fashion the details of measurement specifications, derivative methods, and analytic limitations) facilitates cooperation and understanding—and hence create the desired pathway of tangible quality improvements. Unfortunately, despite best intentions and efforts in this direction, traditionalists (categories of stakeholders to

Table 6–2 *Differences in Quality/Outcomes Measure Preferences and Perspectives*

Measure characteristic	*Physicians*	*Administrators*
Simple	+	+++
Nuanced	+++	+
Valid	+++	+
Reliable	+++	++
National	+	+++

Martha Radford, MD (personal correspondence).

remain unnamed in this regard for politically expedient reasons) continue to be stalwart and obstructionist in accepting any notion of self-measurement and comparison.

In spite of these issues, the fortunate trend in the healthcare market place is in the direction of encouraging a broad range of stakeholders to utilize OMs with the sole purpose of improving quality of care. These stakeholders include consumers, purchasers, health plans, regulators, clinicians, and health systems.[6]

To highlight this issue further, a report from members of the RAND Corporation centering on the state of quality of healthcare in the United States was published in the June 26, 2003, issue of the *New England Journal of Medicine*.[10] The quality indicators used in the study were derived from RAND's Quality Assessment Tools system and represent the leading causes of illness, death, and utilization of health care, as well as preventive services related to these causes.

RAND Corporation: Follow-up Report on Quality

The RAND Corporation has produced a national report card that describes the quality of health care in the United States. The report was developed by a team of experts who conducted a comprehensive examination called the Community Quality Index Study. This research assessed the extent to which recommended care was provided to a representative sample of the US population for a broad range of conditions in 12 metropolitan areas. Some of the key findings include:[28]

- Overall, adults received about half of recommended care.
- The level of performance was similar for chronic, acute, and preventive care.
- Quality of care varied substantially by condition.
- Performance was similar in each of the metropolitan areas studied.
- No community had consistently the best or worst quality.

The findings of this study were meant to provide policy makers and providers with a real-time snapshot of the quality of care in the United States. Transparent acknowledgment by the researchers of their intentions to spark public interest with the purpose of influencing public policy and legislative initiatives permitted a "soft landing" in many hearts of well-intentioned providers and healthcare organizations that were highly disappointed with these obvious results, but were nonetheless openly honest that they could and in fact needed to do a better job of taking care of patients.

Methods of Measurement

Rather than provide extensive detail on measurement methods, which is beyond the scope of this chapter, it will be more informative to those not familiar with OMs to learn from a real-life example. The American College of Cardiology has developed an explicit framework for evaluating OMs.[11] Another excellent example is illustrated in Table 6–3, which highlights the framework of measurement attributes used by the

Table 6–3 *Attributes Used to Evaluate Diabetes Measures*

Attribute	Definition
1. Importance of topic area addressed by the measure	
a. High priority for maximizing health of person or population	The measure addresses a process or outcome that is strategically important in maximizing the health of persons or populations. It addresses an important medical condition as defined by high prevalence, incidence, mortality, morbidity, or disability.
b. Financially important	The measure addresses a clinical condition or area of healthcare that requires high expenditures on inpatient or outpatient care. A condition is financially important if it has either high per-person costs or if it affects a large number of people.
c. Demonstrated variation in care and/or potential for improvement	The measure addresses an aspect of healthcare for which there is a reasonable expectation of wide variation in care and/or the potential for improvement. If the purposes of the measure are internal quality improvement and professional accountability, then wide variation in care across physicians or hospitals is not necessary.
2. Usefulness in improving patient outcomes	
a. Based on established clinical recommendation	For process measures, there is good evidence that the process improves health outcomes. For outcomes measures, there is good evidence that there are processes or actions that providers can take to improve the outcome.
b. Potentially actionable by the user	The measure addresses an area of healthcare that potentially is under the control of the physician, healthcare organization, or healthcare system that is assesses.
c. Meaningful and interpretable to the user	The results of the measure are reportable in a manner that is interpretable and meaningful to the intended user. For example, physicians must be able to use the information generated by the measure to improve patient care. Healthcare organizations must find the information useful for decision-making purposes. When measures are used to compare healthcare systems, users should be able to understand the clinical and economic significance of differences in how well systems perform on the measure.

National Quality Forum (NQF) to establish national consensus on a standardized set of diabetes care quality improvement measurements.

In developing outcome measures, paying heed to validity and reliability is critical to the process. Without these and other key attributes (listed in Table 6–4), the likelihood that the OMs that are produced will have significance and meaning to other users is unlikely.

As can be seen from this information, the process is complex, labor-intensive, and highly detailed. One can sense that the development of OMs is not for the faint of heart, nor something that should be naively "tried at home." On the contrary, OM development requires time, expertise, close monitoring for new changes

Table 6–3 *Continued*

Attribute	Definition
3. Measure design	
a. Well-defined specifications	The following aspects of the measure are well defined: numerator, denominator, sampling methodology, data sources, allowable values, methods of measurement, and method of reporting.
b. Documented reliability	The measure will produce the same results when repeated in the same population and setting (low random error). Tests of reliability include (a) test-retest (reproducibility); test-retest reliability is evaluated by repeating administration of the measure in a short time frame and calculating agreement among the repetitions; (b) inter-rater: agreement between raters is measured and reported using the kappa statistic; (c) data accuracy: data are audited for accuracy; and (d) internal consistency for multi-item measures; analyses are performed to ensure that items are internally consistent.
c. Documented validity	The measure has face validity—it should appear to a knowledgeable observer to measure what is intended. The measure also should correlate well with other measures or the same measures.

in science, and health services research evidence that can necessitate technical changes to OM specifications.

Risk Adjustment

Various methods are used to adjust for severity and other characteristics of measurement subjects in an attempt to normalize comparisons between populations. Risk adjustment techniques are highly desirable but also add expense and complexity to the development of OMs. These risk adjustment methods are often either generated from the measurement process, or more commonly, the methods are utilized using existing, published methods. Examples of such methods include the Charlson Morbidity Index[12] (for co-morbidities based on ICD-9 disease and condition codes); Apache III (for risk assessment of patients in critical care settings); the all patient refined-diagnosis related groups (APR-DRG system (groups patients into four stratified categories based on DRG and ICD-9 classifications); and the Society of Thoracic Surgery (STS) Database for Cardiac Surgery[13] (developed by STS for purposes of evaluating cardiac surgical outcomes at surgeon and facility levels). Typically, these risk adjustment methods are based on statistical models developed by researchers and focus on identifying specific clinical parameters.

Another critically important reason for using OMs that are risk-adjusted is to compare performance between providers. If done effectively, such measures are much more likely to be both meaningful and influential to providers who are willing to change practice based on results that are consistently subpar. Open and honest dialogue targeting efforts to improve care will ensue, rather than devolving to the

Table 6–4 *Criteria for Choosing a Generic Outcome Measure*

Domains of health	Choice of domains affects the treatment effects observed.
Range of health	Range of measure affects the coverage of the spectrum of the performance and change in health status.
Clinical relevance	The interpretation of score will be difficult if numbers do not have a logical ordering and connection to reality.
Level of emphasis	The emphasis determines the relative weight of each domain in the measure.
Sensitivity	The inability of the measure to detect change in health status will miss important subtle changes.
Reliability	Unreliable measures yield inconsistent, uninterpretable results.
Validity	Valid measures provide information about the dysfunction of interest—validity.
Practical considerations	The burden of administration influences responses from patients and providers and amount of information obtained.

Kane RL. *Understanding Healthcare Outcomes Research.* Sudbury, Mass: Jones and Bartlett Publishers; 2004.

unfortunate scenario of a provider who claims, "My patients are sicker, so of course my outcomes can be expected to be worse than others." While never perfect, carefully crafted risk-adjusted OMs can successfully mitigate and neutralize such "cop outs."

Sources of Outcomes Data

There are many and extensive sources that provide vast amounts of information and data within the public domain of the federal government. Examples include the *CDC Source Book,* the AHRQ Healthcare Cost and Utilization Project (HCUP), and others sources at the end of this chapter.

The Agency for Healthcare Research and Quality has redesigned its interactive HCUPnet software tool[14] to make it easier to obtain hospital care trend data for the nation and for individual states. The data represent 90 percent of all hospital stays in the nation and are drawn from 36 states.

HCUPnet's databases include statistics on the conditions for which patients were hospitalized, the diagnostic and surgical procedures they underwent, patient death rates, hospital charges, hospital costs, length of stay, and other aspects of inpatient care. The data is for all patients, regardless of type of insurance or whether they were insured.

For example, using HCUPnet to research the impact of the obesity epidemic on hospital care and costs shows that more than 58,000 surgical procedures for obesity were performed in 2001. In addition, the data shows that between 1993 and 2001:

- The number of patients admitted for treatment of diabetes with complications—a condition often linked to obesity—rose 23 percent, from 373,666 to 461,161.

- The number of lower extremity amputations, a diabetic complication, increased 14 percent from 99,522 to 113,379, and the average hospital charge for this procedure increased 38 percent, from $24,332 to $33,562.
- Admissions for heart attack—which obese persons have a higher risk of suffering—rose 13 percent, from 682,763 to 773,871, and charges increased 61 percent—from an average of $19,178 per hospital stay to $30,875 per stay.
- Knee replacements, also more common among obese patients, increased roughly 29 percent, from 282,177 to 363,536, and the average hospital charge rose 38 percent, from $18,352 to $25,309.

Many of these databases are compiled from administrative sources using ICD-9 codes from aggregated insurance claims submitted by providers to various payors and purchasers of health care. Some data sets are internally kept by healthcare provider organizations (e.g., the American College of Surgeons National Surgical Quality Improvement Program,[15] or NSQIP, and the STS database for cardiac surgical outcomes). Others rely on measures and data constructed by detailed and laborious medical record abstraction (e.g., the Medical Outcome Study, or MOS, managed by AHRQ), while more recent innovative approaches have incorporated prospective, point-of-care methods to assist with the simultaneous enhancement of patient care and data collection (e.g., the American Heart Association's *Get with the Guidelines*[16] program focusing on improving cardiac and stroke care in hospitals). The Dartmouth Atlas[17] elegantly displays both quantitative and graphical information on a vast quantity of outcome data using geo-demographic maps of the United States. The examples of these detailed databases (e.g., the Organization for Economic Co-operation and Development (OECD) database alone is daunting) soon seem to be virtually endless when one begins to explore this vast topic of OM on a global, international basis.

Cost Considerations

Generally, outcomes measurement is an expensive proposition, no matter what methods are used. Not only should the cost of actually collecting and analyzing the data be determined, hundreds of hours of serious and at times heated discussions between experts in a particular field have typically made the development of outcomes not just labor-intensive but also time-intensive. New discoveries obtained in the process of OM will also necessarily tempt a pedantic researcher or health services administrator to continually refine or revise a specific OM method for the purpose of achieving the (in truth and practice unattainable) goal of perfection. The potentially endless temptation to drill down, data mine, and collect more granular data elements using more sophisticated computer algorithms and code for analyses should be carefully tempered with the voice of knowing when to quit—that is, when the primary goals of the OMs are generally (but not entirely) achieved. Because of these inevitable economic and practical limitations, the measurement team must be both skillful and credible in managing the dialogue among an emotionally charged group, especially if members within this group are being compared to one another by external agents (e.g., CMS, JCAHO, etc.) for the purpose of public reporting and accountability. If monetary bonus payments and other financial (and nonfinancial) incentives are to be awarded utilizing specific measures, the best of intentions can rapidly degenerate to mistrust between stakeholders that will, in the end, defeat the purpose of the effort, as witnessed through the dramatic failure of the Cleveland Health Quality Choice program[18] that occurred between 1991 and 1997 comparing hospital Medicare mortality rates for acute myocardial infarction, heart failure, gastrointestinal hemorrhage, chronic obstructive pulmonary disease, pneumonia, or stroke.

On the other hand, OM has several success stories such as the Statewide Planning and Research Cooperative System[19] (SPARCS) of the New York Department of Health, which is a comprehensive patient data system established in 1979. SPARCS continues to be a major management tool assisting hospitals, agencies, and healthcare organizations with decision making regarding financial planning and monitoring of inpatient and ambulatory surgery services and costs. This public reporting system has been credited several times over the years of being the driving force behind improving cardiac surgical outcomes for coronary artery bypass graft (CABG) and other cardiac surgical procedures.[20] Other states, such as Pennsylvania (via the Pennsylvania Health Care Cost Containment Council, or PHC4)[21] have also developed similar systems that are achieving significant improvements in quality of care.

Barriers/Challenges

Unfortunately, there have been many disappointments with OMs (such as the previously mentioned Cleveland Health Quality Choice program). Often, these disappointments resulted in polarizing (and hence paralyzing) conflict between clinicians versus purchasers rather than clarifying issues related to improving quality of care. This has led to what is referred to the "Cycle of Unaccountability" (mentioned earlier in this chapter).

According to Kazandjian,[22] the limitations of OMs are not acknowledged, especially by those who use OMs for accountability:

> In all situations, however, the question of changing outcomes is often met with unrealistic strategies that do not address the causes of the outcome but rather the observed symptoms of it. In other words, the statement that changing outcomes is the goal is, I believe, incorrect and misleading. *In operational terms, one cannot change outcomes.* Outcomes are reflections or consequences that in themselves cannot be changed but would respond to changes in the antecedents to those outcomes, which include processes, inputs into those processes, and the environment within which those processes took place. Thus, from a measurement point of view, changing outcomes should not be a goal but an initial screening approach, whereby the observations about outcomes would lead us to the exploration of

processes and contextual issues within which those processes took place. Outcomes have already happened—they cannot be reversed. But what led to those outcomes can be modified to yield better outcomes the next time around.

Causality is often multifactorial, as demonstrated by the Stroke PORT study presented earlier in this chapter. It is very easy to assume that a specific health outcome can be attributed to one or two variables identified through simple linear regression or other commonly used statistical techniques. Often, limited expertise, analytical resource constraints, plus a traditional "we've always done it this way" mindset of administrators (and some health services researchers focused on OM development) have limited the capability of gaining proper insights needed to solve such problems. Again, the United Way has excellent insights:

- Developing a sound outcome measurement system takes time—to plan, to try out, to adjust, and to implement. It easily could take an agency seven months or more of preparation before collecting any data, and it easily could take three to five years or more before the findings from a program's outcome measurement system actually reflect the program's effectiveness. Rushing the development process decreases the likelihood that the findings will be meaningful.

- There are many things outcome measurement does not do. It does not eliminate the need to monitor resources, activities, and outputs; tell a program whether it is measuring the right outcomes; explain why a program achieved a particular level of outcome; prove that the program caused the observed outcomes; by itself, show what to do to improve the outcome; or answer the judgment question of whether this is an outcome in which resources should be invested.

- Measuring and improving program-level outcomes does not, by itself, improve community-level outcomes. Except in rare instances, an individual program does not serve enough individuals to affect communitywide statistics, regardless of how successful the program is. In addition, community-level conditions are the result of a constellation of influences (e.g., economic conditions, environmental factors, demographic trends, public- and private-sector policies, cultural norms, and expectations) that are far beyond the scope of influence of individual human service programs.

Opportunities

In order to overcome these and other barriers, appropriate incentives must be created that link the need for accountability for quality improvements that are known from scientific and health services research to lead directly to improvements in outcomes. Such linkages have been deemed by the Medicare Payment Advisory Commission[23] (MEDPAC) and other policy-setting groups to be the correct pathway, rather than attempting to enforce compliance through threats of punishment and negative incentives. Therefore, the growing need for both trust and cooperation on the part of clinicians, health systems, managed care organizations, and other entities are necessary for success. With the development of more sophisticated information systems and public dissemination of OMs, the ever-expanding movement of patients who wish to be a part of the decision-making process will demand improvements in OMs and other quality measurements. Those "medical interest groups" who choose to ignore these forces will be left behind economically in the long run.

An excellent example of this is the CMS special demonstration project[24] designed to improve quality of care by rewarding providers who provide top quality care based on superior performance in a variety of standardized quality measurements. This project is designed to simplify and consolidate measurements, making them henceforth more patient centered. CMS believes that by creating the appropriate financial and nonfinancial incentives, it can speed a thus far slow evolution on the part of healthcare providers to provide evidence-based care to Medicare beneficiaries with high impact diseases such as heart failure, AMI, and CAP[25]:

Quality of Care Measures

Under the demonstration, top performing hospitals will receive bonuses based on their performance on evidence-based quality measures for inpatients with: heart attack, heart failure, pneumonia, coronary artery bypass graft, and hip and knee replacements. The quality measures proposed for the demonstration have an extensive record of validation through research and are based on work by the Quality Improvement Organizations (QIOs), the Joint Commission on Accreditation of Healthcare Organizations (JCAHO), the Agency for Healthcare Research and Quality (AHRQ), the National Quality Forum (NQF), the Premier system. and other CMS collaborators.

Hospital Scores

Hospitals will be scored on the quality measures related to each condition measured in the demonstration. Composite quality scores will be calculated annually for each demonstration hospital by "rolling-up" individual measures into an overall quality score for each clinical condition. CMS will categorize the distribution of hospital quality scores into deciles to identify top performers for each condition.

Financial Awards

CMS will identify hospitals in the demonstration with the highest clinical quality performance for each of the five clinical areas. Hospitals in the top 20 percent of quality for those clinical areas will be given a financial payment as a reward for the quality of their care. Hospitals in the top decile of hospitals for a given diagnosis will be provided a 2 percent bonus of their Medicare payments for the measured condition, while *hospitals in the second decile will be paid a 1 percent bonus. The cost of the bonuses to Medicare will be about $7 million a year, or $21 million over three years.*

Improvement Over Baseline

In year three, hospitals that do not achieve performance improvements above demonstration baseline will have adjusted payments. The demonstration baseline will be clinical thresholds set at the year one cut-off scores for the lower nineth and tenth decile hospitals. Hospitals will receive 1 percent lower DRG payment for clinical conditions that score below the nineth decile baseline level and 2 percent less if they score below the tenth decile baseline level.

Further federal legislative initiatives, increasing regulatory pressure from state and federal regulators, market-driven forces (especially from consumers), and the advancement of diagnostic, therapeutic, and information healthcare technologies are considered major forces that will speed improvements in care that lead to more meaningful OMs to be used by individual patients in making their own healthcare decisions, choices, and spending. Several conceptual models of public disclosure of quality information have been developed[26] that highlight the strategic intent of such a process.

Conclusions and Thoughts for the Future of OMs

The science and sociology of OM is becoming ever the more complex and interactive in the current environment. Careful and disciplined attention to the details of OMs as outlined in this chapter are essential ingredients for the achievement of successful healthcare quality and patient safety improvements that are needed by this country's healthcare system. With the rapidly expanding use of health information technology promoted by the new federal Office of the National Coordinator for Health Information Technology;[27] the extent to which OMs are used by patients, healthcare providers (especially hospitals and physicians), governments, researchers, and policymakers will expand exponentially over the next five years. Rapidly accessible OM-based tools for accurate clinical, ethical, and economic decision making and interpretation will be needed and demanded by all of these stakeholders. Retrospective lookbacks at care documented via traditional administrative claims data are destined to be replaced by virtual, real-time, and interactive information systems that efficiently and simultaneously document the process of care and the data elements critical to measuring and enhancing the effectiveness of that care. Those individuals and organizations creating dramatic, frame-shifting positive tensions for change identified by the Institute of Medicine's *Crossing the Quality Chasm* will require ongoing skill-building and technical training designed to successfully manage the conflicts arising from the tensions created by good OMs. This high road must and will lead all who cooperate in using OMs properly to achieve safe, effective, efficient, timely, equitable, and patient-centered care.

Study/Discussion Questions

1. Review Table 6–2 (Differences in Quality/Outcomes Measure Preferences and Perspectives). Identify and discuss some generic and disease-specific root causes of the differences in OM perspectives and preferences between physicians and administrators. How would you address and resolve these differences? Formulate your answers from both points of view as well as from that of a neutral third party.

2. Review at least two online OM resources listed in the Suggested Readings/ Web Sites section that follows. Discuss in detail similarities and differences between these resources in terms of: (a) Types of OMs, (b) Time frames of OMs, (c) Frame of reference, and (d) Methods of OMs. Summarize these differences in a descriptive table and state strengths and limitations of each resource analyzed.

3. Review in detail the Centers for Medicare & Medicaid Services (CMS) special demonstration project described near the end of this chapter. Discuss critical success factors and barriers to implementation. What can be done to mitigate failures and achieve intended success? What are some unintended consequences for the US healthcare system (positive and negative) that might arise out of this and similar initiatives?

Suggested Readings/Web Sites

Organization/Acronym/ Internet address	Resources available for OM	Description of measurements
Agency for Healthcare Research and Quality (AHRQ) (www.ahrq.gov/data/hcup)	Healthcare Cost and Utilization Project (HCUP)	Online query system to analyze health statistics and information on hospital stays at the national, regional, and state level
AHRQ (www.qualitymeasures.ahrq.gov)	National Quality Measures Clearing-house (NQMC)	Public repository for evidence-based quality measures and measure sets
Centers for Disease Control (CDC) (www.cdc.gov)	Data and Statistics	Data from birth and death records, medical records, interview surveys, direct physical exams, and laboratory testing that form key elements of the national public health infrastructure
Centers for Medicare & Medicaid Services (CMS) (www.cms.hhs.gov/ researchers/pubs)	Annual Data Compendium	Historical, current, and projected data on Medicare enrollment and Medicaid recipients, expenditures, and utilization; data pertaining to budget, administrative, and operating costs, individual income, financing, and healthcare providers and suppliers

Organization/Acronym/ Internet address	Resources available for OM	Description of measurements
World Health Organization (WHO) (www.who.int/research/en)	WHOSIS	Guide to epidemiologic and statistical information available from WHO
Organization for Economic Co-operation and Development (OECD) (www.oecd.org)	Statistics, Data, and Indicators	Measurement and analysis of the performance of health care systems in member countries and factors affecting performance designed to help decision makers formulate evidence-based policies to improve their health systems' performance
American Cancer Society (ACS) (www.cancer.org)	Annual Cancer Statistics	Tracks cancer occurrence, including the number of deaths, cases, and how long people survive after diagnosis
Pennsylvania Health Care Cost Containment Council (PHC4) (www.phc4.org)	Annual Report and interactive databases	Independent state agency that promotes healthcare competition through the collection, analysis, and public dissemination of uniform cost and quality-related information of PA hospitals

References

1. United Way of America. Outcome Measurement Resource Network. Available at: http://national. unitedway.org/outcomes/resources/What/ndpaper.cfm. Accessed on May 21, 2005.

2. Iezzoni L, ed. *Risk Adjustment for Measuring Healthcare Outcomes*, 3rd ed. Chicago: Health Administration Press; 2003.

3. Scandinavian Simvastatin Survival Study Group. Randomised trial of cholesterol lowering in 4,444 patients with coronary heart disease: The Scandinavian Simvastatin Survival Study (4S). *Lancet*. 1994;344:1383–89.

4. European Research Group on Health Outcomes. Choosing a Health Outcome Measurement Instrument. Available at: http://www.meb.uni-bonn.de/standards/ERGHO/ERGHO_ Instruments.html. Accessed on September 10, 2004.

5. Closing the Quality Gap: A Critical Analysis of Quality Improvement Strategies: March, 2004 Fact Sheet. Available at: http://www.ahrq.gov/clinic/epc/qgapfact.htm. Accessed on September 10, 2004.

6. Galvin RS, McGlynn EA. Using performance measurement to drive improvement: A road map for change. *Med Care*. 2003;41:I-48–I-60.

7. Berwick DM, James B, Coye MJ. Connections between quality measurement and improvement. *Med Care*. 2003;41:I-30–I-38.

8. http://www.clinpol.mc.duke.edu/ProjectDir/Stroke/SPProg/Applications/Isim/isim.html. Accessed on September 10, 2004.

9. Radford M. Personal correspondence.

10. McGlynn EA, Asch SM, Adams J, et al. The quality of health care delivered to adults in the United States. *N Engl J Med*. 2003;348:2635–45.

11. Krumholz HM, Baker DW, Ashton CM, et al. Evaluating quality of care for patients with heart failure. *Circulation.* 2000;102(12):2443–56.

12. Charlson ME, Pompei P, Ales KL, MacKenzie CR. A new method of classifying prognostic comorbidity in longitudinal studies: Development and validation. *J Chronic Diseases.* 1987;40(5):373–83.

13. The Society of Thoracic Surgeons National Database. Available at: www.sts.org/doc/8406. Accessed on September 10, 2004.

14. Agency for Healthcare Research and Quality. HCUPnet, Healthcare Cost and Utilization Project. Available at: www.ahrq.gov/HCUPnet. Accessed on January 12, 2005.

15. American College of Surgeons National Surgical Quality Improvement Program. Available at: www.nsqip.org. Accessed on September 10, 2004.

16. American Heart Association. Get With the Guidelines. Available at: http://www.american heart.org/presenter.jhtml?identifier=1165. Accessed on September 10, 2004.

17. The Dartmouth Atlas of Health Care. Available at: www.dartmouthatlas.com. Accessed on September 10, 2004.

18. Baker DW, Einstadter D, Thomas CL, Husak SS, Gordon NH, Cebul RD. Mortality trends during a program that publicly reported hospital performance. *Med Care.* 2002;40:879–90.

19. New York State Department of Health. Statewide Planning and Research Cooperative System (SPARCS). Available at: http://www.health.state.ny.us/nysdoh/sparcs/sparcs.htm #datainfo. Accessed on January 12, 2005.

20. New York State Department of Health. State Health Department Releases Reports on Cardiac Surgery. May 6, 2004. Availabel at: http://www.health.state.ny.us/nysdoh/commish/2004/cardiac_release_05-06-2004.htm. Accessed on September 10, 2004.

21. Pennsylvannia Health Care Cost Containment Council (PHC4). Available at: http://www.phc4.org/. Accessed on September 10, 2004.

22. Kazandjian VA. *Accountability through Measurement.* Milwaukee: ASQ Quality Press; 2003.

23. Medicare Payment Advisory Commission. Report to Congress: Medicare Payment Policy. March 2004. Available at: www.medpac.gov/publications/congressional_reports/Mar04_Entire_reportv3.pdf. Accessed January 12, 2005.

24. Centers for Medicare & Medicaid Services. Rewarding Superior Quality Care: The Premier Hospital Quality Incentive Demonstration: Fact Sheet. Available at: http://www.cms.hhs.gov/quality/hospital/PremierFactSheet.pdf. Accessed on March 12, 2005.

25. Jencks SF, Huff ED, Cuerdon T. Change in the quality of care delivered to Medicare beneficiaries 1998–1999 to 2000–2001. *JAMA.* 2003;289(3):305–312.

26. Marshall MM, Shekelle PG, Leatherman S, Brook RH The public release of performance data what do we expect to gain? A review of the evidence. *JAMA.* 2000;283(14):1866–74.

27. US Department of Health and Human Services. Office of the National Coordinator for Health Information Technology (ONCHIT). Available at: http://www.hhs.gov/onchit/framework/. Accessed on January 12, 2005.

28. RAND Health. The First National Report Card on Quality of Care in America. RAND Corporation, 2004. Available at: www.rand.org/RB/RB9053-1. Accessed May 17, 2004.

Chapter 7

Basic Tools for Quality Improvement

Walter H. Ettinger

EXECUTIVE SUMMARY

Quality improvement, or performance improvement, is the methodology by which clinical quality and safety are improved. Developing tools to engage in performance improvement in health care can be divided into five key areas: people, information management, infrastructure, work processes, and culture. This chapter explores these five areas in detail.

LEARNING OBJECTIVES

1. To understand the drivers behind performance improvement.
2. To recognize the importance of information management in health care.
3. To be aware of managing continuous improvement.

KEYWORDS

Performance Improvement

Information Management

Evidence-Based Medicine

Six Sigma

Introduction

Implicit in the goal of providing high quality and safe healthcare is the concept of quality improvement, also known as performance improvement. This chapter will use the term *performance improvement* because it has a broader connotation and can be applied to the improvement of all aspects of healthcare services. Essentially, performance improvement is the methodology used to improve the quality and safety of healthcare.

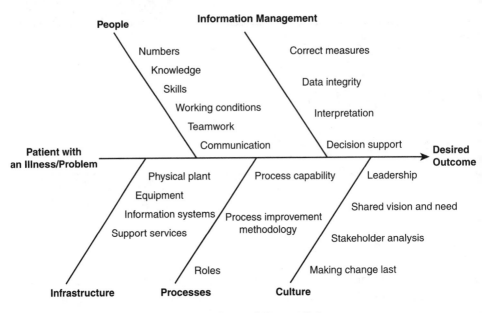

Figure 7–1 *Five Drivers of Clinical Quality and Patient Safety*

The performance improvement methodology described in this chapter is based on ideas that have been promulgated by the leaders of the quality movement in healthcare and other industries. This chapter attempts to synthesize the ideas of performance improvement efforts into a template. The template is based on five drivers of clinical quality (people, information management, infrastructure, work processes, and culture) that should be assessed, measured, and managed as part of performance improvement efforts.

The template illustrated in Figure 7–1 is a tool that can be used for most performance improvement efforts. The systematic assessment of the contributions to a desired healthcare outcome of each of these drivers, as well as the interactions among the drivers, is an essential step in understanding how to improve the likelihood of the outcome of the healthcare service to be improved.

People

Although contemporary management theory stresses a systems-based approach to quality improvement, the individuals who provide healthcare services are the bedrock of quality health care. Moreover, the issues surrounding people are complex and often the most difficult to assess and improve. The numbers, knowledge, skills, working conditions, and interactions of the people who deliver healthcare are critical to assuring and improving quality.[1, 2, 3, 4, 5] One must carefully assess and manage these issues.

At the most basic level, high quality health care requires adequate staffing levels. Most healthcare organizations are under pressure to cut costs, and personnel costs account for the majority of expenses. Given these pressures, one must maintain staffing at a sufficient level to assure safe and effective care.[6]

A high level of skill and knowledge are also important for quality health care. Organizations should not compromise on requirements to maintain skills and knowledge of physicians, nurses, and other professionals. Physician board certification and re-certification are empirically associated with better outcomes, yet hospitals often do not require board certification as a criterion for medical staff membership.[7] Healthcare organizations should maximize the educational level of their nurses by creating incentives for nurses to obtain bachelor's and masters' degrees. Educational level of nurses is associated with better outcomes.[8] The need for appropriate knowledge and skills goes beyond clinicians. Managers responsible for operations must have knowledge of the drivers of clinical quality and the skills to improve quality.

Working conditions can increase the likelihood of mistakes that can adversely affect quality. Frequent disruptions, long hours, and lack of sleep are risk factors for errors that need to be assessed and addressed during quality improvement efforts.[1, 4, 9] One method is to have an independent observer assess working conditions by trailing healthcare workers during their work. The observer can make suggestions as to how to reduce disruptions and variation in the work environment.

To provide high quality, safe health care, providers must work as a team and communicate effectively.[5] Practice and review are means to improve teamwork.[10] Communication is enhanced by use of checklists, readbacks, and timeouts. The Joint Commission on Accreditation of Healthcare Organizations (JCAHO) is mandating improved teamwork and communication among providers as criteria for accreditation.

Information Management

The second driver of clinical quality and patient safety is information management. The assessment and improvement of the quality and timeliness of information is an important aspect of performance improvement efforts. In short, information management is the transformation of data into knowledge and the use of knowledge to improve decision making.

Information management has three dimensions. The first dimension is measurement. Quality metrics can be divided into four categories: outcomes, process measures, resource utilization, and patient perception (see Table 7–1). One must carefully choose what is to be measured.[11, 12] Simply put, if something is not measured, it will not be managed and improved. Moreover, the metrics that one chooses must be important to the patient and reflect the patient's expectations. For example, both providers and patients consider wait time an important quality metric for the provision of emergency department services. But beyond measuring time-to-service, providers must understand what patients consider as acceptable wait time. If a hospital undertakes

Table 7–1 *Dimensions of Information Management*

I. Measurement
    Categories of quality metrics and examples
    Outcomes (mortality rate, morbidity rate, health related quality of life)
    Process of Care (occurrence rate, time)
    Resource Utilization (length of stay, cost per case)
    Patient's Perception of Care (satisfaction, willingness to recommend provider)
   Characteristics of a Good Metric
    Importance: Is it important to the patient (or their representative) or the process of care?
    Validity: Does it truly measure the outcome or process of interest?
    Reliability: What is the variability of the measure?
    Adjustment: Does it take into consideration confounding factors?
    Comparability: Are there benchmarks (goals)?
    Sensitivity to change: Can the metric be moved in response to performance improvement efforts?

II. Interpretation
    Interpret the mean and variation
    Determine defect rate and absolute number of errors
    Use confidence intervals to determine if differences are meaningful
    Trend the data and monitor over time

III. Decision support
    Evidenced-based medicine
    Timely reporting of results
    Clinical guidelines

a performance improvement project to improve wait time in the emergency department to less than three hours, and patients expect to be seen in no more than 45 minutes, most patients will not feel they are receiving quality care. Thus, asking patients or surrogates what is critical to quality from their perspective is important.

Beyond the choice of what is to be measured, the metric itself must be accurate, reliable, timely, appropriately adjusted for confounding characteristics, and comparable to internal or external benchmarks. Metrics must also be sensitive to change when performance improvements are undertaken.

The second dimension of information management is interpretation. Correct interpretation of data is critical—and pitfalls are common. A focus on mean (average) values without paying attention to variation is a common mistake. For example, the JCAHO and Centers for Medicare & Medicaid Services (CMS) have identified the time it takes for a patient to go from presentation to hospital until angioplasty as a marker of quality for care of patients with acute ST segment elevation myocardial infarction. The standard is to achieve "door to balloon inflation time" of less than 90 minutes. Hospitals report their mean and median times for a cohort of patients. Unfortunately, this ignores variation and can lead to false assumptions about performance. A hospital can improve its mean time while still having an unacceptable number of patients whose individual time to angioplasty exceeds 90 minutes. Therefore, the defect rate (number of patients who do not meet the standard) must also be reported. The goal of performance improvement

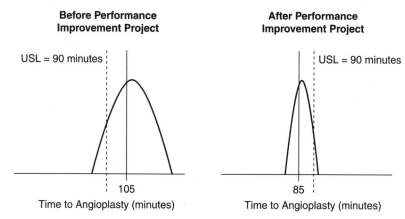

Figure 7–2 *Mean and Standard Deviation of Time from Emergency Department to Angioplasty. Note that after the performance improvement project, the mean time changed 20 minutes but the variance in time was reduced. Therefore, the number of patients whose time was more than 90 minutes decreased from 70% to 3%.*

Table 7–2 *Number of Errors Versus Rate of Filling Correct Orders for a Hospital Pharmacy that Fills 1,300,000 Medication Orders per Year*

Percent Correct	Errors
69.1%	401,700
93.3%	87,100
99.4%	7,800
99.98%	260
99.99966%	4

is to improve both the mean time to angioplasty and the number of patients who do not receive angioplasty within 90 minutes (see Figure 7–2).

Another common error in the interpretation of information occurs when one focuses on percentages alone and not absolute numbers. Many healthcare processes have relatively low error rates but high absolute number of errors because of the high number of times the process occurs. This concept is illustrated in Table 7–2. The pharmacy of a large medical center fills 1,300,000 medication orders a year. If the pharmacy correctly dispenses 99.4 percent of the medications correctly (a high percentage rate), the absolute number of errors is still 7,800, or 21 per day.

All measures have an inherent degree of variability and are estimates of a true rate. One must know whether the apparent change in a measure reflects a true change or is simply a chance variation. Two techniques are useful in this regard. The first is to use 95 percent confidence intervals around all point estimates. The other technique is to

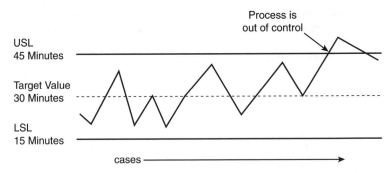

Figure 7–3 *Control Chart for Administration of Antibiotic Prior to Open Heart Surgery*

use control charts to trend data. Information about the stability of a process and whether changes in values are within desired limits are ascertained from control charts (see Figure 7–3). Control charts plot results over time. An upper and lower specification limit is set. If performance falls outside the specification levels, the process is out of control and needs to be examined for the causes of unacceptable performance.

The third dimension of information management is the provision of information at the time that it is needed, to enable a correct decision to be made about diagnosis and treatment. This dimension of information management is decision support. The Evidenced Based Medicine (EBM) movement is the bedrock of decision support.[13, 14] EBM is the use of the best current evidence, combined with clinical expertise and a patient's values, in making decisions about the care of individual patients.[14] Evidence-based medicine can be supported through the use of database resources that are available on hand-held devices, in paper form, and online. In the most sophisticated settings, EBM is imbedded in computer systems that can be used at the time of ordering and documentation. Other examples of decision support include timely reporting of critical laboratory values, use of clinical guidelines, and pre-printed order sets.[15] All of these tools are useful in enhancing performance and improving quality.

Infrastructure

Infrastructure refers to the attributes of the physical environment where clinicians deliver healthcare services. Areas of infrastructure that one should assess and improve as part of performance improvement include: physical plant (e.g., space, lighting, noise level); equipment (availability, function, compatibility, and standardization); and information systems (software and hardware). Well-known examples of technology that have been shown to improve clinical quality are programmable IV pumps, alarm systems, and computerized physician order entry. An additional

Table 7–3 *The DMAIC Process*

Phase	Description
Define	Define the objective of the process improvement initiative; determine the deliverables; identify the critical outcome *(Y)*; build a high level process map
Measure	Determine data collection methods and data integrity; measure the *Y;* determine the critical drivers of the process *(X's)* and measure *X's;* measure the process capability.
Analyze	Identify the quantitative and/or qualitative relationships between *X* and *Y*; use cause and effect diagrams, graphical analysis, and correlation analysis; determine which inputs *(X's)* to change.
Improve	Identify the solutions to improve the process; test solutions (pilot project).
Control	Validate solution and sustainability; use dashboard, control charts, and continuous improvement; celebrate success.

aspect of infrastructure that is often overlooked is the availability of support personnel to help assess and interpret data and to assist with process improvement.

Processes

The fourth driver of clinical quality and patient safety are the processes used to deliver health care. Perhaps the most important aspect of performance improvement is process improvement. The methodology for process improvement can be quite simple or rigorous and complex, such as Six Sigma Management System.[16, 17, 18]

A process is any group of activities that takes an input, adds value to it, and provides an output. All healthcare services are the result of processes. For any given procedure, service or transaction, there are inputs *(x)* and outputs *(y)* such that $y = f(x^1, x^2, x^3 . . .)$. In order to understand how well a process is working, one needs to measure the output *y* and the inputs *(x^1, x^2 . . .)*. To change the performance of a process, one must identify and change the critical inputs.

Most process improvement techniques use a continuous improvement cycle. Although there are different versions, one of the most rigorous is the Define, Measure, Analyze, Improve, Control (DMAIC) methodology (see Table 7–3). The DMAIC methodology begins by defining the outputs of importance (so-called critical **y**'s), mapping the process to be improved; measuring the output; determining the performance of the process; determining the critical inputs that affect the process; creating and optimizing a solution that changes the critical inputs to improve the process; and assuring the process change is sustained.[17, 18] The DMAIC methodology can be used either in a qualitative fashion or quantitative fashion.

A detailed discussion on how to apply the methodology of process improvement is beyond the scope of this chapter. However, four critical concepts of process improvement will be elaborated: process mapping, roles, throughput yield, and continuous improvement.

Process Mapping

Regardless of the methodology used for process improvement, the creation of a high-level process map is a sine qua non successful process improvement. A high-level process map illustrates the five to 10 important high-level process steps and defines the beginning and end of the process in question. A useful tool for creating a high-level process step is to use a modification of the Suppliers, Inputs, Process, Outputs, Customers (SIPOC) map. A SIPOC map identifies the process steps, person performing a process step, the inputs, variables that affect the process, outputs, and measure of output. An example of a process map for the ordering and administration of antibiotics to patients with pneumonia is shown in Figure 7–4.

Roles in Process Improvement

There are three key roles in process improvement that one should hone efforts: executive sponsor, process improvement team, and facilitator. The executive sponsor is the clinical leader or senior manager who is responsible for giving the process improvement team their charge, assuring that the process improvement team has adequate resources, and ultimately assures accountability for implementation of the team's recommendations. The executive sponsor sets a timeline for completion of the work of the process improvement team.

Step 1 Patient examined	Step 2 Chest x-ray ordered	Step 3 Chest x-ray interpreted	Step 4 Diagnosis made	Step 5 Antibiotic ordered	Step 6 Antibiotic dispensed	Step 7 Antibiotic administered

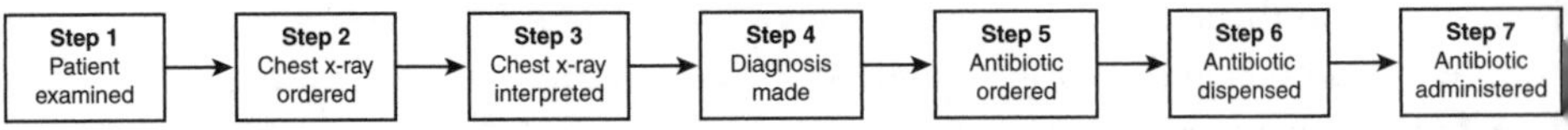

	Input	Process Step	Output	Person
1.				
2.				
3.				
4.				
5.				
6.				
7.				

Transfer the steps in the process map to the column titled process step. Fill in the inputs, outputs, and the person performing the tasks.

Figure 7–4 *High Level Process Map*

The process improvement team is made up of people who are involved in actually delivering the healthcare service that is targeted to be improved. The team should be multidisciplinary and of manageable size (no more than 10 members). Members of the team must be freed up from other duties to allow them to devote the necessary time to do the team's work.

The process improvement facilitator is an individual trained in process improvement methodology. The facilitator clarifies roles and expectations, provides structure, facilitates communication, offers ideas for solutions, and assures that work is completed between meetings.

Rolling Through-Put Yield

Every process has a capability. The process capability is a quantification of how often the process results in a desired outcome. The process capability is the product of the yield or capability of each step in the process. For example, if a process has five steps with the following yields: 0.98, 0.90, 0.97, 0.94, 0.97, the process capability is 0.78. Thus, the process will fail 22 percent of the time despite the fact that all of the individual process steps have a success rate of 90 percent or better. There are two key concepts in through-put yield illustrated in this example. First, the more steps in a process, the lower its capability. Thus, reducing the number of steps in a process should be one of the goals of process improvement. Second, process improvement efforts should focus on the steps with the highest defect rate in order to improve the overall process capability.

Continuous Improvement

Once a process improvement team has completed its work and the new process is in place, a group of people who are responsible for different parts of the process should monitor and adjust the process to assure continuous improvement in the outcome. Nearly all processes, and the individuals who carry out the processes, will follow a learning curve. A learning curve is a plot of process capability versus time. Inevitably, it takes a period of time for a process to be operating at maximum capability. People will make errors as they learn the new process and unanticipated consequences occur that must be dealt with by adjusting the process. The continuous improvement group should meet frequently to monitor progress, make adjustments, and solve unanticipated problems.

Organizational Culture

The fifth driver of clinical quality and patient safety is organizational culture. Much has been written about the importance of culture on organizational performance, yet in many performance improvement efforts, cultural issues are ignored or, at best, acknowledged but not actively managed.[19, 20, 21] Clinical quality and patient safety can be dramatically improved with relatively straightforward changes in processes of care and the use of proven technologies and practices.[13] Yet most healthcare organizations have been slow to adopt the practices that improve clinical outcomes and reduce preventable injuries. While there are many reasons for the failure to implement change, the existing cultures of healthcare organizations and the failure of healthcare leaders to change the culture are major barriers to performance improvement. Thus, it is important that one develop an active strategy to manage change (cultural issues) as part of a performance improvement process.

Culture is often talked about, but not easily understood or measured. The definition of culture as defined by Edgar Schien is a good starting place:[20]

> [A] pattern of shared basic assumptions that the group learned as it solved its problems of external adaptation and internal integration, that has worked well enough to be considered valid and therefore to be taught to new members as the correct way you perceive, think and feel in relation to those problems.

Implicit in this definition is that culture is stable, deep, and difficult to change. Culture is broad and affects all aspects of an organization including strategy, structure, systems, and processes. An organization's culture can be analyzed at three levels:

Symbols	Signs, logos, styles of dress, etc.
Norms	Shared rules that guide behavior
Assumptions	Beliefs, often unspoken, that pervade, and underpin social systems

Organizational culture is difficult to measure. Schien believes that surveys and other instruments are not sufficient, but that an anthropologic approach is more complete and accurate. Others have empirically shown that at least certain dimensions of culture can be measured with instruments that have psychometric validity.[19, 22]

To understand culture, one must get beyond what is visible and know and understand the basic beliefs of an organization or group. Some key questions that reveal basic assumptions are:[23]

- What activities are considered important?
- Who gets promoted?
- Who and for what does a person get rewarded?
- Who fits in and who does not?
- Who exercises authority and makes decisions?

The concept of organizational culture is made more complex by the presence of subcultures within the organization and the fact that professionals such as physicians, nurses, and other healthcare providers have their own professional cultures that often conflict with those of the organizations in which they work.

A large body of work (outside of healthcare) supports the hypothesis that managing culture and its change is essential for improving performance. Specifically, organizations that have implemented quality initiatives have, by and large, fallen short of their objectives.[19, 21] Sixty to 70 percent of failures are due to cultural barri-

Table 7–4 *Characteristics of High-Performing Organizations and Non-High Performing Organizations*

High Performing	Average or Low Performing
• Optimistic staff and leaders	• Bureaucratic
• Open to change and innovation • Focus on both customers and staff by leaders • Process oriented • Commitment to excellence • Measure and share information	• Reactive • Focus on self by managers and leaders • Risk averse • Widespread emphasis on control • Lack of information at managerial level

ers. The successful implementation of quality improvement programs depend in large part on having the improvement strategies imbedded in culture change. A study by McKinsey of 40 organizations found a strong relationship $(r^2 = 0.70)$ between percent of predicted change achieved in a change initiative and the level of change management effectiveness.[24]

General Electric, one of the world's most admired companies, has quantified the value of culture and change management in process improvement. They use the equation: $Q \times A = E$, where Q is the quality of the technical solution, A is the acceptance of employees who must institute the change, and E is the effectiveness of the results of the improvement effort.

There does not seem to be an optimal type of organizational culture. However, certain features of culture are associated with success. Kotter and Heskett found that organizations with cultures that facilitate rapid adaptation changes in the environment had a better record than those that were less adaptive.[21]

In their book, *What Really Works: The 4+2 Formula for Sustained Business Success*, Nohria, Joyce, and Robersen found that one of the essential four characteristics of consistently high performing companies is a performance-oriented culture.[25] Organizations that are performance oriented set high expectations, inspire employees to do their best, and push decision making and responsibility down the organization. Table 7–4 lists the characteristics of high performing versus non-high performing organizations.

Managing Culture in the Context of Performance Improvement

The preceding evidence suggests that successful performance improvement requires a cultural strategy to improve outcomes. The goal of a cultural strategy in a performance improvement project is not to change the organization's culture but rather to overcome any cultural barriers to change. Organizational cultural transformation is a major undertaking that must be led by the chief executive officer and takes years to be successful. Therefore, in undertaking performance improvement efforts, the cultural strategy should focus on effectively dealing with cultural issues relative to a specific project. The following five-step strategy can be used to address cultural issues as part of performance improvement projects:

(1) Identify a Leader

Leadership of a change initiative is a sine qua non for success. The leader of the project is often the executive sponsor, but can also include other executives such as the CEO of the organization. Physician leadership is important. Department chairs, division chiefs, or chief of staff can fulfill the role singly or in a group. The role of the leader is to state importance of the project and to continually advocate for change and success.

For example, a performance improvement team was charged to improve the care of patients with myocardial infarction at a large medical center. The leaders of the change initiative were the chairman of the Department of Medicine and the chief of Interventional Cardiology. Together they stated that the goal of the project was to be in the 95th percentile in all process measures and outcomes for care of patients with myocardial infarction within one year. They staked their reputation on achieving the desired results and continued to publicly and privately advocate for the project until the goals were met.

(2) Creating a "Shared Vision and Shared Need"

A shared vision is the desired state of affairs in the future. In the preceding example, the change leaders laid out a specific measurable goal and timeline (performance at the 95th percentile in one year) that was lofty but achievable. The leaders of this project appealed to the desires of the clinicians caring for such patients by stating, "We have an excellent medical staff. We want the measures of process and outcomes to show the world just how good we are."

The flip side of a shared vision is a shared need for change. The latter states the rationale for change. Such a rationale can be to avoid a negative outcome (e.g., a clinical performance improvement initiative to avoid liability) or to create a positive outcome (e.g., "We want our scores to affect just how good we are.") or a combination of the two. Recent research indicates that motivation for change is greatest if individuals feel cognitive dissonance between their beliefs and the current state of affairs.[26] Getting people on the same page as to where they are and where they want to go is important.

(3) Identifying and Addressing Cultural Obstacles

The most important part of a cultural strategy is to identify key stakeholders in the process, identify the role of stakeholders in the process, identify potential obstacles of the stakeholders, and propose potential solutions to overcome the obstacles.

The stakeholder analysis tool shown in Figure 7–5 provides a useful framework for identifying and addressing cultural barriers. Start by listing all key individuals or groups that have a stake in the healthcare process that is being improved. This list includes people who are involved in the provision of care, interested parties,

Names	Role	Source of Resistance	Against	Neutral	Supportive

List key stakeholders in the process. Identify roles (approver, controller, resource, or interested party). Determine if the individual is for or against the proposed change and list sources of resistance as Technical, Political, or Cultural.

Figure 7–5 *Stakeholder Analysis*

power brokers, and those that must provide resources. Next, the process improvement team determines the role that the stakeholders play in performance improvement. "Approvers" are those who must approve and support the project to move forward. "Controllers" are individuals who provide resources such as space, people, and dollars. A "resource person" is an individual who will provide needed expertise to the project, and lastly an "interested party" is someone who should be kept informed and who can informally enhance chances for success or failure. Note that roles can change over the life of a project.

The third step in the stakeholder analysis is to determine the initial level of support for the project. Is the individual against the project, neutral, or supportive? If a person is against a project or is neutral, and the team believes their support is essential, the reason(s) for their resistance is identified. The source of resistance can be classified into one or more of three categories:

Technical: Resistance or objection due to inadequate skills, personal, technology, or physical plant. In theory, technical resistance is the easiest type of resistance to identify and overcome. In developing a process to care for stroke patients in the emergency room, the radiologists resisted the change because a neuroradiologist had to be available 24 hours a day, seven days a week. The department of radiology had only one neuroradiologist in the department and that person could not take calls every day.

Political: Resistance based on a threat or challenge to power and authority. The power can be over a group (e.g., union leaders) or individual power. A common source of political resistance is the autonomy that physicians exert over their individual practice.

Cultural: Resistance based on norms of behavior or basic beliefs and values. Cultural resistance is the most difficult to overcome because it often resides below the surface and is unspoken. A commonly held belief in medical centers is that nurses should not challenge decisions made by physicians. Thus, this belief is a cultural barrier to improving safety and promoting teamwork.

(4) Rapid Cycle Improvement

During performance improvement efforts, problems are identified that have symbolic meaning that should be rapidly fixed. These types of problems include those that have been repeatedly brought to the attention of management but never addressed, such as chronic shortages of supplies or equipment, or issues that seem to put patient quality or safety further down on the priority list. Leaders of a performance improvement project can gain credibility and support by cutting through red tape, solving such problems, and getting them off the table. In one performance improvement project designed to speed the movement of critically ill patients from the emergency department to the intensive care units, the performance improvement team noted that elevators were often full or took up to 10 minutes to come to the ground floor where the department was located. This issue was a "hot button" for staff and had been an issue for years. The leader of the project solved the problem by allocating funds to have a card reader installed on a freight elevator so that the emergency department personnel could call an elevator immediately. The leaders also had the freight elevator spruced up to make it acceptable for patients. The improvements took six weeks. The benefits of this "rapid cycle improvement" were not only that patient care improved but the performance improvement team and emergency department staff had renewed faith that the hospital really did care about patient care issues.

(5) Celebration

An important component in change management is celebration. Leaders of performance improvement should publicly embrace success by publicizing success internally. Thanking members of a performance improvement team in staff meetings, medical staff meetings, and Board of Trustee meetings is one such way of celebration. Leaders should publish the results of successful performance improvement initiatives internally and encourage the publication of such efforts in peer-reviewed literature. As previously noted, "What gets rewarded?" is an important measure of an organization's culture. If an organization wants to create a culture of quality and safety then it must reward those who do the work.

Conclusion

Performance improvement is the methodology by which clinical quality and safety are improved. Five key drivers all should be assessed and managed in performance improvement efforts: the people doing the work; the flow and interpretation of information; the infrastructure that supports the work; the processes that underlie the work; and the cultural milieu in which the work is performed. Achieving and sustaining improvement in quality requires a systematic and sustained effort by leaders of an organization as well as by the people who are delivering the care to patients.

Case Study

One of the drivers of clinical quality and patient safety was identified as the processes used to deliver health care, which includes Six Sigma Management Systems. A significant aspect of performance improvement, Six Sigma is defined by the International Organization for Standardization as a, "statistical business-improvement approach that seeks to find and eliminate defects and their causes from an organization's processes, focusing on outputs of critical importance to customers."

Fairview Health Services in Minneapolis implemented a Six Sigma initiative to improve a number of processes in the hospital system. For example, emergency department cycle times were analyzed. They wanted to reduce the amount of time from when the patient entered the emergency department to when the patient was discharged. The average at the beginning of the project was 162 minutes and their goal was set at 120 minutes over a five-month period, and then to 90 minutes within one year.

They measured patient length-of-stay in the emergency department, patient and employee satisfaction, as well as the number of patients leaving without being seen. The strategy to improve the process was a quicker turnaround for imaging and lab times, a decrease in time to bring patients to rooms, and to improve the distribution of employees in the emergency deparment. Action plans were developed and the benefits they hope to see include increased patient and employee satisfaction as well as increased productivity and reduced cost per unit.

Study/Discussion Questions

1. What are the drivers of performance measurement?
2. How does the interpretation of data affect performance measurement?
3. What is evidence based medicine?
4. What type of problems should be a priority for rapid cycle improvement?

Suggested Readings/Web Sites

Centers for Medicare & Medicaid Services (http://www.cms.hhs.gov).

Center for the Study of Healthcare Management. *Deploying Six Sigma in a Healthcare System.* (http://www.csom.umn.edu/Assets/8260.pdf).

References

1. Chassin MR, Becher EC. The wrong patient. *Ann Intern Med.* 2002;136:826–33.

2. Gawande A. *Complications.* New York: Pan Books Limited; 2002.

3. Sexton JB, Thomas EJ, Helmreich RL. Error, stress, and teamwork in medicine and aviation: Cross-sectional surveys. *BMJ.* 2000;320:745–49.

4. Volpp KGM, Grande D. Residents' suggestions for reducing errors in teaching hospitals. *NEJM.* 2003;348(9): 851–55.

5. Sutcliffe K, Lewton E, Rosenthal MM. Communication Failures: An insidious contributor to medical mishaps. *Acad Med.* 2004;79(2):186–94.

6. Aiken L, Clarke SP, Sloane DM, Sochalski J, Silber JH. Hospital nurse staffing and patient mortality, nurse burnout, and job dissatisfaction. *JAMA.* 2002;288(16):1987–93.

7. Brennan TA, Horwitz RI, Duffy FD, Cassel CK, Goode LD, Lipner RS. The role of physician specialty board certification status in the quality movement. *JAMA.* 2004;292(9): 1038–42.

8. Aiken LH, Clarke SP, Cheung RB, Sloane DM, Silber JH. Educational levels of hospital nurses and surgical patient mortality. *JAMA.* 2003;290:1617–23.

9. Lanchigan, C, Lockley SW, Cronin JW, Evans EE, et al. Effect of reducing intern's weekly work hours on sleep and attentional failures. *NEJM.* 2004;351(18): 1829–37.

10. Pisano GP, Bohmer RMJ, Edmondson AC. Organizational differences in rates of learning: Evidence from the adoption of minimally invasive cardiac surgery. *Manag Science.* 2001;47(6): 752–68.

11. Ittner C, Larcker DF. Coming up short on nonfinancial performance measurement. *Har Bus Rev.* 2003;81(11):88–95.

12. Weinberg N. Using performance measures to identify plans of action to improve care. *Jt Comm J Qual Improv.* 2001;27(12):683–88.

13. Leape LL, Berwick DM, Bates DW. What practices will most improve safety? *JAMA.* 2002; 288(4):501–7.

14. Sackett DL, Rosenburg WMC, Gray JAM, Haynes RB, Richardson WS. Evidence-based medicine: what it is and what it isn't. *BMJ.* 1996;312;71–72.

15. National Guideline Clearinghouse. Available at: www.guideline.gov. Accessed on August 24, 2004.

16. Ettinger W, Van Kooy M. The art and science of winning physician support for Six Sigma change. *Physician Exec.* 2003;29(5): 34–38.

17. Ettinger WH. Six Sigma: Adapting GE's lessons to heath care. *Trustee.* 2001;54(8):10–15.

18. Harry M, Schroeder R. *Six Sigma: The Breakthrough Management Strategy Revolutionizing the World's Top Corporations.* New York: Doubleday; 2000.

19. Cameron K, Quinn RE. *Diagnosing and Changing Organizational Culture.* Reading, Mass: Addison-Wesley Publishing Co; 1999.

20. Schein EH. *The Corporate Culture Survival Guide.* San Francisco, Calif: Jossey-Bass Publishers; 1999.

21. Kotter JP, Heskett JL. *Corporate Culture and Performance.* New York: Kotter Associates, Inc.; 1992.

22. Nieva VF, Sorra J. Safety culture assessment: A tool for improving patient safety in healthcare organizations. *Qual Saf Health Care.* 2003;12 (Suppl 2): ii17–23.

23. Watkins M. *The First 90 Days.* Boston, Mass: Harvard Business School Press; 2003.

24. LaClair J, Rao R. Helping employees embrace change. *The McKinsey Quarterly.* 2002, Number 4. Available at: www.mckinseyquarterly.com. Accessed on September 9, 2004.

25. Joyce W, Nohria N. *The 4+2 Formula: For Sustained Business Success.* New York: Harper Collens; 2003.

26. Lawson E, Price C. The psychology of change management. *The McKinsey Quarterly.* 2003, Number 2. Available at: www.mckinseyquarterly.com. Accessed on December 1, 2003.

Stakeholders in Quality Improvement

Chapter 8

The Provider's Role in Quality Improvement

Physicians and Quality Improvement

Stephen T. Lawless
Roy Proujansky

EXECUTIVE SUMMARY

This chapter reviews current efforts related to the physician provider that are being designed and implemented to enhance patient care quality. The context for this discussion is the provider's role in a system of care delivery, and interwoven in this narrative is the characterization of the skills that physicians must develop and master to enable these efforts.

LEARNING OBJECTIVES

1. To understand the current changing environment of care and how it is forcing the shift from the classic individualistic model the provider has evolved from, to a systems model of care.
2. To understand the evolution of Clinical Practice Guidelines and how this evolution is fostering provider participation.
3. To understand the limitations and roadblocks and areas of focus required to foster provider accountability within the context of a system.
4. To understand the rationale and changes needed in order to promote future change.

KEYWORDS

Physician
Quality Assurance
Culture
Systems

Introduction

Physicians and clinical services account for 22 percent of total healthcare spending, but physicians' decisions and recommendations affect a far larger percentage of the total expenditures of healthcare.[1] Hence, there is perhaps no actor more prominent in the entourage attempting to enhance healthcare quality than the physician provider, whose role ultimately will be the implementation of meaningful change. In addition, change for physician providers will not be the historic individual and autonomous approach that has characterized previous incremental and slowly advancing quality efforts in healthcare. Rather, closing the quality chasm will require physician change as part of a system redesign for healthcare delivery with the patient at the center, benefiting from a diversity of efforts in the surrounding environment. These efforts will include advances in information technology, implementation of best practices and evidenced-based approaches to care, and physician profiling and performance measurement that should lead to effective and efficient care with a reduction in medical errors and enhancement of patient safety. These changes will be striking and will not only require the acquisition of new technical skills, but physician providers will now need to excel in communication skills, proficiency with team behaviors, resilience and tolerance of change, and accountability.

Systems of Care and the Role of the Provider

The overarching principle for the evolution of the care model to one of higher quality is the requirement to move away from a provider-centric model to a model of systems of care, with the provider as a key member of the system. The key implications to the provider of such a paradigm shift are an awareness of the activity of the rest of the system, an understanding of how provider actions influence the system, and the development of behaviors that enhance system (and hence, patient), rather than individual (physician), effectiveness and safety.

What is a system of care? The model for a healthcare system was outlined by Avedis Donabedian.[2] Donabedian's model demonstrates that in order to have a system of care, there needs to be a coordinated and organized linking of inputs, processes, and outputs (see Figure 8–1).

Healthcare is probably even more complex than what Donabedian proposed. It cannot be interpreted that a system is just a straight-line path. In fact a healthcare system involves a two-part system that is not parallel but rather in a continuous loop series.[3] This loop variation of the Donabedian model recognizes the importance of input controls to processes to outcomes. This variation links hospital/manager controlled processes to provider controlled processes. Inputs (energy, supplies, and materials) link management controlled processes (ancillary and nursing services) and result in outputs (beds, patient types, care hours, and laboratory and imaging

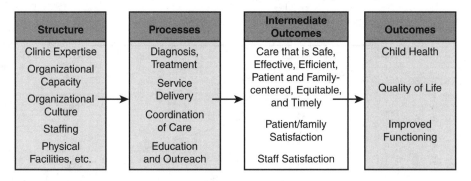

Figure 8–1 *Donabedian's Model*

services). These management outputs then become the clinical inputs that the provider controlled processes (medical service) utilize to produce outputs (diagnoses, treatments, medical records, outcomes, satisfaction) that feed back to the management systems as refining inputs.

In this model, structure includes the organizational and participants skills, resources, and physical characteristics through which health care is delivered. Process refers to the activities and steps required diagnosing and treating illness and coordinate care. Outcomes are the result of healthcare structures and processes. These results include patient; provider; operational short-term, immediate, and long-term; and performance. Without a strategic plan and ongoing organized links among structures, processes and outcomes, a healthcare system will not function.

There are many implications of the shift from a provider-centric to systems approach to care delivery. One such implication is a shift from the isolated analysis of treatment results to a more comprehensive assessment of the quality of the patient care experience. While excellent treatment outcomes will always be a critically important goal of healthcare delivery, the systems approach will additionally account for other aspects of the care experience that impact on overall satisfaction. As is taught in the concept of Six Sigma,[4] any outcome is very dependent on both the number of steps and the overall efficiency of each of those steps. Even if each process step is successful 95 percent of the time (in most schools this would qualify as an A+ grade) the number of steps in order to have process completion can result in an overall failing grade (see Figure 8–2).

For instance, our own analysis of a specialty clinic process has demonstrated this Six Sigma effect. We demonstrated that operational processes do impact the perception of medical care (in the short-term). We asked patients and their families to rate the efficiency of sequential steps of the clinic visit process from pre-registration to various wait times to post-encounter visit closure. When any step in the queue was rated as less than "the best" by patients, there was a correlation with the overall visit

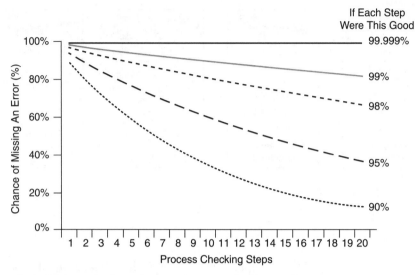

Figure 8-2 *Six Sigma Analysis of Process Complexity on Chance of Error*

satisfaction with the medical encounter, irrespective of the actual physician interaction component of the visit. And, in addition, there was a cumulative negative impact if multiple steps performed less than optimally (see Figure 8–3).

The systems concept can be expanded to encompass the environment of care delivery as well as the level of satisfaction of both patients and providers. That there would be a relationship between patient satisfaction (with their care experience); provider satisfaction (satisfaction with their professional work experience); and other aspects of the healthcare environment (outcomes, medical malpractice liability occurrence) might or might not seem intuitive but is supported in the literature.[5]

When we analyzed our practices own data, we found a strong suggestion that there was both a positive correlation between patient satisfaction and provider reported self-satisfaction. In addition, patient and provider satisfaction were lower as a function of the actual number of malpractice claims adjusted for expected clinical risk (based on the type of physician encounter). This association implies but does not prove a cause-and-effect relationship between any two or more of the variables (see Figure 8–4).

This data suggests that many aspects of systems of care cannot be taken for granted or ignored as important considerations in the design of care delivery models and also raise some important questions. Can a dissatisfied physician (e.g., depressed, inadequately rested, unsatisfied with work environment) deliver an excellent care experience? The literature cites numerous stresses that can influence physician's performance including family issues, work hours, burnout, decreasing patient encounter time, to loss of clinical control due to Managed Care.[5–12] An interesting, timely, and newly identified stress involved IT Stress, whereby 67 percent of faculty report that keeping up with technology as a stress is

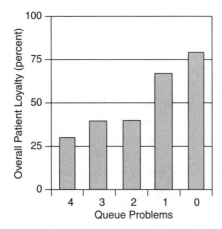

Figure 8–3 *Impact of Number of Clinic Queue Errors on Patient Loyalty*

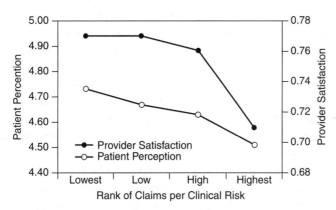

Figure 8–4 *Relationship of Claims History to Patient Perception of Service Delivery and Provider Self-Satisfaction*

greater than that of research, publishing, teaching load, and promotion but not as great as time pressure, household demands, or institutional red tape.[13]

Are some patients dissatisfied even prior to their encounter with their physician and can this be recognized and addressed as part of the care process? Does malpractice liability in the short- or long-run serve to mitigate or intensify the issues influencing provider and patient satisfaction? While answering these questions is not primarily the goal of this chapter, the issues help to elucidate the vital and non-silo role of the provider as part of a larger system that includes interdependent structures and processes.

Maintenance and improvement of a system involves formulating a strategy, creating a culture, and being sure that what a system hopes to accomplish has the technical and structural infrastructure to accomplish its goals. Without a system strategy many results can be meaningless. Without a culture (defined as shared values and beliefs that interact with an organization's structures and control systems to produce behavioral norms[14]) system results will not have a lasting impact. Without the technical attributes, a system will see many false starts before success. And without the proper structures in place, a system will not have the ability to capture and disseminate learning.[15]

Moving toward a system of higher quality will require physicians to have a greater awareness of the system's components as well as a better understanding of how provider behavior influences and is influenced by the rest of the system. When physicians work in a system, they accept that their purpose as leaders is not to fix quality problems and make quality improvements. Rather, their main purpose is to establish an environment in which quality improvement will thrive. Among the many roles physicians play is that of leader. When physicians assume leadership, they must not only lead the specific mechanisms and tools that will allow them to reassure, understand, and improve care but must also acquire the skills and abilities that will allow them to lead departments, office practices, and complex healthcare institutions. This body of knowledge permits physicians to work as leaders in a system of care, not just as members of the system.[16]

According to the Institute of Medicine,[17] in order to achieve a comprehensive safety program, trained personnel are needed along with mechanisms both to capture and report adverse and near-hit detection. Physicians must demonstrate commitment to system thinking. Small, multidisciplinary, fast-moving work teams, driven by front-line staff members supported and sponsored by senior leaders regularly assemble to respond to trends in safety reports.[18] Tools are available from other industries that can be adapted to healthcare in order to teach physicians teamwork. For example, Crew Resource Management is defined as using "all available sources of information, equipment, and people to achieve safe and efficient flight operation—encompasses team training, simulation, and interaction. It is used heavily by the FAA, NASA, and the Military. It has as its goals: safety, efficiency, and morale." [19]

Systems of Care, the Provider, and Patient Safety

System failures that result in errors can be classified as active or latent errors. Latent errors come from design failures; active failures come from people involved in immediate situational contact. System designs often delay the detection and correction of latent errors. Resolution of system errors due to information flows can be achieved by making information timely, accurate, and widely accessible. Reducing steps, rapid and accurate communication, utilizing interdisciplinary rounds, and using clinical pathways or guidelines all facilitate system flow.[20]

Despite 35 percent of physicians and 42 percent of the public reporting an error in care of their family or self, only 5 percent of physicians and 6 percent of the public identified medical errors as serious problems. Physicians identified nurse staffing and overworked, stressed, and fatigued staff as being significant causes of medical errors. The public identified the key factors resulting in errors being physicians not taking enough time and being overworked, the healthcare team not acting like a team, and understaffing.[21] Solutions to any of these causes need a system approach.

In a study of intensive care units, only 33 percent of nurses rated the quality of collaboration and communication with physicians as high or very high. In contrast, 73 percent of physicians rated collaboration and communication with nurses as high or very high. Specific issues brought up in the intensive care unit included a lack of nurses speaking up, lack of disagreement resolution, and apparent input not well received as relates to clinical care.[22] This, despite evidence that clearly demonstrates how collaboration and teamwork can result in improved quality of care, decreased patient length of stay, decreased nursing staff turnover, increased quality of care, increased family reports of being kept informed, and overall, reports of physician communication and performance.[23,24] Physician improvement in interactions and respect for nursing also leads to effective communication and directly impacts patient care and work flow provided by nurses.[25]

Physician lack of clear communication and team orientation with other physicians also contributes to the perception of patient safety. When physicians utilize consultants, compliance with recommendations to care averages only about 44 percent to 75 percent based on the clinical severity of the patient.[26,27]

A properly functioning system depends on communication. To be effective, physician and hospital executives need to move from autocratic leadership styles to consultative and group consensus methodologies. The essential task in creating effective hospital and physician networks is to foster collegiality.[28] The lack of emphasis on communication and its impact on system safety in healthcare today is not unlike the situation at NASA around the time of the Columbia Shuttle disaster. The culture of NASA that resulted in system strain is highlighted in Figure 8–5.[29]

At NASA, cultural traits and organizational practices detrimental to safety that were allowed to fester are not dissimilar to what physicians are accustomed. Traits

- Intense pressure to stay on schedule
- Making improvements that atrophy with time
- Heavily matrixed organization
- Budget allocation limitations
- Incomplete and misleading information
- Poor management judgments

Figure 8–5 *Reasons for System Strain at NASA Prior to the Columbia Shuttle Disaster*

including reliance on past success as a substitute for sound practices, fostering barriers to communication of critical safety information, stifling the integration of dissent, and professional differences of opinion result in preventing the evolution of an informed chain of command and decision makers.[29]

The image of the physician as the lone professional is not merely historically obsolete; actually, at the beginning of the twenty-first century, it can be misleading. The age of the organizational physician has arrived, not only because more physicians work in an organizational setting, but because the institutional environment in which these organizations themselves function has also changed. More research is needed to see the impact of this movement.[30]

Leaders must generate this sense of common purpose and find ways to draw hospitals and physicians together. The leader that can actively engage physicians in the process and co-opt their frustration and anger will begin to build the trust necessary to convince doctors of the propriety and economic sense of a system of care. Hospital administrators must be willing to include all levels of physicians, not just department chairpersons, in the power structure and cede much of their ability to control to an integrated administrator/physician team.

It is striking that the major failures within a healthcare system are not usually brought to light by the quality assurance or improvement programs, nor by incident reporting; clinical profiling; mortality and morbidity review; credential, risk, and claims management; or the external announcement by regulators, inspectors, accreditation, and oversight.[31]

Complex systems, like those in healthcare, often discover system failures only when they become major disasters. When a crisis does hit, chances are that there was some prior build-up of many smaller bad risks to a point where a minor event tips things over and sends an avalanche of problems crashing down.[32]

Systems of Care, the Provider, and Information

A physician's role within a system of care is more complex than ever before. The physician role is now increasingly complicated by increased expectations, guidelines, recommendations, professional societies, specialty groups, health plans, and advocacy organizations.[33] In order to facilitate the physician's role, medical information systems are being developed in order to collect the data needed to establish the standard of care. In some current and future managed-care systems, hospitals will look at national and local practice patterns to ensure high-quality care. The aim will be to reduce statistical variation as much as possible without compromising physician autonomy. The difficulty in establishing quality standards is that there is such variability in practice patterns that conflict between physician and management invariably occurs over what is the proper standard. While 70 percent of physicians believe that practice guidelines will improve care (especially younger physicians, those working less than 20 hours/week and those paid a fixed salary), many do not think it will reduce the cost of care.[34]

As more data is being captured and organized, the strengths and weaknesses but more important, the contextual framework by which data can be used to evaluate system and physician performance has been in a constant state of refinement. The story of "Clinical practice guidelines" (CPG) demonstrates this evolution well.

The problem with CPG is in balancing a doctor's judgment against national guidelines. Regulatory tools for profiling physicians, practice protocols, and guidelines are praised because they subordinate the physician's personal assessment to a standard outside personal judgement. However, outcomes research and CPG cannot substitute for either clinical experience or clinical sense. The naïve initial models of CPG did not recognize this and assumed that there was a right and wrong way regarding care decisions. Unfortunately, every physician probably felt this way, each had their own way—which was the "right way." While appropriate perhaps for a single-stage decision, they were doomed for failure in a healthcare system.

When even patient and disease progression was recognized as having significant variability, a better model that incorporated decision points in the care process gained popularity. These decision points involved expert and consensus opinion. These consensus development groups consisted of people who were experts (both real and self-proclaimed) in the appropriate area and who had credibility with the target audiences.[35] Unfortunately, the development of consensus CPGs still did not address the creation of a practice culture. These CPGs often had so many complex stages with decision point options (still relying on physician discretion) that often physicians and caregivers felt they were in a jumbled maze (see Figure 8–6).

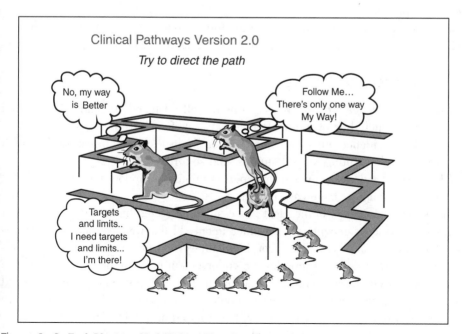

Figure 8–6 *Each Physician Might Believe Their Way Is the "Right" Way*

The advent of unprecedented data access ushered in by the growth of Informatics and searchable databases offered the chance to take a fresh look at CPG development. Simultaneously there was the realization that ideal performance evaluation measures involves an evidence-based assessment of the literature. This evidence-based review should provide the standard specifications that earmark satisfactory performance.[36] Each evidence-based review and subsequent CPG now is characterized as both the type of recommendation forthcoming (Standard, Guideline, Practice Option, or Practice Parameter) and the classification of evidence supporting those recommendations.[37]

A. Types of Recommendations

Standards—Generally accepted principles for patient management that reflect a high degree of clinical certainty (i.e., based on Class I evidence or, when circumstances preclude randomized clinical trials, overwhelming evidence from Class II studies that directly addresses the question at hand or from decision analysis that directly addresses all the issuers).

Guidelines—Recommendations for patient management that can identify a particular strategy or range of management strategies and that reflect moderate clinical certainty (i.e., based on Class II evidence that directly addresses the issue, decision analysis that directly addresses the issue, or strong consensus of Class II evidence).

Practice options or advisories—Other strategies for patient management for which the clinical utility is uncertain (e.g., based on inclusive or conflicting evidence or opinion).

Practice parameters—Results, in the form of one or more specific recommendation, from a scientifically based analysis of a specific clinical problem.

B. Classification of Evidence

Class I—Evidence provided by one or more well-designed randomized controlled clinical trials, including overviews (meta-analysis) of such trials.

Class II—Evidence provided by one or more well-designed clinical studies such as case-controlled studies, cohort studies, and so forth.

Class III—Evidence provided by expert opinion, nonrandomized historical control subjects, or one or more case reports.

The scrutiny and rigor of the ideal process is highlighted by the fact that a recent review of 79 patient safety practices resulted in only 11 that were considered evidence-based medical practices.[21] The rigor but paucity of true evidence-based recommended processes does not prohibit the endorsement of many nationwide systemic processes that empirically appear sound but lack Class I evidence as experienced when The Leapfrog Group identified computerized physician order entry, intensive care unit staffing by intensivists, and evidence-based hospital referrals.[38]

Basing performance measures purely on current statistical databases are of limited utility.[39] The statistical models used to evaluate doctor performance are too primitive to provide much more than a rule-of-thumb about doctor performance. Existing performance measures try to compare standardized treatment patterns with individual doctor variation, but there are too many unmeasured variables both in national averages and individual treatment patterns to provide reasonable accuracy.

Administrative databases might not take into account factors like a patient's coexisting illness, socioeconomic status, hereditary health history, patient compliance or desire for care, or patient use of medication. This is not to say that databases cannot be created to measure these criteria, but the present state of the art does not allow for compensating factors. Potentially, a doctor who "got a bad draw from the deck" by receiving very sick patients might look deficient, even if the doctor provided extraordinary care. The process limits a doctor's autonomy since it subordinates a doctor's judgment and discretion to a statistical package. Even risk-adjustment methodologies are still in their infancy and are relevant to the population, not individual patient level.[40,41] Even when matured, risk-adjustment measures, CPGs, and physician and system evaluation will need to incorporate both patient feedback[42] and additional measures of professional competence. These competencies include expert judgment, management of ambiguity, professionalism, time management, learning strategies, and teamwork.[43] Taking this into consideration, perhaps a more evolving approach is needed before CPGs are endorsed (see Figure 8–7).

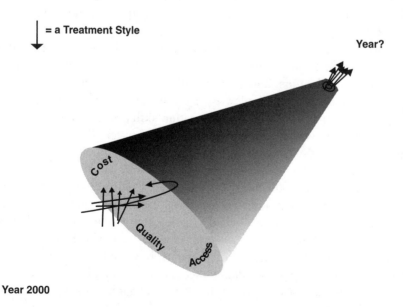

Figure 8–7 *The Cone Model for CPG Evolution*

Systems of Care, the Provider, and Feedback Loops

There is an urgent need for proper evaluation of physicians as it relates to their efforts and leadership with healthcare quality. Job enhancement is known to be impacted by skill variety, task identity, task significance, and coinciding with autonomy and feedback.[44] Technology alone will not be able to address fundamental problems responsible for many of the major issues in medicine today.[45] A feedback system requires the support of senior management, effective clinical leadership, data support, a change in culture, coordination, infrastructure, adoption, and innovation to reduce threats and fears. This involves the creation of an evaluation system model based on the earlier described Donabedian model.[2]

However, many misconceptions hinder the encouragement and acceptance of this quality feedback approach. This feedback is based on a reporting system that has to be nonpunitive, confidential, independent, based on expert analysis, timely, system-oriented, and responsive.[46] While there is no definitive link between this type of reporting system and malpractice risk of litigation,[46] physicians still practice and assume a defensive posture when it comes to either giving or receiving feedback on performance. At the same time litigation does not result in quality improvement, and in fact litigation (or practicing defensive medicine) can impede quality and safety.[47] There is also increasing evidence that physician attributes can be acquired and modified and are not stagnant.[48]

Physician evaluation relates to the setting of goals and expectations and an acceptance of accountability for one's performance and value-added creation as a result of one's action given those goals and expectations. Work published by James Reason[14] creates a framework on which the culpability for unsafe acts or process failures often is discovered to occur at the system rather than the individual physician level (see Figure 8–8).

Evaluation also involves competence and proficiency. The common tools that can be used to assist in a classic evaluation (case reviews, peer reviews, satisfaction surveys, honors, publication, and administrative impact) are not adequate to evaluate a physician as a system leader. An assessment of competence as relates to knowledge, overall patient care, communication skills, professionalism, practice-based learning, improvement, and a determination of system-based practice impact is needed.[49]

Physicians also need to be brought into the process by which a system (including structures, processes, and outcomes) are evaluated. Quality management processes will need to rely heavily on the use of statistical techniques and trend analysis to determine causes of variation in clinical practice and patient outcome. Physicians who are trained based on the application of scientific methods should be willing to accept these techniques. Sources of variation must be traced to nonphysician as well as to physician factors. Improved data collection and availability will allow physicians to have more than just anecdotal information about how they practice relative to their peers.

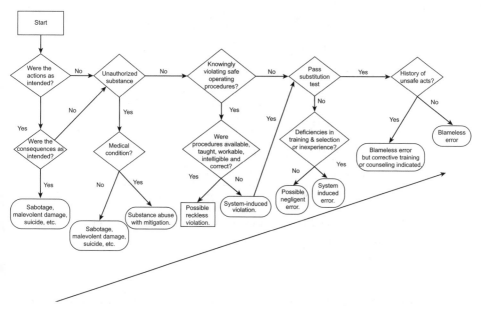

Figure 8–8 *A Process Flow Diagram That Assists in Determining the Culpability of Unsafe Acts*

Sound clinical and financial data should permit objective analysis of practice patterns that affect the delivery of patient care. The key is for hospital managers, physician managers, and physicians to work together so that meaningful information can be used to support optimal clinical decision making and evaluation. The accelerated movement toward managed care budgeted systems is outpacing the availability of databases on healthcare utilization patterns and patient outcomes. This underscores the fact hospital management and the medical staff need to come to agreement about what is appropriate to review and how this data should be utilized.

Finally, there is a strong desire that eventually a system of physician evaluation that was in fact a directed 360° process rather than just a reporting of data or just global feedback will emerge. While the technologic issues of obtaining data in order to evaluate productivity and satisfaction are near at hand, there is also a need to teach the evaluators to be evaluators. Providing feedback should not be left to a 15 minute, setting salary purpose only, required as an end of the year process. Training leaders on how to provide continuous loop feedback is a system process in itself. An internal study that we performed at our institution demonstrated that with minimal formalized training of physicians as evaluators, the level of face-to-face agreement between the physician supervisor and physician staff regarding that staff physician's performance showed significant variation (see Figure 8–9). Of concern was the fact that in all aspects of this evaluation, except for the dimension of "personal effectiveness," the evaluator rated the staff physician higher than the staff physician rated themselves.

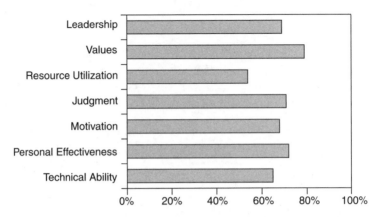

Figure 8–9 *Level of Agreement Between Physician Supervisor and Physician Staff on Physcian Staff Performance During an Annual Review*

The concern is that feedback is muddled due to the desire to retain expensive, revenue-generating staff and may come at the cost of long-term performance improvement. Other studies have evaluated physicians as educators, noting significant differences among attending faculty members and identifying strengths and weaknesses. Many educators' self-perception differed significantly from resident assessment.[50] How these differences are communicated back to the educators and the setting of action plans to facilitate improvement would be an essential next step in the progression to a 360° evaluation system.

Skills of the Next Generation of Providers

It is naïve to think that the creation of a true physician culture of safety and continuous quality improvement would appear with current efforts. Strategies that ease work pressures include increased use and enhanced scope of nonphysician clinicians, adoption of information technology and disease management programs to reduce errors, and thoughtful practice design.[33] Novel programs like "extra pay for quality performance"[1,51] are still in their infancy and have yet to be evaluated as to whether they foster the needed stimulus for quality improvement. These efforts set the infrastructure for change but do not in themselves change the culture. In order to promote a new culture there needs to be endorsement by senior physician management, effective clinical leadership, data support, coordination, infrastructure, adoption, and innovation to reduce actual threats to process change.[52]

The effort will take years but needs to start with a multifaceted approach that involves the current physicians in practice and those physicians in various stages of training. This long-term perspective should not overshadow the sense of urgency as a driver for change. This effort will fail if there is no sense of urgency, vision, or under-communication. Obstacles to the new vision must be addressed and there needs to be systematic planning for and the creation of short-term wins. Declaring victory too soon and not anchoring changes in the corporation's culture will assure frustration and failure.[53] Just like the Stockdale Paradox described in the book *Good to Great*,[54] efforts that involve long-term but urgent goals will fail without this sense of urgency—but it will also fail if success is linked to a specific deadline.

Having a system perspective can be taught but there also has to be a change in culture.[53] Systems need to be designed that will provide physicians with the comfort level to optimize, encourage, and nurture change. The emphasis on systems change needs to focus on causes and not just symptoms (a novel concept in medicine, indeed).

The goal is to have physicians informed such that they can become change agents in a culture of safety. This culture will foster respect for all the entities involved in the health care process, gather the right kinds of information, allow blameless reporting, be just and flexible, and provide an environment to encourage continuous learning.[14] The physician managers must be the change agents that seek out cost efficiencies, refine quality and performance measures, and integrate the changes into the resident training program and ongoing quality functions. The administrators and physicians must work through communication and their personal commitment to engage every physician to accept and participate in changes. Communication, training, and commitment are the major tools to achieve the desired changes. There needs to be not just a retraining but a redesign of medical school and residency curriculum that builds interpersonal skills and team leadership.

Leadership must make a substantial time and financial commitment to developing the physician's business competence, understanding of cost effective medical practice, and team-building activities. There needs to be an individualized determination of areas of educational deficiencies, and resources need to be provided to close those gaps. Executive education courses, involvement in organizations such as the American College of Physician Executives, and site visits to other facilities further advanced in strategies should all be part of this educational process. The upfront expense could be significant, but as this process matures, it will become a chief means of driving the needed education throughout the organization. Table 8–1 outlines some potential key competencies and skills that every physician leader should possess.[54]

Academic medical centers and medical schools seem to embrace the potential for a retooling of their educational mission[55] in order to include:

- Quality improvement educational agenda
- A means to measure the continuous quality of education
- Expansion of faculty involvement
- Accreditation processes that encourage physicians to be life-long learners

The current generation of physician and nonphysician leaders must work through communication and personal commitment to engage every physician to accept and participate in the changes. These changes will cause some pain and anxiety, but if planned and implemented openly and professionally, the nation's healthcare system will emerge from the changes ready to provide empowered quality care for another 50 years.

Table 8–1 *Key Competencies and Skills for Physician Managers*

Clinical Credibility

Communication
  • Listening
  • Speaking
  • Writing

Leadership
  • Articulating a vision for the future
  • Creating an environment of shared responsibility
  • Developing the skills of others
  • Framing and facilitating critical conversation

Team Building
  • Embrace a participatory leadership style
  • Developing common goal or purpose
  • Creating a climate of communication and trust
  • Effectively leading meetings
  • Recognizing and encouraging synergy
  • Negotiation and conflict resolution
  • Focusing on interests rather than positions
  • Encouraging others to communicate and resolve conflict
  • Serving as facilitator

Quality Management
  • Articulating a philosophy of continuing improvement
  • Embracing the "good apple" approach
  • Focusing on processes as the cause of problems
  • Empowering the people who do the work to solve problems
  • Using data to gain insight

Study/Discussion Questions

1. What paradigm shift will be required for physicians to change their approach to providing care?
2. How can something like Crew Resource Management and the Columbia space shuttle disaster help improve healthcare delivery?
3. Are risk-adjustment methodologies adequate for performance measurements?

Suggested Readings/Web Sites

NASA (www.nasa.gov).
National Guidelines Clearinghouse (http://www.guideline.gov).

References

1. Federal Trade Commission, Department of Justice. "Improving Health Care: A dose of Competition." July 2004, Chapter 1.

2. Donabedian A. *Explorations in Quality Assessment and Monitoring. Volume I: The Definition of Quality and Approaches to Its Assessment.* Ann Arbor, Mich: Health Administration Press; 1980.

3. Chilingerian J, Sherman D. Managing physician efficiency and effectiveness in providing hospital services. *Health Serv Manage Res.* 1990;3(1); 3–15.

4. Breyfogle F. *Implementing Six Sigma Smarter Solutions Using Statistical Methods.* New York: John Wiley & Sons; 1999.

5. Devoe J, Fryer G, Hargraves J, Phillips R, Green L. Does career dissatisfaction affect the ability of family physicians to deliver high-quality patient care? *J Fam Pract.* 2002;51(3):223–28.

6. Tetrick L, LaRocca J. Understanding, predicting, and control as moderators of the relationship between stress, satisfaction and physiological well-being. *J App Psych.* 1987;72(4):538–43.

7. Gundersen L. Physician burnout. *Ann Intern Med.* 2001;135(2):145–148.

8. National survey of physicians-doctor's opinion about their profession. March 2002.

9. Cameron K, Freeman S. Cultural congruence, strength and type: Relationships to effectiveness. In: Woodman RW, Passmore WA, eds. Research in Organizational Change and Development. Greenwich, CT: JAI Press, Inc.; 1991.

10. Haas JS, Cook EF, Puopolo AL, Burstin HR, Cleary PD, Brennan TA. Is the professional satisfaction of general internists associated with patient satisfaction? *J Gen Intern Med.* 2000;15:122–28.

11. Shanefelt T, Bradley K, Wipf J, Black A. Burnout and self-reported patient care in an internal medicine residency program. *Ann Intern Med.* 2002;136:358–67.

12. Vincent C. Understanding and responding to adverse events. *NEJM.* 2003;348:1051–56.

13. www.gseis.ucla.edu/heri/prtechnology.html "High-tech anxiety."

14. Reason J. *Managing the Risks of Organizational Accidents.* Ashgate, VT: Publishing, Burlington; 1997.

15. Shortell S, Bennett C, Byck G. Assessing the impact of continuous quality improvement on clinical practice: What will it take to accelerate the process. *The Millbank Quarterly.* 1998;76(4):593–624.

16. Reinersten J. Physicians as leaders in the improvement of health care systems. *Ann Intern Med.* 1998;128:833–838.

17. Institute of Medicine. *Patient safety: Achieving a new standard of care.* Washington, DC: National Academy Press; 2002.

18. Herman C, Rowan L. Managing culture: Building a blameless reporting system for the ambulatory care environment. *Group Prac J.* 2004;53(4):9–16.

19. Pizzi L, Goldfarb N, Nash D. *Crew Resource Management and Its Application to Medicine.* Available at: www.ahrq.gov.clinic/ptsafety/pdf/chap44.pdf. Accessed on May 24, 2005.

20. Yourstone S, Smith H. Managing system errors and failures in health care organizations: Suggestions for practices and research. *Health Care Manage Rev.* 2002;27(1):50–61.

21. Blendon R, DesRoches CM, Brodic M, et al. Views of practicing physicians and the public on medical errors. *NEJM.* 2002;347(24):1933–40.

22. Thomas E, Sexton J, Helmeich R. Discrepant attitudes about teamwork among critical care nursing and physicians. *Crit Care Med.* 2003;31:951–59.

23. Surgenor S, Blike G, Corwin H. Teamwork and collaboration in critical care: Lessons from the cockpit. *Crit Care Med.* 2003;31(3):992–93.

24. Majzun R. The role of teamwork in improving patient satisfaction. *Group Pract J.* 1998;47:12–16.

25. Institute of Medicine. *Keeping patients safe: Transforming the work environment of nurses.* Washington, DC: National Academy Press; 2003.

26. Sears C, Charlson M. The effectiveness of a consultation—compliance with initial recommendations. *Am J Med.* 1983;74:870–76.

27. Ballard W, Gold J, Charlson M. Compliance with the recommendations of medical consultants. *J Gen Intern Med.* 1986;1:220–24.

28. Goldsmith J. Hospital/physician relationships: a constraint to health reform. *Health Aff.* 1993;12(3):160–69.

29. Columbia Accident Investigation Board Report/CAIB. Available at: www.nasa.gov. Accessed on May 25, 2005.

30. William ES, Konrad TR, Scheckler WE, Pathman DR. Understanding physician's intention to withdraw from practice: The role of job satisfaction, job stress, mental and physical health. *Health Care Manage Rev.* 2001;26(1):7–19.

31. Walshe K, Shortell S. When things go wrong: how health care organizations deal with major failures. *Health Affairs.* 2004;23(3):103–11.

32. Burton R. System instability, system risk. *Physician Executive.* 2003;29(2):34–8.

33. Mechanic D. Physician discontent—challenge and opportunities. *JAMA.* 2003;290: 941–46.

34. Tregunno D, Baker G, Barnsky J, Murry M. Competing values of emergency department performance and balancing multiple stakeholder perspectives. *Health Serv Res.* 2004;35(4):771–91.

35. Murphy M, Black N, Lamping D, McKee C, Sanderson C, Aikham J, Marteau T. Consensus development methods, and their use in clinical guidelines development. *Health Tech Assessment.* 1998;2(3).

36. Landon B, Norwood S, Blumenthal D, Daley J. Physician clinical performance assessment. *JAMA.* 2003;290(9):1183–89.

37. National Guideline Clearinghouse. Available at: http://www.guideline.gov. Accessed on May 25, 2005.

38. Birkmeyer JD, Dimick JB. The Leapfrog Group's Patient Safety Practices, 2003: The Potential Benefits of Universal Adoption. February 2004. Available at: https://leapfroggroup.org/media/file/Leapfrog-Birkmeyer.pdf.

39. Iezzoni L, Foley S, Heeren T, et al. A method for screening the quality of hospital care using administrative data: Preliminary validation results. *QRB Qual Rev Boll.* 1992; 18(11):361–371.

40. Haga Y. Estimates of physiologic ability and surgical stress (E-PASS) for a surgical audit in digestive surgery. *Surgery.* 2004;135:586–94.

41. Iezzoni L. Identifying complications of care using administrative data. *Med Care.* 1994;32(7):700–15.

42. Hickman G, Federspiel C, Rickert J, Miller C, Gaclat-Jaeger J, Best P. Patient complaints and malpractice risk. *JAMA.* 2002;287(12):2951–57.

43. Epstein R, Hundert E. Defining and assessing professional competence. *JAMA.* 2002;287:226–35.

44. Hackman J, Oldham G, Janson R, Purdy K. A new strategy for job enhancement. *Calif Manage Rev.* 1975;17(4):57–71.
45. Marklis R. Successful patient safety initiatives: Driven from within. *Group Pract J.* 2001;50(10):11–16.
46. Leape L. Reporting of adverse events. *NEJM.* 2002;347(20):1633–38.
47. US Department of Health and Human Services. Addressing the new health care crisis: Reforming the medical litigation system to improve the quality of health care. March 3, 2003. Available at: http://aspe.hhs.gov/daltcp/reports/medialib.htm. Accessed on May 25, 2005.
48. Wright S, Kerin D, Kolodner K, Howard D, Brancoti F. Attributes of excellent attending—physician role models. *NEJM.* 1998;339:1986–93.
49. Surgical competence and surgical proficiencies: definition, taxonomy, and metrics. *J Am Coll Surg.* 2003;196(6):933–37.
50. Claridge J, Calland J, Chandrasckhara V, Young J, Sonfey H, Sherman B. Comparing resident measurements to attending surgeon self-perception as surgical educators. *Am J Surg.* 2003;185:323–27.
51. Rosenthal M, Fernandopolle R, Ryan-Song H, Landon B. Paying for equity: Providers' incentives for quality improvement. *Health Affairs.* 2004;23(2):127–41.
52. Bradley E, Nebster T, Baker D, et al. Translating research into practice: Speeding the adoption of innovative health care programs. *The Commonwealth Fund.* July 2004.
53. Kotter J. Leading Edge: Why transformation efforts fail. *Harv Bus Rev.* 1995;73(2):59–67.
54. Collins J. *Good to Great.* New York: HarperCollins Publishers, Inc.; 2001.
55. Blumenthal D. Training tomorrow's doctors—The medical education mission of academic medical centers. *The Commonwealth Fund.* April 2002.

Chapter 9

Employers Focus on Quality

Vittorio Maio
Christine W. Hartmann

EXECUTIVE SUMMARY

By providing coverage for their employees, employers account for a large proportion of the annual healthcare spending in the United States. Not surprisingly, employers, predominantly private, have become more involved in looking for quality when making healthcare purchasing decisions. The driving force underlining such employers' effort is the strong belief that pursuing quality can to some extent reduce overall healthcare costs. By using their sizeable purchasing power, single employers as well as coalitions of employers have been engaging in several types of activities to make healthcare providers and health plans accountable for the quality of the services they deliver. Thus far, these strategies have demonstrated a potential to reshape the healthcare market. However, those employers presently involved in quality initiatives are facing a number of barriers that could jeopardize the achievement of this goal. Collaborative efforts undertaken by private and public healthcare purchasers are needed to overcome such barriers and inject new vigor and force into the endeavor to improve the quality of care.

LEARNING OBJECTIVES

1. To describe the role of employers in the healthcare quality movement.
2. To define the most common activities adopted by employers.
3. To characterize the extent of employers' initiatives.
4. To list the factors impeding employers' efforts to improve quality.
5. To explain the current impact of employers' strategies.

KEYWORDS

Employer

Business Coalition

Value-based Purchasing

Introduction

Over the course of history, in one way or another, employers have always considered quality to be of prime importance in their corporate equations. Increasingly, employers regard quality in healthcare as part of that equation. As seen in Chapter 1, health care in the United States can no longer be assumed to be of the highest quality or to be uninfluenced by market or social factors, but take a moment now to reflect on the current influence of employers in the healthcare arena. For more than a decade General Electric, General Motors, Ford, and Motorola, just to name a few large employers, have engaged in a number of different strategies aimed at improving the quality of care.

Why should employers become involved in trying to influence quality, when it is the individual employee who interacts with the healthcare system? And if employers become involved, what is it, exactly, that they do? There are actually many compelling reasons for an employer's involvement in the healthcare system, and this chapter focuses on outlining the most important. It begins with a brief discussion of quality as it directly relates to employers, including a summary of the employer's interest in moving the quality agenda forward. Then, an overview of the employer initiatives in the market will be given. Next comes a description of the extent to which employers are currently involved in such initiatives and the barriers they encounter in promoting quality. The chapter ends with some conclusions about the impact of employers' quality movement, as well as a few theories about the future directions of these movements.

Why Are Employers Interested in Improving the Quality of Care?

Since the mid-twentieth century, US employers have played a primary role in the financing of healthcare for workers through the provision of health insurance coverage as a portion of a benefits package. In 2001, the largest percentage (35 percent) of healthcare expenditures were paid by private health insurance (as compared with other sources: federal, state, and local government, and consumer out-of-pocket) and over 90 percent of individuals under the age of 65 received private coverage through employers.[1] In 2003, approximately 98 percent of larger employers (those with 200 or more workers) and 65 percent of smaller firms (three to 199 workers) offer health benefits.[2] Despite double-digit increases in premiums, employers in 2004 continued to offer healthcare coverage to their employees—in effect, their dependents—with little reduction in benefits,[2] and it is predicted that employers, particularly large ones, will continue to offer benefits into the future.[1]

What does this all mean? It means that employers have a strong financial investment in the healthcare system and have the right to expect value for their money (where value is defined as a relationship between cost and quality). It also means that many employees have come to see their employers as agents who are able to use negotiating power to choose better health insurance.[3] Indeed, it is because of the substantial financial expenditure and because the majority of employers offer their employees no choice in health plans that employers, not employees, are seen as being in a position to influence the healthcare market.[4]

There are a number of logical reasons for employers' increasing efforts to improve the quality of healthcare. Prior to the late 1980s, there was no large-scale employer movement of this type, but with a weakening economy and yearly increases in health insurance premiums rising to almost 20 percent by the end of that decade, employers began to fight back.[5] Employers became more involved in developing strategies for the purchasing of health insurance. For example, one employer strategy involved implementing self-insurance plans, whereby employers contracted directly with physicians and hospitals, reducing employers' insurance overhead and eliminating the need for a third party.[5]

Certainly employers are interested in reducing or stabilizing the cost of health care, and this has been shown to be a prime consideration in motivating employers' actions in the marketplace.[6,7,8] However, while the relationship between costs and profits is clear and straightforward, the relationship between profits and quality is often only indirect.[2] Nevertheless, there are a number of other potential reasons for employers' interest in improving quality. Offering health insurance can help employers recruit and retain workers[4,9] and can also increase employee satisfaction.[9,10] In addition, access to high-quality healthcare can increase employees' general health, which results in reduced healthcare expenditures, absenteeism, and disability,[4,10] although no studies have yet shown the direct effect of health insurance on a company's bottom line.[9] Furthermore, healthy and satisfied workers can be more productive.[4,9] Also employers might be interested in measuring and improving healthcare quality simply because they are used to knowing what they are getting for their money when they make a purchase.[10] Finally, employers can be interested in this issue out of a larger sense of compassion and a desire to have a positive, long-term impact on the healthcare system.[11]

It is clear that employers have many reasons to focus on having an impact on the quality of healthcare. To further this end, the establishment of a "business case" for quality aims to highlight the economic value of an employer's focus on healthcare and has been espoused from various perspectives.[9,12] It has been suggested,

> a *business case* for a healthcare improvement intervention exists if the entity that invests in the intervention realizes a financial return on its investment in a reasonable time frame, using a reasonable rate of discounting.[12]

However, from an employer perspective the return on investment in the case of improvements in healthcare quality is not always clear. In other words, there exists a conceptual business case for quality, but an empirical case has yet to be demonstrated.

Value-based Purchasing

The lack of an established business case for quality notwithstanding, some purchasers of healthcare—including private and public employers and public programs (e.g., Medicaid and Medicare)—have invested considerable financial resources and human capital to weave quality considerations into their healthcare purchasing programs. The objective of these purchasing initiatives is to foster accountability in the healthcare system at a reasonable cost. Initiatives designed to do this focus on enabling a healthcare purchaser to influence the quality of healthcare through contracting measures or purchasing power. These types of strategies have gained much ground in recent years and are collectively termed value-based purchasing (VBP).

What exactly is VBP? It refers to an organized attempt by purchasers "to ensure and improve the quality of health programs when negotiating costs with providers and insurers."[7] More specifically, when it comes to employers, VBP describes a set of strategies that are pursued by employers singlely as well as by groups of employers acting in unison. Groups of employers (often called business coalitions) joined together to achieve a common purpose before the existence of the VBP movement, but they are especially important in the history and current practice of VBP, due to the nature of the healthcare market. Under the auspices of a coalition, the purchasing power of employers is increased through collective action, and there are many local and regional coalitions around the country that are focusing on VBP activities.

National business coalitions exist as well, the most notable being The Leapfrog Group, a coalition of more than 150 public and private organizations including some of the nation's largest healthcare purchasers. Its mission is to have purchasers endorse a set of targeted initiatives aimed mainly at improving patient safety and the quality of care. Today, there even exist coalitions of coalitions, such as the National Business Coalition on Health (NBCH), whose mission is to foster and facilitate employer members' interest and involvement in VBP.

As can be seen, the concept of VBP is very broad and encompasses a considerable variety of initiatives. The most common VBP strategies can be classified into the following six categories: 1) collecting and analyzing information and data on quality; 2) selective contracting with high-quality plans or providers; 3) partnering with plans or providers to improve quality; 4) promoting Six Sigma quality; 5) educating consumers on quality issues; and 6) rewarding (or penalizing) health plans and/or providers through the use of financial and nonfinancial incentives—or disincentives.[7] In the following section, each of these aspects of VBP is explained in detail.

Collecting and Analyzing Information on Quality

In order to be able to factor quality into healthcare purchasing decisions, data on which to base decisions about quality must first exist. Therefore, one of the goals for most employers engaged in VBP efforts is to collect information on the quality of care. This information is then used in some manner to guide purchasing decisions. Data that is meaningful and valuable to the employer must be accessible, reliable, valid, and in a form that can be used. It must also pertain to the performance of the health plans or providers of interest to the employer.

Both private and public purchasers of healthcare are interested in collecting or analyzing data on quality.[7] For employers interested in collecting this data, various standardized methods exist, such as the National Committee for Quality Assurance (NCQA) accreditation status measures—including the Health Plan Employer Data and Information Set (HEDIS)—and consumer satisfaction measures, such as the Consumer Assessment of Health Plans Survey (CAHPS). A recent survey of members of NBCH has shown that data on quality from a variety of standard data sets, including HEDIS, were pursued by 90 percent of the respondents.[4] In addition, Maxwell et al. found in a survey of *Fortune 500* companies that virtually all reported collecting some type of data on health plan quality.[13] Overall, employer collection of different types of data on quality is on the increase.[7]

Selective Contracting with High-Quality Plans and Providers

An infrequently used but effective method for conducting VBP involves employers directly contracting with health plans or provider networks for services. This type of activity is more common when a group of employers pools its purchasing agreements and contracts selectively with only certain plans or providers, based on quality and performance measures. One of the best documented examples is that of the Buyers Health Care Action Group (BHCAG) in Minnesota. This coalition uses the combined purchasing power of its members to foster competition on price and quality among a group of healthcare providers and allows the process to be driven by consumer choice.[14,15]

The BHCAG purchasing program, launched in 1997 and called Patient Choice, helps the employees of participating members choose among competitive provider "care systems," which are groups of physicians, hospitals, and other healthcare providers that have gathered together to provide defined health services.[16] Each year, care systems bid on a standardized benefit package and, based on these bids, are grouped into high-, medium-, and low-cost tiers. Thus, BHCAG's employers are free to offer any care systems to their employees and determine contribution levels based on cost-effectiveness of the systems. In addition, employees are provided with information on the cost, quality, and service differences among the care system choices to further inform decision making.

Partnering with Providers or Plans to Improve Quality

Instead of using a selective contracting process to choose certain plans or providers while eliminating others, another VBP effort involves trying to "raise the level of all boats" by partnering with health plans and providers to improve performance through continuous quality improvement initiatives.[7,17] This involves close collaboration between employers and health plans or providers. After the performance of health plans and providers is measured and feedback is provided, employers work together with plans and providers to improve performance. These types of efforts can even extend beyond just the employer/health plan/provider realm, reaching out to other stakeholders in government, public health, education, and consumer sectors. An example of this strategy is the Health Improvement Collaborative of Greater Cincinnati—a nonprofit coalition of hospitals, physicians, employers, insurers, community members, government representatives, public health agencies, and consumers—whose objective is to establish a common ground for fostering continuous health improvements among all stakeholders.[18]

Promoting Six Sigma Quality

A number of employers have focused at least some of their VBP efforts around the adoption of disciplined quality improvement formulas. These are directly related to extensively used business strategies such as Six Sigma.[19] As seen in Chapter 7, the principle foci of Six Sigma are on reducing process variation and improving process capability. In the case of VBP, this means that employers use Six Sigma as a rigorous and structured process to identify and help eliminate clinical and operational issues in the services of providers. General Electric and Motorola are employers that have pioneered the application of Six Sigma methodologies to contracting negotiations with health plans and providers.[19,20]

Educating Consumers on Quality Issues

One of the most widely recognized VBP initiatives is that of educating consumers about quality issues. Although it takes many different forms, it generally involves providing consumers with information on or material (e.g., report cards) about the quality of health plans, providers, hospitals, and other healthcare facilities, in order to enable them to make educated choices.[21] Some experts hold that employers and other purchasers of health care will not be able to achieve significant improvements in quality until consumers themselves become actively involved in making decisions about health care.[22,23]

It seems natural to assume that providing consumers with information about quality will lead them to become active participants in the selection process, thus directly inspiring healthcare delivery systems to improve. However, the data on whether consumer involvement actually has this effect remains unclear. A national survey showed that quality information was used by only 12 percent of consumers, and that only 4 percent used this information when making a decision about choosing a physician or hospital, and 9 percent did so when choosing a health plan.[24] Other research suggests that consumers are increasingly factoring quality information into decisions about plan selection, but cost considerations are still the most important.[25,26,27]

Rewarding (or Penalizing) Health Plans
and Providers through Financial
and Nonfinancial Incentives (or Disincentives)

A final VBP method involves rewarding or penalizing health plans or providers for their performance on certain quality measures.[7,20,28] This can be achieved through the insertion of financial incentives or disincentives in contacts and involve premium rebates or the withholding of payment.[29] A well-documented example of this comes from the Pacific Business Group on Health (PBGH). In 1996, this California coalition of only large employers negotiated with thirteen of the state's largest health maintenance organizations (HMOs) based on over two dozen performance guarantees—at risk was 2 percent of the annual premium paid by PBGH members.[30] The results of the project were somewhat surprising. Of approximately $8 million at risk for meeting PBGH performance targets, about $2 million was given back to PBGH by the HMOs because they did not achieve their goals.

Currently, a large number of incentive and reward programs to improve quality of care are underway across the country. The Leapfrog Group has established a public, Web-based national database of such programs, with the object of raising awareness regarding quality initiatives among healthcare purchasers, providers, and health plans. As of July 2004, this compendium listed seventy-seven programs, including those with both financial (e.g., rewarding providers with quality bonuses) and nonfinancial (e.g., rewarding providers with public recognition) incentives. One of the newer initiatives, the Bridges to Excellence program, is supported by a group of large employers and is aimed at tying physician incentive payments to performance. The effort was initially launched in several target markets across the nation to encourage improvements in three distinct areas: diabetes care, cardiovascular care, and patient care and management.

To What Extent Are Employers Engaged in Value-based Purchasing Activities?

In the decade and a half since the first implementation of VBP initiatives, the number of organizations involved, the types of activities pursued, and the public awareness of the issues have all increased dramatically. Forums for the exchange of information and experience as well as for education, interaction, and debate have been organized across the United States. These are frequently aimed at ensuring that purchasers are kept abreast of the varying techniques and tools available, at improving the performance of health plans and providers, and at investigating avenues for collaboration among purchasers. As mentioned earlier, the number of coalitions with members interested in pursing VBP activities is growing as well. In addition to The Leapfrog Group, national coalitions include the National Business Coalition on Health and the National Business Group on Health, and some of the larger local and regional ones include the Pacific Business Group on Health, the Florida Health Care Coalition, Gateway Purchasers for Health, and Buyers Health Care Action Group.

Despite this growing interest in VBP, the extent to which employers are firmly committed to embracing and implementing these strategies remains unclear. Results of surveys suggest that while employers and coalitions do consider quality and are involved in some data collection, as a group they act on cost.[31–35] For instance, in one survey of thirty-three large employers purchasing insurance for 1.8 million covered lives, the majority of respondents stated that they collect performance data on health plans in the form of HEDIS measurements, consumer satisfaction levels, and NCQA accreditation. However, only a few were found to place significant emphasis on quality information in the decision-making process, and instead, costs were found to drive employers' decisions.[34] In another survey, some 350 small employers of a Rhode Island coalition were found not only to purchase health insurance based on cost and premium rates rather than on quality performance but also were not familiar with quality measures (HEDIS, CAHPS, etc.).[36]

Recent data also shows that a trend found in earlier research toward employers shifting more of the financial burden of healthcare onto employees is not abating.[37] Large employers are in more favorable positions to implement VBP strategies due to their large market share in some regions of operation. Nevertheless, these large employers tend not to engage in activities such as direct contracting, which has more of a straightforward influence on the quality of care, but instead focus on sharing quality information with employees and educating them about their choices. Some employers also encourage employee selection of higher quality plans by providing financial incentives. Final decisions in these types of scenarios, however, are left up to the employee.

As pointed out previously, private purchasers of healthcare only comprise a portion of the total purchaser pie. Public organizations—state and local governments as well as federal entities such as the Department of Defense, among others—have a large stake in the healthcare system, but the evidence regarding adoption of VBP activities among these entities remains equivocal.[38,39] There is evidence showing that more and more public purchasers are in the process of implementing certain VBP strategies, such as requiring health plan performance measurement with regard to certain outcomes. However, as with large employers, public purchasers have been slow to implement more demanding techniques, including direct contracting.

Legislative efforts can provide increasing momentum for adoption of VBP practices in the future. The Medicare Modernization Act of 2003 (MMA), for example, sets both voluntarily and mandatory standards regarding quality demonstration programs, electronic prescribing, medication therapy management, and others.[40] Some of the standards set in the MMA directly reflect those espoused by The Leapfrog Group and, thus, can facilitate employers' ability or willingness to incorporate these types of measures and data into VBP efforts. However, the role of legislation has yet to be fully explored, and more research is needed on the direct and indirect effects of this type of initiative on the quality of healthcare, the market, and the adoption of VBP strategies.

Barriers to Pursuing Quality

As discussed, the evidence regarding the implementation of VBP activities is mixed. Although there exists a core of committed organizations, VBP has yet to be adopted by the majority of US employers, either private or public. This raises the question of what types of obstacles exist to increasing the use of established techniques designed to promote the use of quality in healthcare purchasing decisions. Three major categories of barriers to VBP are outlined as follows.

Data Collection

The obvious first step in any VBP endeavor involves some form of measurement of quality indicators and data collection. Without current information regarding the present state of the market, employers cannot evaluate the performance of health plans, hospitals, or providers and, therefore, cannot use quality information to influence or drive purchasing decisions. Not all employers are or need to be directly involved in data collection themselves, but data needs to be available, credible, relevant, and usable to them. Unfortunately, this is not always easily achieved.

For example, while standardized quality indicators exist (HEDIS, CAHPS, and others), employers can feel overwhelmed by the multiple forms and measures that this data can take or entail. Most purchasers, research has shown, are interested in collecting data on a number of topics, but having too much information that does not allow for comparisons across plans or providers can complicate decision making.[41,42] There is increasing interest in NCQA accreditation, because this process integrates several quality characteristics within one relatively simple measure.[34] In this regard, it is noteworthy to mention a recent initiative embraced by a number of large employers using a common Request for Information (eValue8) tool to solicit information about quality from health plans seeking to do business with them.[43] Because it promotes standardization, eValue8 helps employers compare and contrast providers in the selection and payment process.

Reliability and Validity of Data

In addition to concerns about data collection and availability, research shows that purchasers are also unsatisfied with the reliability and validity of the available data.[4,34] Indeed, plans' performance can be rated differently in different report cards, due to a lack of standardization among data collection methods. When faced with information that a plan scores high according to one set of criteria but low according to another, purchasers justifiably question what information to present to consumers and how to make a decision themselves. Also, data that is available might not match employers' needs. The HEDIS tool, for example, aggregates information only on the health plan level and not on the provider level. It also does not include factors related to issues of interest to some employers, such as quality of consumer service or cost of care.

Implementing VBP strategies is certainly not without cost, and for some potential initiators, the costs appear to be prohibitively high.[8] Measuring performance and collecting, cleaning, and analyzing data can be financially burdensome and require the initiation of organizational changes. The benefits of VBP are overwhelmingly long-term, and it can be difficult to justify the investment necessary, when an organization is traditionally focused on a more immediate return on investment.[11] Due to these concerns, large employers and coalitions of employers seem to be in better positions to engage in quality improvement initiatives than small or mid-size organizations working alone.

Consumer Preferences

A final barrier has to do with the nature of consumer preferences. Research indicates that consumers will generally value cost over quality when making healthcare purchasing decisions.[3] Employers committed to pursuing a VBP agenda, therefore, need to invest time and resources in consumer education efforts designed to enhance consumer comprehension of quality information.[11] When consumer focus on cost aligns with the purchaser's tendency toward a focus on the bottom line, the resulting interaction can limit the desire of purchasers to pursue VBP or it can encourage simply the negotiation of lower premiums.

Impact of the Employer's Quality Efforts

How much of an impact are the efforts of committed VBP implementers having, both on the activities of health plans and providers as well as on quality outcomes in healthcare? Unfortunately, the literature does not provide clear-cut answers. Data from surveys conducted in 1993 and in 2001 shows rather similar results.[44,45] In general, providers in both periods perceived purchasers to be focused on cost rather than quality. This does not match changes among managed care organizations and healthcare providers, who are more interested and engaged in quality improvement than ten years ago. In fact, research has shown that managed care organizations are investing resources to reorganize their management and technical structures in order to increase their quality improvement capabilities.[46] However, to what extent these types of changes are due to the influence of employer-based VBP efforts is unclear.

As regards to changes attributable to VBP activities that have resulted in improvements in the quality of care, few studies have been done. Research to assess the impact of the BHCAG activities, mentioned earlier, has shown that over the period studied the quality of care remained stable or improved moderately while the overall healthcare expenditures were kept slightly under the national rate.[15] Until there exists solid evidence on whether purchasers' VBP activities have positive effects on clinical quality or other quality outcomes, VBP strategies will most probably be pursued based on their theoretical ability to effect change.

Conclusions

During the last decades, employers have begun to factor quality into their decision-making process in negotiating healthcare benefits with plans and providers. These quality strategies have the potential to address the need for accountability from the healthcare system. However, although this promising movement has gained momentum among employers, it is still in its infancy. A number of obstacles still undermine these initiatives. It remains to be seen, therefore, whether value-based purchasing is able to produce improvements in the quality arena and change the current health market substantially. The growing interest in quality by public purchasers can have a profound effect in consolidating and increasing the effectiveness of employers' current value-based purchasing initiatives.

Case Study

General Electric

General Electric (GE) provides healthcare coverage to 700,000 individuals in the United States and accounts for $1.5 billion in annual healthcare benefits worldwide.[20] One of the most notable pioneers in the healthcare quality arena, GE has been engaging in a variety of VBP initiatives to hold providers accountable for their services since the early 1990s. Driven by the vision of the corporate healthcare director, Robert Galvin, MD, a leading advocate for value-based buying, GE's goal is to improve the quality of healthcare and get more value for the money it spends. As one of the founding members of The Leapfrog Group, GE has distinguished itself by launching several VBP strategies involving consumers, health plans, and providers at both the national and local levels.

The focal point of GE's VBP initiatives is the pay-for-quality purchasing approach, and GE has been applying Six Sigma to healthcare since 1996. The objective is to encourage health plans and providers to make systematic changes toward quality improvements in access, customer service, and care using rewards and penalties for performance. The company measures and follows performance via the Sigma Scorecard, assessing how a supplier is doing in four areas: member satisfaction, controllership, cost, and quality. Suppliers are required to place a significant amount of their administrative fee (from 10 percent to 25 percent) at risk, linking it to one area or a combination of areas on the scorecard. In addition, GE has been the promoter of the Bridges to Excellence—a program designed to make physicians accountable for their performance—as well as to promote greater patient involvement in healthcare decision making. More details about this initiative may be found at www.bridgestoexcellence.org.

Study/Discussion Questions

1. What are the most important reasons why employers have shown a strong interest in the quality of healthcare over the last decades?

2. Describe and discuss the business case for quality from an employer's perspective. What factors could make the employer's quality movement stronger?

3. Examine and define in your own words the most common VBP strategies that employers have been adopting thus far. To what extent are these initiatives improving the quality of care?

4. Explain the most important barriers affecting an employer's quality efforts. Propose activities that employers could adopt to overcome such barriers.

5. Access the Web site of any employer, business coalition, or supporting organization that is currently involved in quality initiatives. Identify and describe the organization's VBP activities.

Suggested Readings/Web Sites

Becher EC, Chassin MR. Improving the quality of health care: Who will lead? *Health Affairs.* 2001;20:164–79.

Bohmer R, Galvin R, Nembhard I. *Bridges to Excellence: Bringing Quality of Health Care to Life.* Case no. N9-604-030. Cambridge, Mass.: Harvard Business School Publishing; 2003.

Darby M. Health care quality: From data to accountability. *Academic Medicine.* 1998;73:843–53.

Galvin R. Purchasing healthcare: An opportunity for a public-private partnership. *Health Affairs.* 2003;22:191–95.

Galvin RS. An employer's view of the U.S. healthcare market. *Health Affairs.* 1999;18(6):166–70.

Galvin RS, McGlynn EA. Using performance measurement to drive improvement: A road map for change. *Medical Care.* 2003;41:148–60.

Meyer J, Rybowski L, Eichler R. Theory and reality of value-based purchasing: lessons from the pioneers. *Agency for Health Care Policy and Research.* Pub.No. 98-0004, 1997.

Milstein A, Galvin RS, Delbanco SF, Salber P, Buck CR. Improving the safety of healthcare: The Leapfrog initiative. *Effective Clinical Practice.* 2000;3(6):313–16.

Sirio CA, Segel KT, Keyser DJ et al. Pittsburgh Regional Healthcare Initiative: A systems approach for achieving perfect patient care. *Health Affairs.* 2003;22:157–65.

Young DW, Barrett D, Kenagy JW, et al. Value-based partnering in healthcare: A framework for analysis. *J Healthcare Manage.* 2001;46:112–32.
The Leapfrog Group (www.leapfroggroup.org).
The Buyers Health Care Action Group (www.choiceplus.com).
Employer Health Care Alliance Cooperative (www.alliancehealthcoop.com).
The Employer's Managed Health Care Association (www.emhca.org).
The National Business Coalition on Health (www.nbch.org).
The National Health Care Purchasing Institute (www.nhcpi.net).
The Pacific Business Group on Health (www.pbgh.org).
The National Business Group on Health (www.wbgh.org).
The Pittsburgh Regional Healthcare Initiative (www.prhi.org).
The Health Improvement Collaborative of Greater Cincinnati (www.the-collaborative.org).
Bridges to Excellence (www.bridgestoexcellence.org).

References

1. National Center for Health Statistics, CDC. 2003 Highlights from Trend Tables and Chartbook. Centers for Disease Control and Prevention. Available at: http://www.cdc.gov/nchs/hus.htm. Accessed on July 17, 2004.

2. The Kaiser Family Foundation, Health Research and Educational Trust. Employer Health Benefits Survey: 2003 Summary of Findings. Available at: http://www.kff.org/insurance/loader.cfm?url=/commonspot/security/getfile.cfm&PageID=20688. Accessed on July 28, 2004.

3. Peele PB, Lave JR, Black JT, Evans JH. Employer-sponsored health insurance: Are employers good agents for their employees? *Milbank Quarterly.* 2000;78(1):5–21.

4. Fraser I, McNamara P, Lehman GO, Isaacson S, Moler K. The pursuit of quality by business coalitions: a national survey. *Health Affairs.* 1999;18(6):158–65.

5. Bodenheimer T, Sullivan K. How large employers are shaping the healthcare marketplace. First of two parts. *NEJM.* 1998;338(14):1003–7.

6. Goldfarb NI, Maio V, Carter CT, Pizzi L, Nash DB. How does quality enter into healthcare purchasing decisions? *Commonwealth Fund Issue Brief.* 2003;635:1–8.

7. Maio V, Goldfarb NI, Carter CT, Nash DB. Value-based purchasing: A review of the literature. *The Commonwealth Fund.* 2003;636:1–32.

8. Fraser I, McNamara P. Employers: Quality takers or quality makers? *Med Care Res Rev.* 2000;57(Suppl 2):33–52.

9. O'Brien E. Employers' benefits from workers' health insurance. *Milbank Quarterly.* 2003;81(1):5–43.

10. Bodenheimer T, Sullivan K. How large employers are shaping the healthcare marketplace. Second of two parts. *NEJM.* 1998; 338(15):1084–87.

11. Hartmann CW, Goldfarb NI, Maio V, Roumm AR, Nash DB. Improving healthcare quality through value-based purchasing: Lessons from the pioneers. 2004. Unpublished work.

12. Leatherman S, Berwick D, Iles D, et al. The business case for quality: Case studies and an analysis. *Health Affairs.* 2003;22(2):17–30.

13. Maxwell J, Temin P. Corporate management of quality in employee health plans. *Health Care Manage Rev.* 2003;28(1):27–40.

14. Christianson JB, Feldman R. Evolution in the Buyers Health Care Action Group purchasing initiative. *Health Affairs.* 2002; 21(1):76–88.

15. Lyles A, Weiner JP, Shore AD, Christianson J, Solberg LI, Drury P. Cost and quality trends in direct contracting arrangements. *Health Affairs.* 2002;21(1):89–102.

16. The California Healthcare Foundation. Voices of experience: Case studies in measurement and public reporting of health care quality. March 2001. Available at: http://www.chcf.org/topics/index.cfm?topic=CL117&PgNum=2. Accessed on July 28, 2004.

17. Young DW, Barrett D, Kenagy JW, Pinakiewicz DC, McCarthy SM. Value-based partnering in healthcare: A framework for analysis. *J Healthcare Manage.* 2001;46(2):112–32.

18. Young DW, Pinakiewicz DC, McCarthy SM, Barrett D, Kenagy J. Value-based partnering in health care. *Benefits Quarterly.* 2001;17(2):18–25.

19. Chassin MR. Is health care ready for Six Sigma quality? *Milbank Quarterly.* 1998;76(4):565–91.

20. The Milbank Memorial Fund. Value Purchasers in Health Care: Seven Case Studies. 2001. Available at: http://www.milbank.org/reports/reportstest.html. Accessed July on 28, 2004.

21. The Leapfrog Group. The Leapfrog Group Clearinghouse of Patient Safety Communications Tools. Available at: www.leapfroggroup.org/clearinghouse.htm. Accessed July on 28, 2004.

22. Galvin R, Milstein A. Large employers' new strategies in healthcare. *NEJM.* 2002;347(12):939–42.

23. Longo DR, Land G, Schramm W, Fraas J, Hoskins B, Howell V. Consumer reports in health care: Do they make a difference in patient care? *JAMA.* 1997;278(19):1579–84.

24. The Kaiser Family Foundation, Agency for Health Care Research and Quality. National Survey on Americans as Health Care Consumers: An Update on the Role of Quality Information. Available at: http://www.kaisernetwork.org/health_cast/uploaded_files/Brodie12.11.01.pdf. Accessed on July 28, 2004.

25. Spranca M, Kanouse DE, Elliott M, Short PF, Farley DO, Hays RD. Do consumer reports of health plan quality affect health plan selection? *Health Serv Res.* 2000;35(5 Pt 1): 933–947.

26. Feldman R, Christianson J, Schultz J. Do consumers use information to choose a health-care provider system? *Milbank Quarterly.* 2000;78(1):47–77.

27. Schultz J, Thiede CK, Feldman R, Christianson J. Do employees use report cards to assess healthcare provider systems? *Health Serv Res.* 2001;36(3):509–30.

28. Rosenthal MB, Fernandopulle R, Song HR, Landon B. Paying for quality: providers' incentives for quality improvement. *Health Affairs.* 2004; 23(2):127–41.

29. The National Health Care Purchasing Institute. Provider Incentive Models for Improving the Quality of Care. 2002. Available at: http://www.nhcpi.net/monographs.cfm. Accessed on July 28, 2004.

30. Schauffler HH, Brown C, Milstein A. Raising the bar: The use of performance guarantees by the Pacific Business Group on Health. *Health Affairs.* 1999;18(2):134–42.

31. Maxwell J, Briscoe F, Davidson S, et al. Managed competition in practice: "Value purchasing" by fourteen employers. *Health Affairs.* 1998;17(3):216–26.

32. Deloitte & Touche LLP. 1997 Employer survey on managed care. *Medical Benefits*. 1998; 15(10):1–2.

33. Lipson DJ, De Sa JM. Impact of purchasing strategies on local healthcare systems. *Health Affairs*. 1996;15(2):62–76.

34. Hibbard JH, Jewett JJ, Legnini MW, Tusler M. Choosing a health plan: Do large employers use the data? *Health Affairs*. 1997;16(6):172–80.

35. Lo Sasso AT, Perloff L, Schield J, Murphy JJ, Mortimer JD, Budetti PP. Beyond cost: "Responsible purchasing" of managed care by employers. *Health Affairs*. 1999;18(6):212–23.

36. Nelson DJ, Sloan Alday C, Follick MJ. Teaching small employers to buy value. *Business & Health*. 2000;18(7):30–6.

37. Watson Wyatt Worldwide. Creating a sustainable health care program: Eighth Annual WBGH/Watson Wyatt Survey. Watson Wyatt Worldwide. Available at: http://www.watsonwyatt.com/research/resrender.asp?id=W-640&page=1. Accessed on July 28, 2004.

38. Landon BE, Huskamp HA, Tobias C, Epstein AM. The evolution of quality management in state Medicaid agencies: A national survey of states with comprehensive managed care programs. *Joint Commission Journal on Quality Improvement*. 2002;28(2):72–82.

39. Rosenbaum S. Negotiating the new health system: Purchasing publicly accountable managed care. *Am J Prev Med*. 1998;14(3 Suppl):67–71.

40. Clancy CM. Testimony on Health Care Quality Initiatives. Agency for Healthcare Research and Quality, before the Subcommittee on Health of the House Committee on Ways and Means. Available at: http://www.ahrq.gov/news/qtest319.htm. Accessed on March 18, 2004.

41. Eddy DM. Performance measurement: Problems and solutions. *Health Affairs*. 1998; 17(4):7–25.

42. Ginsberg C, Sheridan S. Limitation of and barriers to using performance measurement: Purchasers' perspectives. *Health Care Financing Review*. 2001; 22(3):49–57.

43. The Leapfrog Group. 2004 Health Plan eValue8 Request for Information. Available at: www.leapfroggroup.org/toolkit.htm. Accessed on July 31, 2004.

44. Anonymous. Who knows what employers want? *Business & Health*. 2001;19(4):12.

45. Bergman R. Employers consider cost over quality in health purchases. *Hospital and Health Networks*. 1994;68(5):54.

46. Scanlon DP, Rolph E, Darby C, Doty HE. Are managed care plans organizing for quality? *Med Care Res Rev*. 2000;57(Suppl 2) 9–32.

Chapter 10

A Patient-Centered Approach to Care

Vincenza T. Snow

EXECUTIVE SUMMARY

The Institute of Medicine (IOM) *Crossing the Quality Chasm* report made several fundamental recommendations aimed at instigating sweeping and sustained change in the American healthcare system.[1] As mentioned in Chapter 1, the IOM committee designated six aims for improvement of the current healthcare delivered: patient-centeredness, safety, effectiveness, timeliness, efficiency, and equity. This chapter will discuss how to deliver patient-centered and safe care through the use of patient self-management education, skills, and tools.

Patient self-management, however, is not to be confused with traditional patient education. They differ in some fundamental ways. Patients with chronic illness need support, as well as information, to become effective managers of their own health. Yet, in order for a patient to effectively self-manage, it is essential for them to have more than basic information about their disease. They also need to acquire understanding of and assistance with self-management skills building and they need ongoing support from members of the practice team, family, friends, and community. Patients are the experts on their own lives, and the role of the clinician is to add their medical expertise to what patients know about themselves in order to create a plan that will help patients achieve their goals.[2] Thus, an essential characteristic of patient self-management is to help people understand their health behaviors and develop strategies to live as fully and productively as they can. This chapter will review the theoretical background of self-management, see what the evidence-base for self-management is, and provide real examples of strategies for developing self-management expertise in a doctor's practice.

LEARNING OBJECTIVES

1. To understand what constitutes patient self-management.
2. To review what are the main elements of patient self-management.
3. To understand how patient self-management differs from patient education.
4. To learn how to implement a self-management program in your practice.

KEYWORDS

Patient Self-Management
Patient Education
Patient Self-Efficacy
Patient Safety

Introduction

The Institute of Medicine (IOM) *Crossing the Quality Chasm* report made several fundamental recommendations aimed at instigating sweeping and sustained change in the American healthcare system.[1] The report endorsed the overarching statement of purpose proposed by the President's Advisory Commission that said, "The purpose of the healthcare system is to reduce continually the burden of illness, injury, and disability, and to improve the health status and function of the people of the United States." Using this statement of purpose as a backbone, the IOM Committee designated six "Aims for Improvement" that the committee recommends be embraced by all stakeholders in the heathcare system (see Chapter 1).

This chapter of *The Quality Solution* concentrates on the aims for improvement of patient-centeredness and patient safety, although the other four are embedded in the concept of patient self-management. As Don Berwick put it, "True north is the experience of patients, their loved ones, and the communities in which they live."[3]

Patient-Centered Care and the Chronic Care Model

Making healthcare delivery more patient-centered is obviously not an overnight process. Patient-centered care respects the individual values, cultural diversity, and information needs of each individual patient. To do this, the healthcare teams need to be aware of issues such as health literacy, language barriers, and differing cultural health behaviors and values. Unfortunately, most healthcare providers are not trained to address any of these matters. Moreover, the system is not currently designed to provide the customized care that the IOM report calls for. Berwick, in his "Users Manual for the IOM Report" provides some illustrations of how current care and optimal care, as defined in the report, compare.[2] Some examples are:

1. Current care is based primarily on visits. The new system will provide care that is based on continuous healing relationships.

2. In current care professional autonomy drives variability. The new care is customized according to patients' needs and values.

3. Currently professionals control care. In the new system the patient is the source of control.

4. Currently information is in records. In the new system information and knowledge is shared freely.

5. In current care, "Do no harm" is an individual responsibility. In the new system safety is a system property.

While these simple rules seem to be simple truths, they are very complex to implement and change is a slow and arduous process. So, what can an individual physician or clinician do to help instigate more patient-centered, customized, and open care as described in the IOM report? What is needed is a model for systems change that allows clinical practice to move from eternally reacting—scrambling, even—to events as they occur to a system where care is planned and coordinated in the context of a collaborative relationship between professionals and the patients they serve.

The Chronic Care Model developed by Wagner and others provides a framework for systems change in which care is transformed from the predominantly acute-care system presently in place to a planned-care system in which the patient's needs are anticipated. In this model, clinicians and patients have access to information needed to make clinical decisions at the time of the visit, and during which patient self-management is an essential component.[4] The Chronic Care Model delineates five essential elements needed to implement such systems change. They are:

- Patient Self-Management: Patient self-management is very different from telling patients what to do. Patients should have a central role in determining their own care, one that fosters a sense of responsibility for their own health.

- Decision Support: Treatment decisions need to be based on explicit, proven guidelines supported by at least one defining study. Healthcare organizations should integrate guidelines into the day-to-day practice of the primary care providers in an accessible and easy-to-use manner.

- Delivery System Design: The delivery of patient care requires not only determining what care is needed, but clarifies roles and tasks to ensure the patient gets the highest quality care and follow-up.

- Clinical Information System: A registry—an information system that can track individual patients as well as populations of patients—is a necessity when managing chronic illness or preventive care.

- Organizational Supports: The effort to improve care should be woven into the fabric of the organization and aligned with a quality improvement system. Senior leadership must identify the effort to improve chronic and preventive care as important work, and translate that into clear goals reflected in the health center's policies, procedures, business plan, and financial planning.

- Community Resources: Community programs and organizations that can support or expand a health system's care for chronically ill patients and prevention strategies are often overlooked.

With these elements in place, it becomes an easier task for a healthcare team or system to deliver the kind of planned, patient-centered care called for in the IOM report.

Patient Self-Management versus Patient Education

Patients with chronic illness need support, as well as information, to become effective managers of their own health. After all, the patient lives with their condition 365 days a year while the clinician actually interacts with the patient only a few minutes to maybe a few hours a year. However, most clinicians believe that those few minutes of interaction should be sufficient to create changes in patient behaviors. Moreover, clinicians tend to take it as a personal failure when patients do not change their behaviors. Yet, in order for a patient to effectively self-manage, it is essential for them to have more than basic information about their disease. They also need to acquire understanding of and assistance with self-management skills building and they need ongoing support from members of the practice team, family, friends, and community. Patients are the experts on their own lives, and the role of the clinician is to add their medical expertise to what patients know about themselves in order to create a plan that will help patients achieve *their* goals.[2] Thus, an essential characteristic of patient self-management is to help people understand their health behaviors and develop *strategies* to live as fully and productively as they can.

This, however, is not to be confused with patient education. While patient education is needed to develop self-management skills, it is not a synonym for self-management. The two differ in some fundamental ways, as shown in Table 10.1.

Steps in Self-Management Support

The key aspect of patient self-management is the patient-generated short-term action plan. The action plan should be realistic, where the patient proposes a short—literally a week or two weeks—but fundamental change in behavior. For example, "I will walk around the block after dinner three days a week." Another fundamental concept in self-management is self-efficacy, which is the confidence that a patient can carry out a behavior needed to reach a set goal. Thus, when providing self-management training for patients, they need to be asked how confident they feel about their ability to achieve their goal. If the patient says he will walk three days a week, the professional needs to ask what

Table 10.1 *Traditional Patient Education versus Patient Self-Management*

Traditional Patient Education	Patient Self-Management
Teaches by providing information and technical skills about the disease.	Teaches skills on how to act on problems.
Problems are viewed to reflect inadequate control of the disease.	The patient identifies problems they experience that may or may not be related to the disease.
Education is disease-specific and gives information and technical skills related to the disease.	Education provides problem-solving skills that are relevant to the consequences of chronic conditions in general.
The underlying theory is that disease-specific knowledge creates behavior change, which in turn produces better clinical outcomes.	The underlying theory is that greater patient confidence in his/her capacity to make life-improving changes (self-efficacy) yields better clinical outcomes.
The goal is patient compliance with the behavior changes taught to improve clinical outcomes.	The goal is increased self-efficacy to improve clinical outcomes.
The educator is the health professional.	The educators are health professionals, peer leaders, other patients.

From Wagner EH, Glasgow RE, Davic C, et al. Quality improvement in chronic illness care: A collaborative approach. *J Quality Improve.* 2001;27:63–80.

s the patient's level of confidence, on a scale of one to ten, he will be able to achieve that
goal. If his confidence is low, then the plan needs to be reassessed. Also, contingency
plans need to be made: "If it rains, what will you do instead?" This is important because
self-efficacy theory states that the successful achievement of the action plan is more
important than the plan itself. In other words, it is more important to walk three times
a week for two weeks, than to have an ambitious plan of going to the gym five days a
week—which can quickly fail and lead to frustration. The following is an outline of the
four steps needed to begin working with your patients on self-management skills.

1. Collaborative Goal-Setting: Together you discuss what the goal will be.
   Remember to measure their level of confidence in their ability to achieve this
   goal. Then agree to try it out for a one- or two-week period. In this example,
   the patient said, "I will walk around the block after dinner three days a week."

2. Identification of Barriers and Challenges: At the time of formulating the
   action plan discuss potential barriers and challenges and collaboratively
   identify solutions. In this example, the patient was asked, "What happens
   if it's raining on the days you were going to walk?" The patient responds,
   "I'll go for a stroll around the local mall instead." You ask if this is feasible: Will it be a barrier to have to drive there? The patient says he is confident this will work, so it is agreed to be part of the action plan.

3. Personalized Problem Solving: Provide the patients with solutions to their problems rather than scolding or expressing disappointment if they have trouble fulfilling their plan. For example, at the one-week follow-up the patient recounts, "It was raining so I did go stroll at the mall, but I ended up over-eating in the food court." The response should not be exasperation or pointed looks but rather collaborative problem solving. Suggest avoiding the food court. But after discussion the patient expresses a very low level of confidence in achieving this. Together patient and professional can work out a plan B. What is fundamental is that this will be decided by the patient, always measuring the level of confidence to achieve the new goals.

4. Follow-up Support: Follow-up support can take many forms, from a quick phone call to ask the patient how the plan is going, to e-mail messaging or interactive Web sites for patients to access. This will depend on the patient's preference or technological abilities as well as those of the physicians. However, whatever form the follow-up takes, it is essential to let the patient know the professional supports the patient all the way and is there to help, not scold or chastise.

But, how is it possible to know if any of this works? What is the evidence that implementing any of these recommendations or elements creates change?

The Evidence Base for Patient Self-Management

There is growing evidence that patient self-management, patient activation or empowerment, collaborative goal setting, and problem-solving skills can lead to better patient outcomes. There are several examples in the literature of patient self-management programs that have not only increased patient understanding of their conditions but, more important, demonstrated improvements in patient outcomes and quality of life.

In an arthritis self-management program developed by Lorig et al. at Stanford University, patients attended six self-management classes lead by lay leaders. The classes covered action plans and problem-solving skills, and attempted to improve patient self-efficacy. These patients were compared to controls receiving usual care. After four years of follow-up, the intervention group showed a 20 percent reduction in pain symptoms, improved health behaviors, and growth of self-efficacy as shown by improvements in patient confidence in being able to cope with their chronic illness.[5] In another study derived from the previous, patients with a variety of chronic conditions attended seven weekly classes teaching problem-solving skills and the use of action plans.[6] At the six-month follow-up the participants showed improved control of their symptoms and a reduction in limitations of activities when compared to the control group.

In a study of patient empowerment by Anderson and colleagues at the University of Michigan, patients with diabetes received six weekly sessions of patient empowerment education. The sessions emphasized the whole patient, not just the disease entity; patients generated options and learned to build on their strengths. Failures were treated as learning experiences. After twelve weeks of follow-up, the intervention group showed gains in measures of self-efficacy and reductions in their levels of hemoglobin A1c.[7]

In another study, a self-management program for acute lower back pain was studied in a low income inner-city environment.[8] Patients in the intervention group attended three weekly sessions focused on behavioral changes, increasing self-efficacy, and reducing negative affect. They also received follow-up phone calls at weeks four, six, and eight in order to reinforce skills learned at the sessions, assist in problem solving, and assess goal attainment or the need for setting new goals. Thereafter patients received monthly reinforcing phone calls until month twelve. Compared to patients receiving usual care, patients in the intervention group reported improvements in functional status, self-efficacy, mental functioning, increased physical activity, and reduced fear of movement or reinjury.

In summary, there is good evidence that implementing patient self-management education programs improves a patient's self-efficacy, health status perceptions, and health outcomes.

Doctors Can Make Changes in Their Practice to Improve Patient Self-Management

There are several steps and strategies doctors can use to implement patient self-management support in their practice. The Improving Chronic Illness Care program recommends the following:

- Train providers and other key staff on how to help patients with self-management goals.
- Use self-management tools that are based on evidence of effectiveness.
- Set and document self-management goals collaboratively with the patient.
- Follow up and monitor self-management goals.
- Use group visits to support self-management.

Train Providers and Other Staff to Help Patients with Self-Management Goals

Ideally, doctors would like to be able to train everyone on their healthcare team using a skilled trainer. However this is probably not realistic for most practices. So, once the doctor has identified a self-management team he or she needs to define tasks and roles (e.g., who will set the action plan, who will do follow-up). Let the self-management team select its own leader. As is always the case in improvement strategies, start on a small scale. Test the self-management tool with one provider and the team working with several patients. Provide follow-up education for providers and remind them about the importance of not lecturing their patients and to let patient concerns lead the discussions. Review the self-management tool on an ongoing basis and gradually add layers of competence and complexity.

Use Self-Management Tools
That Are Based on Evidence of Effectiveness

It is important to identify high-quality patient education materials (see Web sites at the end of this chapter). Review materials for reading level and cultural appropriateness. Health literacy is an important barrier to effective self-management and the professional needs to be aware that although patients might be literate, they might be unable to understand or are impaired in their understanding of health related information. Determine if different versions—languages, literacy levels—are necessary to serve the patient. Provide patients with resources, but keep the materials brief and include materials with larger print. Test the materials with a few patients and revise as necessary. Make the materials available to patients, families, and providers by placing them in examining rooms and waiting rooms. Always remember to remove outdated educational materials from the clinic and coordinate patient education with the organization's care guidelines.

Creating a Tool for Setting and Documenting the Patient's Self-Management Goals

A self-management plan needs to include an action plan that explicitly includes goals and describes specific behavior, for example, "I will walk fifteen minutes, three times per week" not "I'm going to start exercising." Work with the patient to define goals. The physician should not prescribe goals or use checklists, but whenever possible include family and caregivers in setting goals. Once the goals are identified, a review of the patient's confidence level on a scale of one to ten will help determine how realistic the goal is and if it needs to be modified. Remember, a realistic goal that is accomplished is much more powerful than an over-enthusiastic one that leads to failure. Then a follow-up plan needs to be instituted. This might require assigning specific staff to do follow-up. With each follow-up, be it a clinic visit, group visit, telephone call, or e-mail, review the goals with the patients. Follow-up also must be documented in the chart and can be inserted on one self-management form.

Develop a form or use already developed tools (see Web sites at the end of the chapter) that will help document in the chart what the patient's self-management plan is. A copy should go in the chart and to the patient so she can keep track of her own progress. When a tool is chosen, go over it with the multidisciplinary team, including all those who will be involved in its use—physicians, nurses, volunteers, among others. Test the tool with a few patients and revise as indicated. Retest with additional patients and different populations.

How to Institute Follow-up Mechanisms and Monitor Self-Management Goals

Staff assigned to this duty might need training in providing follow-up. Have different staff or volunteers do the follow-up. Make sure patients determine the follow-up date, based on dates in the action plan. The method of follow-up can be by phone, e-mail, fax, home visit, clinic visit, and so on. No matter what, never skip scheduled follow-up: Patients will feel uncared for. Test different follow-up mechanisms (calendar, registry, tickler file) and scripts. Be sure the staff assigned to follow-up are able to provide problem solving to patients during the follow-up.

How to Use Group Visits to Support Self-Management

First identify the type of group to set up—is it a support group, an educational group, or a medical visit? Then identify a population to focus on, for example, Hispanic patients, the homeless, or the newly diagnosed. Also assess the target group's cultural/ethnic needs and identify appropriate methods/materials for patient education. A facilitator will need to be identified and trained. This can be a health professional or a lay person/patient depending on the goals set for the group. However, let the group determine the content of sessions. Leaders can monitor the content to assure that critical information is covered. Be mindful of logistics such as space, staffing needs, or billing requirements. Contact local hospitals or health centers to ask if they have been conducting group visits and elicit their "lessons learned" about logistics of scheduling, availability of rooms, and so on. Providing a meal and anticipating a patient's need for transportation and childcare can be very important incentives for patient participation. Publicize the group visits through an appropriate communication channel for the target group. If appropriate for the target group, make reminder calls.

Conclusion

To have a successful self-management program, providers and patients need to work together to define problems, set priorities, establish goals, create treatment plans, and solve problems encountered along the way. In patient-centered care, clinicians plan visits well in advance, based on the patient's needs and self-management goals, taking into account the patients' cultural identity and individuality. There is good evidence that patient self-management; patient activation or empowerment; collaborative goal setting; and problem-solving skills can lead to better patient outcomes. Patients are the experts on their own lives, and the role of the clinician is to add medical expertise to what patients already know about themselves in order to create, together, a plan that will help patients achieve their goals and ultimately help them develop strategies to live as fully and productively as they can.

Case Study

A patient-centered approach to healthcare consists of six goals according to the Institute of Medicine: safety, effectiveness, patient-centeredness, timeliness, efficiency, and equity. As healthcare evolves to focus more on consumer preferences, this approach will be increasingly significant. Some practices around the country have implemented parts or all of these aspects to cater more directly to patient needs.

Thomas Jefferson University Hospital's Department of Family Medicine instituted an open-access policy where there is no priority given to patients who need an appointment, whether or not the matter is urgent. In fact, 50 percent of the appointment slots can be available at the beginning of the work day, allowing patients to schedule appointments according to their own needs and schedule. Furthermore, the staff and physicians operate at a more efficient level as the number of no-shows has greatly decreased.[9]

Study Discussion Questions

1. What is patient self-management?
2. What are the main elements of patient self-management?
3. How is patient self-management different from patient education?
4. How do I start a self-management program in my practice?

Useful Web Sites

Health Disparities Collaboratives (www.Healthdisparities.net).
Quality Tools. Agency for Healthcare Research and Quality (www.QualityTools.ahrq.gov).
Institute for Healthcare Improvement (www.IHI.org).
Initiative for a Competitive Inner City (www.ICIC.org).
National Diabetes Education Program (www.BetterDiabetesCare.nih.gov).

References

1. Institute of Medicine. *Crossing the Quality Chasm: A New Health System for The 21st* Century. Washington, DC: National Academy Press; 2001.

2. Bodenhiemer T, Lorig K, Holman H, Grumbach K. Patient self-management of chronic disease in primary care. *JAMA.* 2002;288:2469–75.

3. Berwick D. A user's manual for the IOM's "Quality Chasm" report. *Health Affairs* 2002;21:80–90.

4. Wagner EH, Glasgow RE, Davis C, et al. Quality impovement in chronic illness care: a collaborative approach. *J Qual Improv.* 2001;27:63–80.

5. Lorig KR, Mazonson PD, Holman HR. Evidence suggesting that health education for self-management in patients with chronic arthritis has sustained health benefits while reducing health care costs. *Arthritis Rheum.* 1999;36:439–46.

6. Lorig KR, Sobel DS, Stewart AL, et al. Evidence suggesting that a chronic disease self-management program can improve health status while reducing hospitalization. *Med Care.* 1999;37:5–14.

7. Anderson RM, Funnell MM, Butler MS, et al. Patient empowerment. Results of a randomized controlled trial. *Diabetes Care.* 1995;18:943–49.

8. Damush TM, Weinberger M, Perkins SM, et al. The long-term effects of a self-management program for inner-city primary care patients with acute low back pain. *Archives of Internal Med.* 2003;163:2632–38.

9. Berry L, Seiders K, Wilder S. Innovations in access to care: A patient-centered approach to care. *Ann Intern Med.* 2003;139:568–75.

Chapter 11

The Health Plan's Perspective

Payer, Provider, and Partner

Michael D. Parkinson
Gregg S. Meyer

EXECUTIVE SUMMARY

The role of the health plan in the delivery of quality healthcare has evolved as health plans themselves have changed over the last few decades. The overarching goals of health plans in this area have remained constant: to ensure quality, efficiency, and optimal service. But the means to achieve those goals is highly dependent on the structure and operations of the plan. The transition of plans from traditional indemnity to staff-model HMOs to looser PPO arrangements—and most recently, to consumer-driven health plans—has resulted in shifting roles in the measurement and improvement of healthcare quality. The emergence of new models to create more direct relationships between purchasers and providers to assure quality will be key determinants of the future role of health plans.

LEARNING OBJECTIVES

1. To understand the significant roles that health plans can play to improve quality.
2. To describe common and emerging health plan benefits and payment methods, and their impact on quality.
3. To understand the strengths and weaknesses of data sources used by health plans to measure and improve quality.
4. To describe innovative models to closely link payment with quality performance.

KEYWORDS

Payment Methods
Incentives
Managed Care
Payment for Performance

Introduction

Health plans have often been at the center of the payer-provider and patient relationship. They help to administer payment for services, monitor quality of providers and care, and in some cases, are accountable as a delivery system. As a result of purchaser dissatisfaction, increasing costs, and quality deficiencies, health plans are under pressure to re-evaluate and reengineer many of the philosophies and practices common to managed care. Aligning payment methods and incentives for consumers and patients, seeking out better providers, and fairly reimbursing providers are all critical goals for health plans in the acceleration of healthcare quality improvement.

History and Role of Health Plans

Paul Starr[1] details the history of American medicine and describes three general kinds of medical benefits: indemnity benefits, which reimburse the subscriber (member or patient) for medical expenses; service benefits, which guarantee payment for services directly to the physician or hospital; and direct services, namely, the provision of health services to the subscriber (member or patient) by the organization receiving prepayment. Health plans serve in all these roles today and each model can have different strategies and approaches for improving healthcare quality.

Health plans or insurers pay providers either directly from premiums collected from health insurance purchasers ("insured" products for individuals and smaller employers), or indirectly by administering payments to providers on behalf of larger purchasers ("self-insured" employers or government). In the former case, the health plan retains the financial risk for delivering and/or paying for necessary healthcare services for an individual or small group. In the latter case, the larger self-insured employer retains the financial risk and the health plan charges a fee to the employer to administer the reimbursement and other aspects of healthcare services. In either case, health plans can have a significant role in promoting healthcare quality through creating financial incentives; building infrastructure to improve outcomes; and providing information to consumers, patients, providers, and payers.

Although the success of programs to improve quality is in the interests of all three actors in the purchaser, payer, and provider triad, the mechanisms to do so differ dramatically for insured versus self-insured purchasers. Insured purchasers benefit from quality improvement indirectly, through the mitigation of rate increases and improved workforce health. For the self-insured the impact of quality improvement programs is far more direct, because the payer acts as a pass-through of all the risks and rewards of quality improvement accrued to the purchaser. For the self-insured purchaser the role that the health plan plays is to help mitigate that risk through value-added programs.

The role of health plans as direct providers (as opposed to administrators of health insurance) began in the early-to-mid twentieth century with the creation of prepaid group practices such as Kaiser Permanente in California and the Health Insurance Plan (HIP) of New York. Prepaid healthcare (as opposed to fee for service) was dramatically expanded in the early 1970s with federal legislation encouraging the development of health maintenance organization (HMOs). Preferred Provider Organizations (PPOs) and Independent Practice Arrangements (IPAs) also were created as less structured but still organized models of managed care. Managed care in all its forms, but particularly in HMOs, was designed to provide comprehensive care less expensively and with higher quality compared to traditional indemnity, fee-for-service plans.

Employer annual health insurance premiums, which reflect the cost of medical care, increased at a rate greater than 10 percent per year in the late 1980s.[2] The subsequent dramatic growth of managed care, a direct response to purchaser's desire to constrain those costs, reduced premium increases to that of overall inflation through the mid 1990s. Cost savings were predominantly achieved through a supply side approach such as controlling or limiting the number, types, and unit costs of healthcare services through plan design, network creation, and provider discounts.

By the late 1990s, double-digit increases returned and with it, a new model of benefit design. Consumer-driven or consumer-directed health plans emerged.[3] These plans combined the better availability of cost, quality, and care information enabled by the Internet; greater cost-sharing by the consumer (via managed care in the 1990s); and greater freedom of choice (with a cost). The designs typically entail either a health reimbursement arrangement (HRA) with a notional account of the employer's money that the employee controls and can roll over from year to year; or premium-tiered or point-of-care benefit plan in which the member pays differential payroll contributions, copayments, or coinsurance for higher quality (and/or lower cost) providers.[4]

The passage of the Medicare Prescription Drug, Improvement, and Modernization Act in 2003 authorized the creation of tax-deductible and tax-free health savings accounts (HSAs) in association with a high deductible plan. Health savings accounts cannot exceed the size of the deductible, and contributions cannot exceed $2,500 per individual or $5,000 per family per year. These accounts are individually owned; funded (by employer or employee); and portable (when moving from employer to employer). In 2003, PPOs were the most common type of plan enrolling over 50 percent of all employees with health coverage. HMOs enrolled 25 percent with Point of Service (POS) and indemnity plans making up the remainder.[5] Consumer-driven plans, just emerging in the marketplace, enrolled less than 5 percent of employees but many have projected significant and rapid growth.[6]

Health plans can promote quality improvement through many mechanisms: credentialing and monitoring of participating providers, creation of value-added care management systems and infrastructure, and dissemination of best-of-breed tools and processes. Perhaps most important, however, payment methods and economic incentives for physicians, hospitals, and consumers are increasingly being used to improve the effectiveness and efficiency of healthcare.

Current Payment Methods and Relationship to Quality Improvement

The IOM *Crossing the Quality Chasm* report[7] summarized four payment methods that health plans (and conceivably consumers) employ and the theoretical incentives that each drives.

Budget approaches such as per capita arrangements that represent a fixed fee for each enrolled person to cover a specified level of healthcare services. Advantages include incentives to control costs; produce care efficiently; create innovations in cost-reducing technologies and practices; and the promotion of disease prevention. Disadvantages include potential for risk selection (avoiding patients who are high utilizers of care); and minimizing or restricting care for those who need to stay within budget. Physician salaries (as opposed to fee-for-service) are a budget approach that dissociate treatment decisions from the physician's potential financial gain. A more recent twist on budget based payment which aims to provide incentives for quality and efficiency is the shared savings model, where providers and plans split any savings achieved when compared with projected budget payments.

Per case payment methods, such as diagnosis related group (DRG) payments for hospitalizations, help control payment rates from the purchasers perspective and can be updated periodically. While this method has been most commonly applied to short-term hospital stays, it could be used to permit providers to design care and allocate payment for a population of patients, such as diabetics. Such payment arrangements would allow for quality enhancing services such as non-face-to-face care management and group visits, which would not be covered under more traditional payment by unit of care models.

Payment by unit of care, or fee-for-service, the dominant form of reimbursement, typically reimburses for a visit, procedure, or inpatient hospital stay (per diem). Payment by unit of care typically offers little incentive to contain total costs and creates potential for overuse. Coordination of care across providers is also challenging and there are no incentives for providing services to manage patients between visits and procedures. The main advantage is that it reduces the incentive for risk selection and increases the probability that physicians can specialize in difficult-to-treat patients.

Blended payment methods cover multiple providers often in nontraditional ways such as through home care, inpatient settings, and outpatient visits. Quality concerns include which provider entity should be held accountable and how to allocate payments between providers.

Principles for Payment Methods to Reward Quality

The IOM *Quality Chasm Report* outlined five principles for better alignment of payment and incentives in order to accelerate quality improvement.[8]

1. Fair payment must be given for good clinical management for all types of patients of differing complexity.
2. Providers must share in benefits of improved quality and rewards should be targeted for the level of the care system where reengineering is required.
3. Promote consumers and purchasers to "buy quality" through the provision of high quality, available information that can be tailored to their needs.
4. Align financial incentives with the implementation of care processes based on best practices and achievement of better patient outcomes.
5. Reduce fragmentation of care by eliminating any payment methods that create a barrier to the coordination of care for patients across settings and over time.

Some specific innovations that the IOM called for further exploration and possible pilot testing included:[9]

- blended or bundled payment methods that pays providers and groups using capitation supplemented with other system-improvement rewards (such as cost or quality outcomes)
- multiyear contracts and bonus incentives versus the usual practice of annual contracts that often makes quality improvement investments difficult due to rapid turnover of plan enrollees
- better risk adjustment and/or more appropriate use of risk-adjustment methods to identify subpopulations of those at risk of high utilization and cost so that care can be improved for their specific needs
- payment for encouraging the use of electronic or other forms of communication between patients and providers that have been shown to improve safety and quality.

Health Plan Data Sources for Quality Improvement

Health plans create or have access to numerous data sources that have been used to differing degrees with different impact on the improvement of the quality of care. They include medical records, administrative claims, patient/consumer surveys, provider or peer expert opinion, and formal accreditation and certification processes.

Medical records. As of 2004, over 90 percent of physician, medical groups, and hospitals did not employ health information technology (e.g., electronic health records, computerized physician order entry) in their practices.[10] While the medical record remains the gold standard for the documentation of clinical information and care practices, paper medical record review is extremely time consuming and labor intensive. Because medical record abstraction and review is so costly, medical claims and pharmacy data are used most frequently to evaluate the quality of healthcare in most health plans. The increasing availability of electronic health records is expected to address many of the barriers in using medical records for quality measurement and improvement.

Administrative claims. Claims data for medical services (e.g., ambulatory visits, hospitalizations, pharmacy), compared to paper medical record review, is very cost-efficient. Claims data collection, analysis, and dissemination is readily performed and increasingly is the primary basis for evaluating the quality and cost of health plans, hospitals, medical groups, and individual physicians. As in all data collection, information collected for one purpose (documenting for payment purposes) should be used with great caution when employed for other uses (such as assessing the effectiveness, efficiency, or appropriateness of care). Comparisons of medical records with claims data often reveal significant differences, which health plans and purchasers should be aware of and reconcile as appropriate.[11-14] Significant barriers to acquiring and displaying meaningful provider-level information include: inadequate consideration of patient and physician characteristics; difficulty attributing care to individual providers; insufficient or unknown adequate sample sizes for detecting effects; and combining data across plans with different administrative rule sets and poor correlation between claims and medical record data. Claims data also suffer from significant data lags that make them less useful for real-time quality improvement efforts.

The choice of whether relatively available and affordable administrative claims data can be used appropriately for quality measurement or that more costly and difficult to obtain medical record (clinical) data is required is not a simple one. Such decisions must be guided by close attention to the purpose to which the quality measurement will be applied (see Figure 11–1). When the purpose of quality measurement is for internal organizational improvement, without public release, administrative claims data is often adequate. In those cases, the administrative claims data often serves a role in the identification of broad trends and generates hypotheses, which can later be efficiently examined with clinical medical records data. When the purpose of measurement is for dissemination of information outside the organization, the demands on data quality, the need to adequately risk adjust, and the costs of data collection rise. This is particularly true when individual providers will be identified. In those cases the implications of misclassification of true performance becomes greater. When the purpose of the quality measurement is for accountability purposes, including steerage of patients, payment, accreditation, or network participation, the need for validity, reliability, and adequate adjustment are such that the costs and efforts associated with obtaining clinical medical records data are clearly justified.

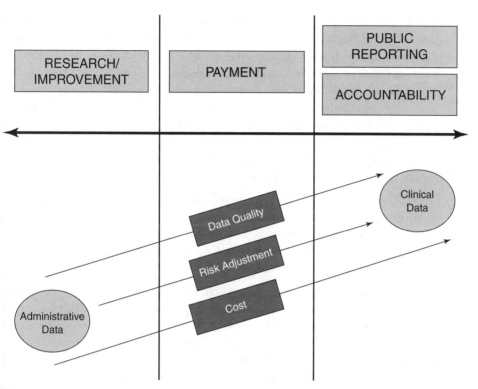

Figure 11–1 *What Is the Purpose of Quality Measurement? The Stakes Get Higher as the Purpose Moves Toward Accountability.*

One of the ongoing challenges in this area is a statistical conundrum between the need to risk adjust and the ability to do so. When measurement is being done at an aggregate level, such as comparing performance between states using administrative claims data, there is a plethora of data (sample size) for risk adjustment but little need to do so, because variations in performance due to differing risk profiles play a relatively small role at such an aggregate level. As one moves toward more granular provider level measurement (e.g., measurement of the performance of individual physicians) the impact of differing risk profiles on performance measures can be substantial.

Unfortunately, however, the availability of an adequate sample size for the necessary risk adjustment is problematic, because the number of cases available for abstraction for any performance measure will be small. A recent study examining the effect of sample size on the validity and reliability of quality measurement at the hospital level found that with the exception of coronary artery bypass grafting, the operations for which surgical mortality has been advocated as a quality indicator are not performed frequently enough to judge hospital quality.[15] It is clear that the accurate (valid and reliable) assessment and improvement of healthcare quality, particularly at the individual physician level, remains a formidable challenge.[16]

Patient and consumer surveys. The standardized and widely utilized Consumer Assessment of Health Plans Survey (CAHPS)[17] are employed to assess a variety of aspects of health plan and provider quality of care issues. Surveys are primarily targeted at a patient's experience of care and customer satisfaction with emphasis on plan and provider access and service. As of 2004, there was no nationally accepted standardized consumer survey instrument for hospitals, medical groups, or individual physicians, though examples of state-level tools were available.[18,19] But it appears that the CAHPS family of surveys, which includes surveys at the plan, hospital, physician, and individual provider levels, are quickly gaining broader acceptance.

Provider survey or peer "expert opinion." Numerous lay publications provide rankings of "best quality" physicians and hospitals based, at least in part, on expert opinion through surveys of nationally recognized physician authorities. While not definitive, these reviews can provide another source of data to be considered in the assessment of quality.[20]

Accreditation and certification. Accreditation of health plans and certification of physicians can occur through a variety of organizations. Health plans, particularly HMOs, can be accredited using the Health Plan Employer Data and Information Set (HEDIS) or for a variety of care management functions through such organizations as the National Committee for Quality Assurance,[21] and URAC.[22] Hospitals are accredited through the Joint Commission on Accreditation of Healthcare Organizations.[23] Certification of physicians is widely recognized as a measure of physician competence and is accomplished through the member boards of the American Board of Medical Specialties.[24] However, accreditation and certification processes, despite being in place for many years, have not sufficiently addressed cost, quality, access, or satisfaction concerns. As a rule, accreditation and certification processes serve to define a "floor" in terms of acceptable performance rather than a mechanism to promote or note excellence.[25]

Public Communication of Quality Data

Quality information is used for internal quality improvement (within the health plan, medical group, or individual practice) as well as for public reporting to provide consumers, employers, and government purchasers with better, more informed choices. Neither internal nor external reporting of quality data has been studied widely but when studied, it is unclear what impact, if any, these activities have had on improving "value-based purchasing" to date.[26,27,28] Content (standardized, valid, and reliable measures of quality by condition); presentation format; rigor; and mode of release must be addressed in order for purchasers and consumers to increase their use of quality information to make informed choices. There is some evidence that voluntary reporting of health plan and provider quality can be ineffective in advancing the goals of systemwide quality improvement and that mandatory reporting might be needed.[29,30] Whether greater consumer education and "ownership" of healthcare dollars and purchasing decisions at the level of individual healthcare services (as compared to the choice of one's health plan) will accelerate the desire for and use of quality information remains to be definitively studied as well.

Changing Relationships Between Payer, Plans, Providers, and Consumers

Health plans, spurred by employers (and their coalitions), government, and consumers are developing innovative quality improvement approaches, payment methods, and incentives. Numerous models have emerged that focus on physicians, hospitals, and consumers, many of which follow the broad principles outlined by the IOM.[31,32,33] Quality incentives are gaining in favor nationally but there is little data to date to suggest which form or focus is most effective in accelerating "structure" (e.g., automation of hospital or physician offices with health information technology); process (e.g., coordination of care between care sites and providers); and outcome (clinical outcome measurements, improved health status, reduced morbidity, and mortality). Characteristics of typical incentives programs offered to providers through the health plan or employer coalition as of 2004 were:

- Bonus payments paid at regular intervals or tying a portion of a provider's payment increase over a multi-year period to the provider's performance on a quality scorecard. Typically the incentives payment were modest—usually 1 percent to 5 percent of total payments.
- Infrastructure incentives (using CPOE in hospitals, acquiring health information systems, and care management tools in office practices) are increasingly being employed by large national employers.[34] Physician recognition programs for chronic diseases such as diabetes or heart disease[35] also have been created to better inform patients about individual provider quality.

Following recommendations from the Institute of Medicine and with the lead of large purchaser organizations such as the Pacific Business Group on Health and The Leapfrog Group health plans, and most recently, the Centers for Medicare & Medicaid Services (CMS) have initiated reimbursement programs to improve quality and service while controlling costs. These pay-for-performance programs to address a pervasive problem in attempting to improve quality, resulted in misaligned incentives. Prior to pay-for-performance programs it was clear that there were programs, such as disease management for heart failure patients, that could improve outcomes and control costs.[36] But the savings from the implementation of such programs accrued to payers—and indirectly, purchasers and patients—while the costs of the programs were borne by the provider. That traditional win–win–lose relationship between plans, purchasers, and providers is an untenable model for the promotion of known quality improvement interventions.

The new programs reward, or at least fail to penalize, hospitals and physicians based on their ability to meet contractual targets for utilization and quality. Under pay-for-performance providers and plans negotiate targets, which in the most sophisticated cases include risk adjustment and protections against secular trends (such as the introduction of new high cost pharmaceuticals). Many pay-for-performance plans develop targets from criteria originally developed for other purposes such as HEDIS while others are negotiated on a case-by-case basis between plans and providers. If those targets are met, providers can receive bonus payments, or more commonly, the return of a percentage of contracted provider revenue that was placed "at-risk" for performance.

Pay-for-performance programs are now estimated to encompass portions of insurance coverage for over thirty million people, with the potential of a significant increase in that number through demonstration programs being piloted by the CMS.[37] The Leapfrog Group has recently created a compendium of such programs.[34] At the present time risk-based programs are being implemented in large physician groups while more straightforward bonus programs are being directed at all types and sizes of providers. The Centers for Medicare & Medicaid Services has $50 million earmarked through the Medicare Modernization Act for fiscal year 2007 to provide pay-for-performance incentives for things such as electronic prescribing. Although pay for performance is relatively new in many markets, its rapid growth has made it one of the dominant trends in the relationship between health plans and quality measurement and improvement. But whether pay-for-performance schemes will prove any better than previous attempts at managing care such as capitation is still unknown. Forces such as lags in data measurement; fragmentation of care; variations in the ability of provider organizations to invest in the infrastructure necessary to do well in such arrangements; and consumer demand for some services, such as high-cost imaging, undermine the potential of these programs to improve quality and rationalize utilization.[31]

More recently there have been some experiments that, if successful, could dramatically change the role of health plans in ensuring and rewarding quality. Traditionally the health plan has served as a mediator between purchasers of healthcare (employers and consumers) and providers of healthcare (physicians and hospitals). Part of that mediation role has been to set the terms by which quality of care will be measured and rewarded. The new programs, such as General Electric's Bridges to Excellence program, aim to fundamentally alter that relationship.[38] These programs create processes ("disintermediation") through which the purchaser provides incentives directly to providers, thus cutting the health plans out of the picture. Under the Bridges to Excellence, physicians are directly rewarded on a capitation basis for their use of electronic medical records, development of disease registries, and successful completion of a diabetes care recognition program.

Consumer- and patient-focused financial incentives, even modest ones, have been shown to be effective in the short run for simple preventive care and distinct, well-defined behavioral goals.[39] Cash incentives (as opposed to coupons, vouchers, and gifts, for example) produce the greatest behavioral effect and demonstrate a dose-response relationship. There is less evidence that economic incentives can sustain the long-term lifestyle or disease management improvements known to be associated with better health and more effective and efficient care utilization. Consumer-driven financing models, which directly align health and medical care behaviors with potential long-term cost savings, will undoubtedly be studied to determine their long-term impact on health and quality outcomes.

Future Considerations for the Role of Health Plans in Quality Improvement

Beyond predicting more change, there is little that can be certain in terms of the evolving role of health plans in healthcare quality. Much more is known, however, about some of the significant forces that will impact this relationship. These forces can be divided into trends in quality measurement; new demands for transparency; development of new consumer-driven benefit models; creation of pay-for-performance programs; and the emergence of new actors in the purchaser, payer, and provider interaction.

Rapid changes in the field of quality measurement are being precipitated by demands for accountability, improvement in the science of measurement, expansion of measurement domains, and the emergence of new organizations devoted to developing and promoting quality measures. Purchasers and patients are driving much of the quality measurement agenda with their insatiable hunger for new measures and public reporting. Improvements in the science of measurement include the development of new models for risk adjustment as well as the increasing availability of electronic data, a trend which could potentially revolutionize quality measurement with the widespread adoption of electronic health records. Among the new measurement domains is renewed attention to measurement of structure by The Leapfrog Group and others, as well as the nascent science of measurement of patient safety. Finally there is the development of new organizations, such as the National Quality Forum for Measurement and the American Medical Association Consortium, as well as new coalitions that include cooperative efforts between CMS, JCAHO, and the American Hospital Association on voluntary hospital quality reporting. The net results of these activities and actors is an increasing array of measures and the attendant concerns with burden of measurement and public release of information.

As those new measures come on line the demands for public release of the information generated from the application of those measures is sure to increase. The IOM, among others, has called for increased transparency in healthcare. But legitimate questions of what benefits will accrue from increased transparency, and at what cost, remain.[40]

New models for consumer-driven benefit designs and payment for performance are also likely to alter the relationships between purchasers, health plans, and providers. Efforts at making consumers the focal points in the relationship among these actors with respect to quality are just developing. In addition, it will be learned whether disintermediation is simply a passing fad or will truly alter the traditional relationships between payers, purchasers, and providers in the next few years.

Among the new, or in some cases renewed and reinvigorated, actors in the interactions between purchasers, plans, and providers with respect to quality are the organizations devoted to developing and vetting quality measures noted in this chapter and the one player that can fundamentally change the game: the federal government. The federal government has taken many roles in the measurement and improvement of healthcare quality but in recent years its potential as a large purchaser is being realized.[41] An array of new demonstration projects sponsored by CMS are illustrative of that trend.[42]

Conclusion

Recent reports from the IOM conclude that there is a chasm between what is and what ought to be in healthcare quality. The challenges in examining and improving quality beg the questions of how that chasm will be crossed and whether each party is ready to take big steps. Interactions between purchasers, payers, and providers have provided some small jumps represented by efforts such as HEDIS and the emergence of payment for performance as a method for health plan contracting. Patients, historically, have not been viewed as major players in the effort to improve healthcare quality. The role of "purchaser" can be moving away from "the plan" and "the employer" toward the "consumer" and the "patient." The health plan's role can change from that of solely or predominantly provider-focused to being more consumer-focused as partners assisting individuals in identifying and improving health risk factors and in seeking out and receiving evidence-based care shown to improve health outcomes and reduce costs. The changing relationships between payer, plan, provider, and consumer including the emergence of consumerism, an expanded role for federal and state government, and direct interactions between purchasers and providers can all provide an opportunity to promote bolder action.

Case Study

Tensions Over the Public Release of Quality Data

Recent events in the Boston marketplace provide a stark example of the intense debates over the release of healthcare quality information and the role of health plans in that process. Purchasers are demanding that health plans post quality and cost data on their Web sites for hospitals, physician groups, and even individual physicians,[43] while the provider community is outraged over the flaws in such data and the potential for real harm that could come from patients using such information to make decisions about where to obtain care.

Health plans in Boston have decided to go forward with plans of making available to their members a Web site that ranks hospital performance in 175 clinical areas. A healthcare column in the *Boston Globe* featured some of the results obtained via the Web site, which relies on a mortality analysis using administrative claims data, ranking acute myocardial infarction care in Boston-area hospitals.[44] To the surprise of the columnist, and no doubt countless readers, the four top hospitals in Boston for care of patients with acute myocardial infarction were community institutions—not the prestigious downtown academic medical centers (two of which have been regularly cited as among the nation's ten best hospitals for cardiac care as ranked in the annual *US News and World Report* survey.[45]

A cursory analysis of the information, however, reveals that these top four hospitals do not perform cardiac surgery. The Web site analysis did not take into account that these institutions routinely (and appropriately) transfer their highest risk patients to downtown academic medical centers further down on the hospital "quality" ranking list for immediate catheterization and revascularization.

Although such misclassification can be dismissed with an attitude that no one pays attention to such information anyway, recent developments in the marketplace are making such rankings harder to ignore. Another area health plan, using the identical Web-based ranking system, has developed a new insurance product, which uses that information to create tiers among hospitals, and in 2005 among individual providers, which are based on "quality" and cost. As a result the stakes in the debate over the public release of quality data have increased as these analyses have gone from a for-your-information status to incorporation into the structure of health plans and tiered premiums and co-pays. This is forcing an urgent search for a middle ground on public reporting and accountability that makes sense for patients, purchasers, plans, and providers.[46]

Study/Discussion Questions

1. What are common payment methods used by health plans and how do they impact quality improvement at the provider level?

2. What are the advantages and disadvantages of using various data sources to analyze and reward health quality improvement?

3. Provide examples of innovative payment methods or incentives currently being employed and try to estimate their likelihood of improving healthcare quality.

4. What is the consumer's role in understanding, seeking, and paying for quality healthcare—particularly given the advent of consumer-driven healthcare and Health Savings Accounts?

5. What are significant obstacles for health plans to improve quality and what strategies can be employed to mitigate them?

6. How has the role of the health plan in ensuring quality evolved as the structure and operations of health plans have changed over time?

Suggested Readings/Web Sites

The Leapfrog Group (www.leapfroggroup.org).

Pacific Business Group on Health (www.pbgh.org).

Center for Studying Health System Change (www.hschange.org).

National Committee on Quality Assurance (www.ncqa.org).

Agency for Healthcare Research and Quality (www.ahrq.gov).

Centers for Medicare & Medicaid Services (www.cms.gov).

The National Quality Forum (www.qualityforum.org).

References

1. Starr P. The social transformation of American medicine. New York: Basic Books; 1982.

2. Iglehart JK. Changing health insurance trends. *NEJM*. 2002;347:956–62.

3. Herzlinger RE, ed. *Consumer-driven Healthcare: Implications for Providers, Payers and Policy makers*. San Francisco: Jossey-Bass; 2004.

4. Rosenthal M, Milstein A. Consumer-driven plans: What's offered? Who chooses? *Health Serv Res*. 2004;39(4 Part II):1055–70.

5. Kaiser Family Foundation. Employer health benefits 2003 annual survey. Available at: www.kff.org/insurance. Accessed on June 4, 2005.

6. Gabel JR, Lo Sasso AT, Rice T. Consumer-driven health plans: Are they more than talk now? *Health Aff*. Web exclusive. 2002; W-3:395–407. Available at: http://content.healthaffairs.org/cgi/reprint/hlthaff.w2.395v1.pdf. Accessed on June 4, 2005.

7. Institute of Medicine. *Crossing the Quality Chasm: A New Health System for The 21st Century*. Washington, DC: National Academy Press; 2001.

8. Ibid. p. 195.

9. Ibid. p. 194.

10. Yasnoff WA, Humphreys BL, Overhage JM, et al. A consensus action agenda for achieving the national health information infrastructure. *J Am Med Inform Assoc*. 2004;11(4):332–38.

11. Maclean JR, Fick DM, Hoffman WK, King CT, Lough ER, Waller JL. Comparison of 2 systems for clinical practice profiling in diabetic care: medical records versus claims and administrative data. *Am J Manag Care*. 2002; 8(2):175–79.

12. Greenfield S, Kaplan SH, Kahn R, et al. Profiling care provided by different groups of physicians: Effects of patient case-mix (bias) and physician-level clustering on quality assessment results. *Ann Intern Med*. 2002;136:111–21.

13. Hofer T, Hayward R, Greenfield S, et al. The unreliability of individual physician "report cards" for assessing the costs and quality of care for chronic disease. *JAMA*. 1999; 281:2098–2105.

14. Garnick D, Hendricks A, Comstock C, et al. A guide to using administrative data for medical effectiveness research. *J Outcomes Manage*. 1996;3:18–23.

15. Dimick JB, Welch GB, Birkmeyer JD. Surgical mortality as an indicator of hospital quality: The problem with small sample size. *JAMA*. 2004;292:847–51.

16. Landon BE, Normand ST, Blumenthel D, Daley J. Physician clinical performance assessment: Prospects and barriers. *JAMA*. 2003;290:1183–89.

17. Consumer Assessment of Health Plans Survey (CAHPS). Available: at www.ncqa.org/ Programs/HEDIS/index.htm. Accessed on June 4, 2005.

18. The Pacific Business Group on Health. Healthscope Quality. Available at: www.healthscope. org. Accessed on June 4, 2005.

19. Massachusetts Health Quality Partnership. Available at: www.mhqp.org. Accessed on June 4, 2005.

20. *US News and World Report Best Hospitals 2004.* Available at: http://www.usnews.com/ usnews/health/hosptl/methodology.htm. Accessed on June 4, 2005.

21. National Committee on Quality Assurance. Available at: www.ncqa.org. Accessed on June 4, 2005.

22. URAC. Available at: www.urac.org. Accessed on June 4, 2005.

23. Joint Commission on Accreditation of Healthcare Organizations. Available at: www.jcaho.org. Accessed on June 4, 2005.

24. American Board of Medical Specialties. Available at: www.abms.org. Accessed on June 4, 2005.

25. Chen J, Rathore SS, Radford MJ, Krumholz HM. JCAHO accreditation of care for acute myocardial infarction. *Health Aff.* 2004;22:243–54.

26. Marshall MN, Shekelle PG, Leatherman S, Brook RH. The public release of performance data: What do we expect to gain? A review of the evidence. *JAMA*. 2000;283(14):1866–74.

27. Goldfarb NI, Maio V, Carter CT, Pizzi L, Nash DB. How does quality enter into healthcare purchasing decisions? *Commonwealth Fund Issue Brief,* May 2003. Available at: www.cmwf.org. Accessed on July 5, 2005.

28. Hibbard JH, Stockard J, Tusler M. Does publicizing hospital performance stimulate quality improvement efforts? *Health Aff.* 2003;22:84–94.

29. McCormick D, Himmelstein DH, Woolhandler S, Wolfe SM, Bor DH. Relationship between low quality-of-care scores and HMO's subsequent public disclosure of quality-of-care scores. *JAMA*. 2002;288:1484–90.

30. Berwick DM. Public performance reports and the will for change. *JAMA*. 2002; 288:1523–24.

31. Epstein AM, Lee TH, Hamel MB. Paying physicians for high-quality care. *NEJM*. 2004; 350:406–10.

32. Rosenthal MB, Fernandopulle R, Song HR, Landon B. Paying for quality: Providers' incentives for quality improvement. *Health Aff.* 2004;23:127–54.

33. Center for Studying Health System Change 2004. Paying for quality: Health plans try carrots instead of sticks. Issue brief no. 82, May 2004. Available at: http://hschange.org/CONTENT/ 675/. Accessed on June 4, 2005.

34. The Leapfrog Group. Rewarding Results and Bridges to Excellence Program. Available at: http://www.bridgestoexcellence.org/bte/bte_overview.htm. Accessed on June 4, 2005.

35. National Committee on Quality Assurance. Physician Recognition Programs for Diabetes and Heart/Stroke. Available at: http://www.ncqa.org/PhysicianQualityReports.htm. Accessed on June 4, 2005.

36. Whellan DJ, Gaulden L, Gattis WA, et al. The benefit of implementing a heart failure disease management program. *Arch Intern Med.* 2001;161(18):2223–28.

37. Family Practice Management. Getting rewards for your results: Pay-for-performance programs. Available at: www.aafp.org/20040300/45gett.html. Accessed on July 19, 2004. The Leapfrog Group. Incentive and reward compendium guide and glossary. Available at: ir.leapfroggroup.org/compendiumresult.cfm. Accessed on August 15, 2004.

38. de Brantes F. Bridges to excellence: a program to start closing the quality chasm in healthcare. *J Healthc Qual.* 2003;25(2):2,11.

39. Kane RL, Johnson PE, Town RJ, Butler M. A structured review of the effect of economic incentives on consumers' preventive behavior. *Am J Prev Med.* 2004;27(4):327–52.

40. Marshall MN, Shekelle PG, Leatherman S, Brook RH. The public release of performance data. What do we expect to gain? A review of the evidence. *JAMA.* 2000;283:1866–74.

41. Tang N, Eisenberg JM, Meyer GS. The role of government in improving health care quality. *Joint Commission J Qual Safety.* 2004;30:47–55.

42. Centers for Medicare & Medicaid Services. CMS demonstration projects under the Medicare modernization act (MMA). Available at: www.csm.hhs.gov/researchers/demos/mma demolist.asp. Accessed on August 3, 2004.

43. Galvin R, Milstein A. Large employers new strategies in health care. *NEJM.* 2002; 347:939–42.

44. Allen S. A new way to rank hospital quality. *Boston Globe.* March 2, 2004.

45. *US News and World Report Best Hospitals 2004.* Heart and Heart Surgery Ranking. Available at: http://www.usnews.com/usnews/health/hosptl/rankings/specihqcard.htm. Accessed on June 4, 2005.

46. Lee TH, Meyer GS, Brennan TA. A middle ground on public accountability. *NEJM.* 2004; 350:2409–12.

Chapter 12

Governmental Perspective

Initiatives to Improve
the Quality of Care
for Medicare Beneficiaries

Stuart Guterman
Rachel Nelson
William C. Rollow
Sheila H. Roman

EXECUTIVE SUMMARY

This chapter describes several areas in which the Centers for Medicare & Medicaid Services (CMS) has undertaken initiatives aimed at improving the quality of care, and attempted to change the traditional role of the Medicare program from a passive payer for health services to an active purchaser of the healthcare that its beneficiaries need. The chapter begins with a description of Medicare's Healthcare Quality Improvement Program (HCQIP) and the evolution from a primarily utilization review function to a more proactive network of organizations aimed at transforming the way that healthcare is delivered to Medicare beneficiaries and all Americans.

An array of activities to collect, analyze, and disseminate information on the quality of care provided by the various types of providers is next discussed, including the most recent initiative supported by the Medicare Modernization Act of 2003 (MMA), which provides some $400 million to encourage hospitals to report a set of quality measures for the purpose of public reporting.

The role of healthcare information technology (HIT) in enhancing the ability of physicians, as well as hospitals and other facilities, to collect and manage the information they need, track their patients, coordinate the care they provide, and avoid mistakes that can increase healthcare costs and—more important—threaten patient safety is then addressed. CMS, and the Department of Health and Human Services (DHHS) of which it is a part, is conducting and developing a number of projects and studies that are intended to encourage the adoption of

HIT to improve the quality and effectiveness, as well as the efficiency, with which healthcare is provided.

Finally, various incentives that can be used both to counter existing barriers to the provision of better quality care and to encourage further improvements are discussed. CMS is conducting and developing a number of projects that will test different approaches, the ability to implement them in the Medicare context, and the impact of both nonfinancial and financial incentives in achieving the ultimate objective, which is to maximize the quality of care while keeping it affordable to the Medicare program.

LEARNING OBJECTIVES

1. To understand Medicare's initiatives to improve the quality of care provided to its beneficiaries.
2. Medicare quality initiatives include the development of quality measures and dissemination of information on providers' performance and financial incentives to encourage quality improvement.
3. Healthcare information technology is crucial in attaining Medicare's quality improvement objectives because it is used to develop and process data on provider performance and monitors the needs and progress of patients.

KEYWORDS

Quality Improvement
Quality Measurement
Financial Incentives
Healthcare Information Technology

Introduction

Previous chapters noted many of the recent reports calling attention to quality deficiencies in the United States healthcare system. With regard specifically to the Medicare program, Jencks and colleagues[1] (2003) found that care provided to Medicare beneficiaries had improved between 1998 and 1999 and between 2000 and 2001, but the rate of improvement was slow (2003). They estimated that, with no change in the trajectory, it could take twenty years for Medicare beneficiaries to receive a threshold of 95 percent performance on measures of recommended care from the nation's healthcare system.

These and similar findings have spurred an acceleration in the pace of activities aimed at improving the quality of care provided to Medicare beneficiaries. Moreover, with Medicare spending passing $300 billion in 2004, there is increasing pressure to improve the effectiveness of the program in purchasing the healthcare its beneficiaries need, so that the best possible outcomes can be achieved for the resources that are expended.

The Quality Improvement Program

Within the overall CMS approach to advancing quality of care for Medicare beneficiaries, the Medicare Healthcare Quality Improvement Program (HCQIP) is the element focused primarily on encouraging and assisting providers to measure, understand, and improve their care delivery processes, practices, and outcomes. Based largely on the methods developed by and the experience of Medicare's utilization and quality assurance case review programs of the 1970s, the HCQIP's key operating components were first established in the early 1980s, marking the beginning of the first of three major evolutionary phases in program history to date.

In the program's first decade, the Peer Review Organizations (PROs) and End-Stage Renal Disease Network Administrative Organizations (ESRD Network) programs functioned as largely separate and independent components of a system relying heavily on a retrospective, case-review paradigm. In the early 1990s, the emphasis shifted to a quality improvement paradigm, and the HCQIP system, of which the PRO (now called Quality Improvement Organizations, or QIOs) and ESRD Network contracts are distinct but related and aligned operating components, was established. Continuing to evolve, the program in 2004 entered its third phase, retaining their quality improvement orientation but emphasizing helping providers to effect changes that will enable them to achieve the HCQIP vision: the right care for every person, every time.

Prior to the establishment of the PROs, Medicare's quality assurance system comprised local associations of physicians that retrospectively reviewed inpatient and ambulatory care services reimbursed by Medicare and Medicaid. Congress had established that initial system, the Professional Standards Review Organization (PSRO) program, by a 1972 amendment to the Social Security Act. The PSROs were highly localized (by 1981, there were 195 separate PSRO review areas in the United States) and focused primarily on utilization review. The PSROs were able to develop hospital discharge data, conduct profile analyses, and review care rendered in settings other than hospitals. But despite their emphasis on utilization review, they were not able to effectively contain the trend of increasing healthcare utilization and spending.

By the early 1980s, growing concern about the viability of the Medicare Trust Funds and the protection of beneficiaries from poor-quality care and inappropriate medical procedures led to the development and implementation of the hospital inpatient Prospective Payment System (PPS), a novel approach to Medicare payment. Because the PPS introduced strong incentives to reduce the cost of each hospital stay, there was concern that the quality of care might suffer without explicit oversight. To provide the necessary quality assurance, Congress decided to replace the PSRO program with the PRO program via the Peer Review Improvement Act of 1982, thus initiating the first phase of the HCQIP.[a]

Program statutory authority and procedural requirements were written into Title XVIII and Title XI of the Social Security Act in order to increase consistency and effectiveness of clinical quality review organizations. Structurally, the program is effected by CMS contracting with a physician-sponsored or physician-access organization in each geographically defined contract regions.[b] Statutory duties include, at a minimum, ensuring that reviewed care provided to beneficiaries in that contract region is medically necessary, provided in the most appropriate setting, and of acceptable quality. The clear assumptions underlying the case review model, and the initial operational design of the PRO program, were: that the vast majority of services meet professionally recognized standards of quality; that implicit case review is a good way to judge quality; and that review-based sanctions of the few sub-standard instances or providers is an effective way to improve the overall level of quality.

By 1991, experience and research findings—including a 1988 Institute of Medicine report—clearly indicated that many services rendered did not meet professional standards; that implicit case review is not reliable as a measure of systematic quality; and that the paradigm on which review and sanction is based is no more effective at improving subsequent performance or system reliability in healthcare than it had proven to be in manufacturing industries. Experience in the program's first phase further indicated that the nature of the relationship established between PRO and provider by the case-review paradigm actively impeded PROs' ability to catalyze meaningful, lasting improvements in providers' overall clinical practices and care delivery systems.

In 1992, adopting the HCQIP name and an operational approach based on the quality-improvement paradigm, the program moved into its second phase, to focus on measuring and improving quality of care via a national program. While retaining their responsibility and commitment to protect the trust funds and individual beneficiaries who feel they have received care of substandard quality—via, respectively, payment monitoring/error reduction activities and a program for investigation of complaints received—the PROs became a centerpiece mechanism of HCQIP. The HCQIP no longer examined individual clinical errors to retrospectively sanction individual instances of substandard quality but now analyzed patterns of care and outcomes, seeking opportunities to proactively and systematically narrow the quality chasm by improving overall performance on explicit, evidence-based measures of clinical quality.

During this second phase, the HCQIP expanded beyond its initial inpatient and primary care measures to include additional clinical settings. In 2000, the HCQIP began to increase its emphasis on measurement and improvement in dialysis facilities, increasing alignment of the ESRD Network's improvement priorities and strategies with those of their PRO colleagues. Their authority also statutorily established in the early 1980s (also in Title XVIII of the Social Security Act), the ESRD Network is specifically responsible for the quality of the care dialysis providers deliver to Medicare enrollees. In 2002, based on prior developmental work, the HCQIP launched national initiatives to improve quality of care in nursing home and home health settings, and emphasized the importance of quality improvement responsibilities by changing the official designation of entities formerly known as Peer Review Organizations to Quality Improvement Organizations.[c]

Although all the data needed for detailed, summative analysis of program results in the second phase is not yet available, it is already apparent that HCQIP has since 1992 seen significant but incremental progress in improving care. Even in advance of final data for the entire seventh QIO contract performance period nationwide, some broad, general observations can be made. For example, within a single given acute-care hospital clinical topic (e.g., pneumonia), rates of some indicators of appropriate care delivery have improved dramatically (although others lag substantially). In other settings, such as nursing homes, aggregate differences in improvement achieved to date suggest that the group of providers to whom QIOs provided more intensive assistance ("identified participants") improved more quickly on focal improvement topics than those with whom the QIOs had only minimal contact during the seventh QIO contract performance period.

Based on experience in prior phases, including results available to date from phase two, the HCQIP in 2004 began to transition into its third phase, which will emphasize assisting providers to achieve transformational (as opposed to incremental) improvement, using four primary strategies: performance measurement and reporting, systems adoption and effective use, process redesign, and organizational culture change.

In practical terms, this means demonstrating efficacy while enhancing efficiency by sharpening program focus on intensively assisting groups of identified participant providers to achieve transformational improvement and then spreading that improvement by a variety of means, including activities specifically designed to create environmental forces conducive to quality improvement. It also means that the program will continue to apply quality improvement principles internally, to program elements dedicated both to quality improvement and to specifically protecting beneficiaries and the Trust Funds. This includes developing and applying enhanced methods to quantify contractor proficiency and measure impact of specific intervention strategies and methods.

Achieving and spreading transformational change—and the measurement methods as well as the process designs, systems, and organizational culture characteristics underlying its achievement—among initial and subsequent groups of identified participants and providers at large is a challenging but, the program believes, attainable objective for its third phase. To accomplish it, the HCQIP plans to leverage alignment of its internal components with one another, and with other environmental forces, including governmental and nongovernmental initiatives also working toward a healthcare system that delivers the right care to every person every time.

In discussing its vision, the HCQIP uses "right care" as shorthand to describe care that is simultaneously safe, effective, patient-centered, timely, efficient, and equitable. To put three of these in contextual perspective: safe hospital care does not subject patients to undue risk of needless harm (e.g., medication not given as prescribed, receiving someone else's surgical procedure); effective, patient-centered nursing home care addresses both the person's medical and psychosocial needs (e.g., prevents development of any pressure ulcers and provides a warm, nurturing home).

During the transition into phase three, HCQIP has projects underway to enhance the healthcare industry's ability to apply the four primary intervention strategies and achieve the vision. Detailing even a representative cross-section of the developmental portfolio would be impractical, but illustrative examples include the set of pilot projects currently developing methods for QIOs to use in helping providers change to more patient-centric cultures and in redesigning processes (including integrating systems adoption/use as appropriate) to improve performance in all six key values of right care, including patient-centeredness.

Ultimately, although its mission is to assist providers to improve care specifically for Medicare beneficiaries, the HCQIP cannot achieve the right care for every beneficiary every time without improving healthcare processes on a systematic basis, and all patients interact with the same systems. Thus, by assisting providers to achieve reliably high-quality performance on topics important to Medicare beneficiaries, HCQIP as part of the overall CMS quality structure is helping to bridge the quality chasm as a whole.

Public Reporting

In November 2001, the Secretary of Health and Human Services announced an effort to encourage improvements in the quality of healthcare through accountability and public disclosure. The objectives of this Quality Initiative are both to empower consumers by providing them with information on the quality of care available to them and to stimulate and encourage providers to improve the quality of the healthcare they deliver by allowing them to compare themselves to their peers and enabling them to identify areas in which quality could be improved.

In 2002, the Nursing Home Quality Initiative (NHQI) was launched, with the publication of a list of indicators relating to services provided in nursing homes. In 2003, the Home Health Quality Initiative (HHQI) provided a similar listing for home health agencies, and a set of activities aimed at providing information on the quality of care provided in hospitals was begun, under the rubric of the Hospital Quality Initiative (HQI). All of these initiatives are part of a comprehensive look at the quality of care that includes the Physician Focused Quality Initiative (PFQI) and ESRD quality activities.

The Quality Initiative builds on previous work, including use of existing data sources and measures, and utilizes collaboration with interested parties and a public process that engages all stakeholders to expand the list of measures beyond what could be obtained directly from claims and other routinely reported data. The focus of this process is to choose measures that are evidence-based, scientifically and clinically sound, and transparent and reproducible. In addition, the process addresses data adjustment needs by building inclusion and exclusion criteria into numerators and denominators as well as risk adjustment as appropriate, and strives to minimize provider burden. The goal of these initiatives is the quarterly publication of national information on measures of quality performance for multiple clinical settings. The information is available at www.medicare.gov, the CMS consumer Web site, after formal consumer testing. Information for professional audiences is available at www.cms.hhs.gov.

Working with measurement experts, the National Quality Forum (NQF), and a diverse group of nursing home industry stakeholders, CMS adopted a set of nursing home quality measures built from resident assessment data that nursing homes routinely collect on residents for payment (the Minimum Data Set, or MDS). After validation of the initial measures and a six-state pilot in spring 2002, the national NHQI was launched in November 2002 and posted to the Nursing Home Compare Web site at www.medicare.gov. The initiative is a four-prong effort designed to improve the quality of care in nursing homes through CMS's continuing regulatory and enforcement systems, new and improved consumer information, community-based nursing home quality improvement programs, and ongoing partnerships and collaborative efforts to promote awareness and support. The NHQI quality measure set was updated in January 2004 and consists of fourteen enhanced quality measures derived from the NQF consensus process (see Table 12–1). The CMS

Table 12–1: *Nursing Home Quality Indicators*

Chronic Care Measures
Percent of residents whose need for help with daily activities has increased
Percent of residents who have moderate to severe pain
Percent of residents who were physically restrained
Percent of residents who spent most of their time in bed or in a chair
Percent of residents whose ability to move about in and around their room got worse
Percent of residents with a urinary tract infection
Percent of residents who have become more depressed or anxious
Percent of high risk residents who have pressure sores
Percent of low risk residents who have pressure sores
Percent of low risk residents who lose control of their bowels or bladder
Percent of residents who have/had a catheter inserted and left in their bladder
Post-Acute Care Measures
Percent of short stay residents who had moderate to severe pain
Percent of short stay residents with delirium
Percent of short stay residents with pressure sores

Centers for Medicare & Medicaid Services. Nursing home quality initiative overview. *Available at http://www.cms.hhs.gov/quality/nhqi/Overview.pdf.* Accessed on June 4, 2005.

anticipates further measure refinements around post-acute measures and nursing home staffing.

The HHQI is an effort to improve the quality of care provided by the nation's home health agencies using the same model implemented for NHQI. Working with the Agency for Healthcare Research and Quality (AHRQ) and a diverse group of home health industry stakeholders, a subset of measures from the Outcomes Based Quality Indicators (OBQI) already in use by home health agencies was chosen. These indicators (see Table 12–2), well known to the home health agencies, are risk-adjusted quality measures derived from the Outcomes Assessment Information Set (OASIS), an outcomes-based data collection instrument used by CMS for payment and quality assurance.

In spring 2003, CMS conducted a pilot of public reporting for home health agencies in eight states using this subset of extensively studied and tested measures. The HHQI national release of the home health quality measures on www.medicare.gov as Home Health Compare occurred in November 2003, when CMS posted a set of eleven quality measures for home health agencies. The HHQI measure set will continue to be refined over time, and CMS has engaged the NQF to review and develop consensus for a larger set of home health quality measures.

The CMS is engaged in a number of initiatives for public reporting of hospital performance measures. The HQI aims to refine and standardize hospital performance

Table 12–2: *Home Health Quality Measures: Outcome-based Quality Indicators (OBQI)*

Percentage of patients who get better at walking or moving around. (Improvement in ambulation/locomotion)
Percentage of patients who get better at getting in and out of bed. (Improvement in transferring)
Percentage of patients who get better getting to and from the toilet. (Improvement in toileting)
Percentage of patients who have less pain when moving around. (Improvement in pain interfering with activity)
Percentage of patients who get better at bathing. (Improvement in bathing)
Percentage of patients who get better at taking their medicines correctly (by mouth). (Improvement in management of oral medications)
Percentage of patients who get better at getting dressed. (Improvement in upper body dressing)
Percentage of patients who stay the same or don't get worse at bathing. (Stabilization in bathing)
Percentage of patients who had to be admitted to the hospital. (Acute care hospitalization)
Percentage of patients who need urgent, unplanned medical care. (Any emergent care provided)
Percentage of patients who are confused less often. (Improvement in confusion frequency)

Centers for Medicare & Medicaid Services. Home health compare. *Available at:http://www.medicare.gov/ HHCompare/Home.asp?dest=NAV\Home\DataDetails#TabTop.* Accessed on June 5, 2005.

measures, data collection, and data transmission in order to construct a prioritized, scientifically sound, and standard quality measure set for hospitals. The HQI has required more developmental work than the NHQI or HHQI, for which CMS had federally mandated, well-studied, and validated clinical data sets with an established data collection and transmission infrastructure from which to draw quality measures for public reporting. Because no regulation for submission of hospital quality data currently exists, all of the hospital initiatives are voluntary.

A starter set of ten well-vetted and evidence-based clinical process of care measures for acute myocardial infarction, heart failure, and pneumonia (see Table 12–3) were identified as the initial public reporting clinical performance measure set on hospitals. These measures were all NQF-endorsed and common to the Joint Commission for Accreditation of Healthcare Organizations (JCAHO) core indicator sets and the CMS Scopes of Work for its Quality Improvement Organizations (QIOs). Collection of this starter set was enhanced by a financial incentive in Section 501(b) of the Medicare Prescription Drug, Improvement, and Modernization Act of 2003 (MMA).

Activities are ongoing to enhance the HQI and expand it beyond the initial set of measures. The QIOs provide technical assistance to hospitals in their data collection and submission. In addition, CMS is working with AHRQ to develop a standardized patient perspectives on care survey (H-CAHPS). Over time, an expanded set of measures will be developed and reported.

Similar to the Hospital Quality Initiative, the PFQI has several developmental components that employ multiple approaches to stimulate the adoption of quality strategies and reporting of quality measures for physician services. The PFQI builds on continuous CMS strategies and programs in other healthcare settings in order to assess the quality of care for key chronic illnesses and clinical conditions that affect many Medicare beneficiaries; support clinicians in providing appropriate treatment

Table 12–3: *Hospital Quality Measures: Original 10 Core Starter Set*

- Acute Myocardial Infarction (AMI)
  Aspirin at arrival
  Aspirin prescribed at discharge
  ACE Inhibitor for left ventricular systolic dysfunction
  Beta blocker at arrival
  Beta blocker prescribed at discharge

- Heart Failure (HF)
  Left ventricular function assessment
  ACE inhibitor for left ventricular systolic dysfunction

- Pneumonia (PNE)
  Initial antibiotic received within 4 hours of hospital arrival
  Oygenation assessment
  Pneumococcal vaccination status

Centers for Medicare & Medicaid Services. Hospital Quality Alliance (HQA) Hospital Quality Measures 2004–2007. *Available at: http://www.cms.hhs.gov/quality/hospital/HospitalQualityMeasures.pdf.* Accessed on June 5, 2005.

of the conditions identified; prevent health problems that are avoidable; and further investigate the concept of payment for performance.

The Doctors' Office Quality (DOQ) project is designed to develop and test a comprehensive, integrated approach to measuring and improving the quality of care for chronic diseases and preventive services in the outpatient setting. The CMS worked closely with key stakeholders, including national physician associations, consumer advocacy groups, philanthropic foundations, purchasers, and quality accreditation and quality assessment organizations to develop and test the DOQ measurement set. The DOQ measurement set is expected to have three components: a clinical performance measurement set, a practice system assessment survey, and a patient experience of care survey. The clinical performance measurement topics include coronary artery disease, diabetes mellitus, heart failure, hypertension, osteoarthritis, and preventive care.

Through the Doctors' Office Quality-Information Technology (DOQ-IT) project, CMS is working to support the adoption and effective use of information technology by physicians' offices to improve the quality of care and safety for Medicare beneficiaries. DOQ-IT seeks to accomplish this by promoting greater availability of high quality affordable health information technology and by providing assistance to physician offices in adopting and using such technology through the infrastructure that is already in place with the QIOs.

The ESRD Quality Initiative incorporates quality improvement activities that began with the Balanced Budget Act of 1997 (BBA). The BBA required CMS to develop and implement a method to measure and publicly report the quality of renal dialysis services provided under the Medicare program. To implement this legislation, CMS funded the development of clinical performance measures based on the National Kidney Foundation's Dialysis Outcome Quality Initiative Clinical Practice Guidelines. Sixteen ESRD measures (five for hemodialysis adequacy, three for peritoneal dialysis adequacy, four for anemia management, and four for vascular access) were developed. The CMS continues to collect this data and the findings are used by ESRD Networks and dialysis providers to improve care.

In 1999, CMS funded the development of dialysis-facility specific measures that could be released to the public. The measures that were selected included nine facility characteristics and three quality measures including dialysis adequacy, adequacy of anemia management, and standardized survival rates. Dialysis Facility Compare on www.medicare.gov was launched in January 2001, and data is updated annually for the 3,500 dialysis facilities in the United States. The CMS currently is exploring additional measures for public reporting in this setting.

The CMS and JCAHO have taken a substantial step to expedite public reporting on hospital quality by their release of a technical manual that aligns all common hospital measures used by the two organizations to assess hospital quality. As the HQI progressed, technical differences between the two organizations in the specifications of the ten measures in the starter set became apparent. Hospitals expressed concern that the lack of alignment in the definitions was a significant obstacle to their ability to collect and report data about their quality of care. To address these concerns, CMS and the JCAHO worked to achieve complete alignment of all of their common hospital performance measures and released a common technical manual for national hospital quality measures in September 2004. It is expected that the organizations will continue to work together to assure that alignment will continue into the future.

The CMS has undertaken other activities to approach the goal of moving toward a single comprehensive set of quality measures to be used by all stakeholders. For the DOQ Project, CMS has collaborated with multiple stakeholders to define a set of ambulatory care measures that will have national application and multiple users. The Center also is attempting to ensure that the process for developing new measures and maintaining existing ones is sufficiently fluid and dynamic to respond to evolving science, evidence, and practice as well as to changes in the healthcare environment.

In the future, CMS expects to be working toward a national set of measures that extends beyond the traditional view of clinical measures of diseases and conditions in setting-specific care to a broader and more cross-cutting view that creates an environment of safety, quality, and accountability to patients. These types of measures are expected to focus on coordination of care, self-management, medication management, and systems of care delivery (both at the system level and the point of care). They would utilize additional sources of data that extend beyond retrospective chart abstraction and administrative data, such as information technology and surveys. Additionally, CMS will be working on how to best measure quality in rural settings with special emphasis on public reporting of small numbers of cases. The Center will also continue to evaluate how to make quality information most accessible and usable to the consumer of healthcare, including the impact of presentation and language, understandability of different types of measures, framing of measures (e.g., with a positive or negative tone), and use of composite measures.

Healthcare Information Technology (HIT)

Over the past couple of years, CMS has developed an explicit approach to the promotion of improvements in healthcare quality through the promotion of adoption and effective use of healthcare information technology (HIT). There are two premises underlying this approach: that substantial improvement in quality, as envisioned by the Institute of Medicine's *Crossing the Quality Chasm* report with its six goals (safety, timeliness, effectiveness, efficiency, patient-centeredness, and equity) is not possible without provider adoption and use of HIT; and that simply promoting HIT adoption is not sufficient to improve quality in this way—systems that are adopted must have the requisite functionality, and they must be embedded in redesigned care processes.

The evidence for the first premise is growing. In the hospital setting, there are several studies that indicate that computerized physician order entry (CPOE) and medication delivery systems reduce medication errors. In the ambulatory setting, there are a number of studies that demonstrated that e-prescribing, e-lab test ordering and results management, and e-registries have a positive impact on safety, efficiency, and effectiveness. And there are two large studies that project a substantial improvement in quality and cost on the basis of adoption of interoperable electronic health records (EHRs).

Nationally, there is movement toward the setting of explicit goals for HIT adoption and use. The MMA envisions widespread adoption of e-prescribing by 2009. In spring 2004, the US President called for action to ensure that most Americans have electronic medical records within ten years, and he created an Office of the National Coordinator for Health Information Technology (ONCHIT) to coordinate efforts to achieve that goal. In response to its mandate, ONCHIT issued a strategic framework in summer 2004 that called for progress in four areas: EHR adoption; interconnecting clinicians (electronic data exchange); personalizing care (personal health records and information to support choice of provider and treatment); and population health (data availability to support quality measurement, public health, and research). To contribute to the adoption of these goals, CMS identified and began deployment of six strategies: promoting data standards and standardized data outputs; reducing regulatory barriers to HIT adoption; promoting the availability of high quality, affordable HIT systems; providing assistance to clinicians to support HIT adoption and effective use; providing financial incentives; and providing an infrastructure for data exchange.

Data standards include vocabularies and messaging rules that enable data to be exchanged among providers. Government can play an important role in promoting data standards, which can enable HIT systems vendors to reduce development costs, and for clinicians purchasing such systems to more easily interface new and old systems and more easily convert from one system to another. The federal government has, through the Consolidated Health Informatics (CHI) initiative, developed recommendations for data standards in a number of areas. The CMS is requiring its contractors, where appropriate, to use such standards.

The government can also create specifications for standardized outputs from HIT systems. The CMS has worked with the American Medical Association to develop a set of physician office-based clinical quality measures. These measures are specified such that they can be coded into HIT systems. Similarly, CMS is exploring adopting requirements for a standardized data set that would be used in information exchange among clinicians and that would be the core clinical information in a personal health record (PHR).

Current law and regulations prohibit hospitals and health plans from offering hardware or software to independent physicians participating in their networks or delivery systems. The CMS is exploring language in a proposed rule that will reduce such barriers as they pertain to e-prescribing.

Although there are dozens of EHRs and related systems available on the market, there are a much smaller number that have functionality to enable clinicians to substantially improve clinical quality, and these systems have often been prohibitively expensive to many physician offices. The CMS has, in concert with other federal agencies and private sector organizations, sought to stimulate the market to offer high quality, affordable systems.

One way to accomplish this is to promote information on the functionality of systems. The CMS has participated in the development of three sets of recommendations regarding functionality—those of the Ambulatory Patient Safety Task Force; those produced in 2003 by the Institute of Medicine; and the standards adopted by HL7. These are being used by a private sector effort to develop a systems certification program.

Another initiative in this regard is the VistA–Office EHR project. The CMS is funding a private developer to produce a version of the Veterans Health Administration's EHR that meets the needs of small- to medium-sized physician offices. The resulting system—which is being developed with input from other federal agencies such as AHRQ, the IHS, and HRSA—will be in the public domain and is expected to be picked up by private developers who will offer support services.

Medicare's QIOs are contracted in each state to offer assistance to providers in measuring and improving quality. In 2003, the California QIO (Lumetra) was contracted to lead the DOQ-IT project, the purpose of which is to develop a methodology that QIOs can use in providing assistance to physicians in three respects.

1. Adoption of HIT—making the decision to purchase a system, and selecting among vendors.

2. Implementation—making the necessary initial process changes to gain the efficiencies of a system and to use it to measure clinical quality.

3. Care management—making the process changes needed to better manage patients with chronic disease and to promote their self-management.

The DOQ-IT methodology is being piloted nationally beginning in November 2004 and is expected to be available for implementation in all states in the QIO Eighth SOW, in August 2005.

Other efforts to facilitate and encourage the use of improved information systems to improve the quality of healthcare are being developed and implemented throughout the government. As described in a separate section, CMS is using its waiver authority to conduct an array of demonstrations that seek to improve quality by aligning payment incentives with quality improvement initiatives, several of them directly or indirectly involving the use of HIT. The CMS also is participating in meetings of a national alliance of private sector purchasers and payers that is exploring coordinating financial incentives for HIT adoption and use.

ONCHIT is developing and implementing a strategy by which the federal government will promote information exchange among clinicians and individuals. This strategy will rely on local information exchange authorities that are linked by an infrastructure that allows for exchange among them.

CMS's QIO program has a national data warehouse that has the authority to receive data from providers on clinical quality measures. The warehouse has data from virtually all hospitals eligible for payment under Section 501(b) of MMA. The data are not limited to Medicare beneficiaries, as the QIOs have been designated as oversight entities under HIPAA. In 2005, the warehouse will be able to receive clinical quality measurement data from physician offices. The QIOs are working with EHR vendors to promote their ability to produce such measures electronically.

Incentives to Promote Quality under Medicare

All of the activities discussed thus far have the effect of providing incentives to improve the quality of care. The development of quality measures focuses attention on the factors that are being measured, and in itself can encourage improvement in those factors, as well as quality overall. The collection of data on quality measures can further enhance quality improvement, by putting in place a process by which, in producing the required information, providers must become more aware of their performance; in addition, the availability of data allows for analyses—both by individual providers and by payers or other entities—that can clarify the relationship between the measures being collected and the performance of the healthcare system.

The dissemination of information on quality performance can lead to improved quality in two ways. It gives purchasers—including patients (and those who help them make healthcare decisions) and third-party payers—the ability to make better choices as to which types of health care to purchase; which features to look for in that healthcare; which providers to buy it from. It also gives providers themselves a strong incentive to improve aspects in which they are deficient (at least in a relative sense)—no one likes to find their name at the bottom of a list that says "quality" at the top—as well as making data available that can help them figure out how to improve their own performance.

In addition to collecting and disseminating information on quality for various types of providers, CMS is designing, developing, implementing, and conducting an array of projects that provide financial incentives intended to encourage improvements in the quality of the healthcare available to Medicare beneficiaries. These projects involve a variety of organizations that provide or coordinate healthcare, and they use a wide range of incentive structures to encourage quality improvement. Many of these projects are conducted under Medicare's demonstration authority, which allows CMS to conduct and sponsor innovative projects to test and measure the effect of potential program changes; these demonstrations study the likely impact of new methods of service delivery, coverage of new types of service, and new payment approaches on beneficiaries, providers, health plans, states, and the Medicare Trust Funds.

In July 2003, CMS unveiled the Hospital Quality Incentive demonstration. This three-year project involves some 280 subscribers to the Premier Perspective™ system that are voluntarily participating in an experiment to explore the use of quality measures to reward hospitals based on the quality of care they provide to their patients.[d] The project is tracking hospitals' performance in five clinical areas: acute myocardial infarction (AMI), heart failure, community-acquired pneumonia, coronary artery bypass graft (CABG), and hip and knee replacement. Some thirty-four measures are used across the five clinical areas to determine aggregate quality scores for each participating hospital in each area.[e]

Based on these scores, hospitals in the top decile in each clinical area are to receive a 2 percent bonus to their Medicare payments for discharges in the diagnosis-related groups (DRGs) that correspond to the clinical area; the hospitals in the next decile are to receive a 1 percent bonus to their DRG payments.[f] In addition to the potential for rewards and penalties, individual hospitals' performance on each of the thirty-four measures will be posted on the www.cms.hhs.gov Web site.

In November 2004, the Physician Group Practice demonstration was announced. This demonstration, mandated by Section 412 of the Benefits Improvement and Protection Act of 2000 (BIPA), is intended to encourage improved coordination of Medicare services, reward physicians for improving health outcomes, and promote efficiency through investment in administrative structure and process. The participants in this project are eleven large, multispecialty group practices (200 or more physicians) around the country; it provides a unique reimbursement mechanism through which providers are rewarded for coordinating and managing the overall healthcare needs of a non-enrolled, fee-for-service patient population.

Under this three-year demonstration, each participating physician group will be paid on a fee-for-service basis and can earn a bonus from savings derived from improvements in patient management. Annual performance targets will be established for each group based on average total Medicare base-year expenditures for beneficiaries assigned to the group, adjusted for health status and local area expenditure growth. The bonus amount is based on the difference between the target amount for each year and actual Medicare expenditures for the assigned patients in that year. The Medicare program retains any savings up to 2 percent of the target amount, and 20 percent of any additional savings. The remaining 80 percent of any additional savings will be available for the bonus, and distributed on the basis of the amount of savings and improvements in process and outcome measures based on data collected from the group. In the first year, for instance, 70 percent of the bonus amount available to the practice will be distributed based on the amount of savings, and 30 percent on the basis of the quality measures. By the third year, 30 percent of the bonus payment will be based on savings and 70 percent on quality.

Section 649 of the MMA requires the Secretary of Health and Human Services to conduct a three-year Medicare Care Management Performance demonstration program in which physicians will be paid to adopt and use HIT and evidence-based outcome measures to promote continuity of care, stabilize medical conditions, prevent or minimize acute exacerbations of chronic conditions, and reduce adverse health outcomes. This project was still in the design phase as of November 2004. The statute limits the program to four sites that meet specified eligibility criteria. Payment can vary based on performance, but total payments must be budget-neutral. QIOs could help enroll physicians, evaluate their performance, and provide technical assistance. The Secretary is required to submit a Report to Congress with appropriate recommendations no later than one year after projects conclude.

Another project mandated in the MMA is the Medicare Health Care Quality Demonstration programs described in Section 646 of the legislation. This provision mandates a five-year demonstration program under which projects can be approved that examine health delivery factors that encourage delivery of improved quality in patient care, including:

- Incentives to improve healthcare safety, quality, or efficiency
- Use of best practice guidelines
- Examination of variations in utilization and outcomes measurement and research
- Shared decision making between providers and patients
- Culturally and ethnically sensitive healthcare delivery

These projects can involve the use of alternative payment systems for items and services provided to beneficiaries, and they can involve modifications to the traditional Medicare benefit package. The provision includes a budget-neutrality requirement over the five-year duration of the program.

Under this provision, the National Institutes of Health (NIH) can be directed to evaluate current medical technologies and improve the foundation for evidence-based practice; the Agency for Healthcare Research and Quality (AHRQ) can be directed to use this program as a laboratory for the study of quality improvement strategies; and CMS can be directed to provide the data necessary to analyze and evaluate the projects conducted under this program (subject to the applicable provisions of the Health Insurance Portability and Accountability Act of 1996). In addition to projects that tie payment to the achievement of performance as measured by explicit quality indicators, CMS is conducting several projects that aim to improving the quality of care by directly purchasing services that are thought to lead to improved coordination and quality of care, as follows:

- The Medicare Coordinated Care demonstration (mandated by Section 4016 of the BBA) is designed to test whether care coordination programs applied in the Medicare fee-for-service context can reduce hospitalizations, improve health status and other outcomes, and reduce the healthcare costs of chronically ill Medicare beneficiaries. This project involves fifteen sites and approximately 17,000 beneficiaries.
- A demonstration to provide Disease Management for Severely Chronically Ill Medicare Beneficiaries (Mandated by Section 121 of BIPA) is intended to test whether applying disease management and prescription drug coverage in a

fee-for-service context for beneficiaries with advanced-stage illnesses such as congestive heart failure, diabetes, or heart disease can improve health outcomes and reduce costs. Organizations participating in this demonstration are at risk for any increase in overall Medicare spending for beneficiaries enrolled in the project. This demonstration is being conducted at three sites and can enroll up to 30,000 beneficiaries.

- A Care Management for High-Cost Beneficiaries demonstration will focus specifically on high-cost Medicare beneficiaries in a fee-for-service context. This project will focus on provider-centered coordination of care for these beneficiaries, who are the most in need of well-coordinated care. Approximately four to six organizations will be selected to participate in this demonstration.

Although it is not a demonstration project, the Medicare Health Support Program, mandated in Section 721 of the MMA, will be the largest of CMS's initiatives in the area of disease management. Unlike the demonstrations described here, this pilot project will require that participating organizations take responsibility for an entire population with the specified conditions (congestive heart failure, complex diabetes, and chronic obstructive pulmonary disease). About ten sites will be selected in the first phase of the program, each of which will serve 15,000 to 30,000 beneficiaries in their geographic area. These organizations will be at risk for their disease management fee, based on their success in improving the coordination of care and reducing Medicare spending for their assigned populations.

Conclusion

The Medicare program is responsible for ensuring access to appropriate, high-quality healthcare for some 41 million people—almost one-seventh of the United States population. Moreover, as the country's largest payer for healthcare, Medicare is in a position to lead and influence the rest of the healthcare sector. For these reasons, it is incumbent on CMS, which runs the Medicare program, to address the fact that the nation's health system, while by far the most expensive in the world, does not produce the kind of care that Americans believe they have a right to demand.

The initiatives described in this chapter are all aimed at addressing this problem. The collection and dissemination of information through the Quality Initiative will focus the attention of patients and providers on the quality of care; enable patients to understand what constitutes good care and to demand that they get it; and help providers to identify areas in which they can improve. Technical assistance available to providers through the Quality Improvement Program will provide help for them to accomplish that improvement and apply it to increasing the efficiency and effectiveness of the care they provide. The provision of incentives will encourage providers to improve care and help counteract the adverse incentives in the current healthcare system.

With these initiatives, CMS is attempting not only to transform the Medicare program, but also to lead the way toward a healthcare system that will be better able to identify, analyze, and implement potential improvements in the way healthcare is provided.

Case Study

The Centers for Medicare & Medicaid Services (CMS) operate the Medicare program, which covers 42 million elderly and disabled Americans, as well as carrying out the federal government's role in the operation of the Medicaid program, which covers 43 million poor and medically indigent people, and State Children's Health Insurance programs, which covers 4 million children. These programs paid out a total of almost $470 billion in benefit payments in fiscal year 2004. The size and importance of these programs, the vulnerability of the populations they cover, and the projected increases in their payments, make it imperative that they find ways to improve both the quality of care and the efficiency with which it is provided. To accomplish these goals, the Medicare and Medicaid programs have implemented an array of Disease Management initiatives to improve the coordination of care provided to their chronically ill populations. The objective is to provide these populations with more appropriate care and to eliminate unnecessary and duplicative care that they might otherwise receive.

One such initiative is the Medicare Health Support Program, implemented as a pilot in 2005. Under this program, which was enacted in the Medicare Modernization Act of 2003, participating organizations will be responsible for improving the coordination, appropriateness, quality, and cost of care provided to the entire Medicare population with congestive heart failure or complex diabetes in a specified geographic area. This will encourage participating organizations to develop innovative approaches to disease management, case management, or care coordination for the entire population for which they are responsible, perhaps including different approaches for different segments of their population. Participating organizations are at risk for their performance. From this pilot, Medicare hopes to learn more about how to implement these programs, as well as which approaches might be successful in different circumstances and for different subgroups. Subject to the findings from the evaluation of the pilot, the Secretary of Health and Human Services can choose to expand the program after two years. More information on this program can be found at www.cms.hhs.gov/medicarereform/ccip.

Study/Discussion Questions

1. How has the government's approach to quality for the Medicare program evolved from the 1960s to today?
2. What are the stakeholder and environmental challenges government faces in seeking to implement a robust quality measurement and improvement system for Medicare?

3. What role does the government play with regard to encouraging and implementing innovation in quality improvement? Why?

Suggested Readings/Web Sites

Epstein AM, Lee TH, Hamel MB. Paying physicians for high-quality care. *NEJM.* 2004; 350(4):406–10.

Hsia DC. Medicare quality improvement. *JAMA.* 2003; 289(3):354–56.

Institute of Medicine, Board on Health Care Services. *The Future of Public Health.* Washington, DC: National Academies Press; 1988.

Institute of Medicine, Committee on the Quality of Health Care in America, *Crossing the Quality Chasm: A New Health System for the 21st Century.* Washington, DC: National Academies Press; 2001.

Jencks S. The right care. *NEJM.* 2003; 348(22):2251–52.

Jencks SF, Huff, ED, Cuerdon T. Change in the quality of care delivered to Medicare beneficiaries, 1998–1999 to 2000–2001. *JAMA.* 2003; 289(3):305–12.

Kerr EA, McGlynn EA, Adams J, Keesey J, Asch SM. Profiling the quality of care in twelve communities: Results from the CQI study. *Health Aff.* 2004; 23(3):247–56.

McGlynn EA, Asch SM, Keesey J, Hicks J, DeCristofaro A, Kerr EA. The quality of health care delivered to adults in the United States. *NEJM.* 2003; 348(26):2635–45.

Schoenbaum SC, Audet AJ, Davis K. Obtaining greater value from health care: the roles of the US government. *Health Aff.* 2003; 22(6):183–90.

Steinberg EP. Improving the quality of care—can we practice what we preach? *NEJM.* 2003;348(26):2681–83.

References

1. Jencks SF, Huff ED, Cuerdon T. Change in the quality of care delivered to Medicare beneficiaries, 1998–1999 to 2000–2001. *J Am Med Assoc.* 2003; 289(3):305–312.

Notes

a. The Peer Review Improvement Act is Title I, Subtitle C, of the Tax Equity and Fiscal Responsibility Act of 1982 (Public Law 97-248). Subsequent legislation has elaborated on the mandates of the program and expanded the responsibilities of these organizations (now the QIOs) to a fuller array of healthcare delivery settings.

b. Within parameters established by statute, the Secretary of Health and Human Services can by regulation establish the specific contract regions. There currently are fifty-three contract regions: one for each US state, the District of Columbia, US Virgin Islands, and Puerto Rico. Guam, American Samoa, and the Northern Marianas Islands are included in the contractual jurisdiction of the contract for Hawaii.

c. Although called on to function as quality improvement organizations, ESRD Networks retain their original name to facilitate differentiation of the HCQIP program contractors/components. Among the several differences in program structure, the ESRD Networks have a slightly different relationship with the providers with whom they work and a name change was not warranted.

d. Premier, Inc. is a group purchasing organization of about 1,500 hospitals. About 500 of those facilities currently track and support data on indicators of the quality and efficiency of care through the Premier Perspective™ system.

e. Quality indicators include process measures, such as prescription of aspirin for AMI and CABG patients and timely administration of antibiotics for pneumonia patients, as well as outcome measures, such as in-hospital mortality rate for AMI and CABG patients and post-operative hemorrhage or hematoma for CABG and hip and knee replacement patients.

f. In the third year of the project, there is the prospect of reductions in payments for hospitals with scores below minimum thresholds. Thee thresholds will be developed based on the distribution of quality scores during the first year of the project. If all hospitals improve sufficiently, they can avoid the potential reduction in payments.

Looking Toward the Future of Quality Improvement

Chapter 13

Role of Information Technology in Measuring and Improving Quality

Thomas N. Ricciardi
Kevin Tabb

EXECUTIVE SUMMARY

The late 1990s brought an explosive change in society with the mass dissemination of information via the Internet and advanced applications for personal computers. Healthcare has begun to take advantage of these advances in numerous ways, including the improvement of quality. This chapter examines issues around the evolving role of information technology (IT), including its potential to restructure the relationships between the major stakeholders in the healthcare industry, as well as barriers to its use. We review some of the key quality domains including both financial and clinical benefits of IT. Focusing on the needed infrastructure to support the adoption of electronic health records and quality measurement systems in the physician office, we discuss architecture for successful IT implementations. The chapter also addresses healthcare IT standards, interoperability, and privacy concerns. The Office of the National Coordinator for Health Information Technology has issued a new framework to spur the "Decade of Health Information Technology," which will result in increased momentum to effectively implement and use IT. These efforts also need to take human factors, organizational issues in healthcare, and clinical workflow engineering very seriously; the "technology problem" is usually the easiest component of any quality improvement effort. Finally, we demonstrate the potential power of IT for clinical management of quality care through a brief case study.

LEARNING OBJECTIVES

1. To understand the evolving role of information technology in healthcare.
2. To understand the main areas of academic inquiry, policy organizations,

standards bodies, and national policy efforts targeted to the dissemination of information technology in healthcare.

3. To be able to describe recent advances in the use of technology to collect and aggregate information in order to measure healthcare quality.

4. To nnderstand at a high level the needed components and architecture to support quality improvement in the physician office.

5. To list the challenges to implementing IT solutions in practice, including some unintended consequences of technology.

KEYWORDS

Information Technology

Privacy

Quality Measurement

Data Warehousing

Population Health

Financial Incentives

National Health Information Network

Introduction

In recent years, more attention has been given in the healthcare sector to the consequences of practicing medicine in a paper-based world. In *Crossing the Quality Chasm,* the Institute of Medicine reports that ". . . IT must play a central role in the redesign of the healthcare system if substantial improvement in healthcare quality is to be achieved in the coming decade."[1] It is becoming increasingly evident to those who seek care under the current system that medicine is far behind almost any industry in the investment in IT. Patients are astounded when confronted with the lack of communication and automation they see when seeking care, in contrast to what they have come to expect—for example, when checking into an airline flight or even ordering fast food. In fact, medicine spends only a small number of dollars per employee on IT, compared to all other industries; some of the most technologically advanced sectors such as financial and securities industries exceed healthcare IT spending by an order of magnitude. Physicians in general do not have full and complete access to patient information during the decision-making process. Lost or unavailable charts, lack of access to images and test results, incomplete histories, allergy lists, and so on are commonplace at the point of care whether it be the physician office, emergency department, inpatient setting, or any other care setting in medicine.

Electronic Health Records and Medical Informatics: Some Definitions

Electronic health records (EHR)—also called electronic medical records (EMR) or computerized patient records (CPR)—are the equivalent of the longitudinal chart record for a patient. Office-based physicians have begun to adopt EHR as a part of their overall strategy to compete, in part by having better benchmark information about quality and outcomes in their own practices.[2] Electronic health records systems are a new source of valuable real-world intelligence for the entire healthcare industry because they collect and maintain clinical information captured in the physician practice during the care delivery process—including patterns of medication use, safety, treatment, and efficacy. The Institute of Medicine recently issued a report stating the use of electronic health records is critical to data collection and population analysis of the quality, safety, and efficiency in healthcare delivery.[3]

Still, far fewer than 20 percent of physician offices in the United States use EHR to collect and manage clinical information about their patients. This, in spite of the demonstrated benefits of EHR for better care quality by decision support; error and adverse events prevention; interaction checking; and disease management and preventive care reminders. A combination of issues surround healthcare economics, including reimbursement, work flow, and who "foots the bill" versus who actually benefits clinically and economically from the adoption of technology. Lack of availability of user-friendly systems that are easy to incorporate into the clinical workflow, as well as a lack of a cultural fit between computing systems and the practice of medicine, have all conspired against the widespread adoption of information technology (IT) in medicine. With the exception of a few forward-looking physicians and healthcare systems that have invested in IT, clinicians have largely continued to practice medicine based on whatever incomplete information is available from paper charts, the patient, or caregivers and relatives.

Medical informatics is the application of computer technology to the practice of medicine[4] The study and practical application of medical informatics in the clinical domain is important because medicine has been slow to adopt the use of computer technology for the purpose of documenting, storing, and communicating clinical information about patients. Traditionally, the main thought leaders in medical informatics have been academicians, who have often sketched the vision of what computers can do for medicine and created many applications in pilot form or demonstration mode to try to spur their incorporation into practice. The related field of bio-informatics is the application of computers to the collection, management, and analysis of genomic, proteinomic, and other bio-marker data derived primarily from biomedical research. Increasingly, clinical- and bio-informatics are becoming more closely intertwined as advanced molecular markers for disease become available in the diagnosis, treatment, and prevention of disease. This will lead to the increasingly important endeavor of "personalized medicine," which is an attempt to tailor diagnosis, treatment, and prevention to the specific individual patient based on his or her phenotype and genetic makeup. But perhaps even more important from both a cost and quality standpoint, medical informatics and healthcare IT will enable population-based approaches to quality and outcomes assessment, disease management, preventive care, and medical error reduction.

This chapter will bring together current knowledge on healthcare IT and medical informatics as applied to the improvement and measurement of clinical quality. Key quality domains—including financial and clinical benefits of IT—will be reviewed. High-level architecture for IT implementation is needed to support quality improvement in the physician office. This discussion will include an overview of healthcare IT standards, interoperability, and privacy concerns. These stem from important national efforts to encourage technology adoption in the practice of medicine. Finally, we will demonstrate the potential power of IT for clinical management of quality care through a brief case study.

Technology, Quality Improvement, and the Business Case

Historically, investment in information technology to improved quality of care has been grounded in fervent arguments based on compassion and intuition. Little data or clear methods for measurement of the impact of IT on quality and quality improvement existed to bolster these arguments. This has started to change over time as a significant rise in health costs has forced healthcare executives to focus on management effectiveness and return on investment (ROI). The barriers to initial and ongoing cost of investing in IT are substantial, particularly in the financially challenged environment that healthcare organizations are facing. As healthcare IT needs and solutions have evolved into much more complex initiatives, the cost of implementing IT projects has skyrocketed. It is reported that healthcare information technology (HCIT) in the United States alone is estimated at $41 billion and is growing at a compound annual rate of 7 percent.[5] Although this only represents a tiny percentage of the total healthcare spent in the United States, this percentage is growing rapidly.

The implementation of any single IT project in the healthcare setting can be prohibitively expensive. Kaiser Permanente is currently in the midst of implementing a major IT project—implementation of systemwide electronic health records—that they expect will have permanent effects on their ability to measure and improve quality of care. They estimate that they will spend over $3.2 billion on IT in this initiative over the next ten years. Clearly, huge expenditures like these will have to be justified by more than improved quality for quality's sake alone.

The vast majority of patients, clinicians, and policy makers all seem to intuitively agree that pursuing improved health quality is both important and worthwhile. However, defining what "worthwhile" means, and proving this quantitatively from a business perspective has proved more challenging. Not only has financial proof been difficult to achieve, but frequently the clinicians responsible for implementing quality improvement are not well trained or qualified to justify quality initiatives on financial grounds. Clearly, quality improvement investment will need to be justified by a quantifiable and parallel ROI. Additionally, it is only in the last few years that a small number of tools measuring and standardizing the cost of quality have been introduced.[6] A large number of industry vendors, government agencies, and nonprofits have all been involved in developing the business case for quality, recognizing that as the high cost of quality programs and their IT components are increasingly scrutinized, the rate of adoption of these programs is directly affected by the financial case presented.

Much of the "case for quality" is based on the development of evidence-based guidelines in medicine, published research on efficaciousness of therapy, and the direct and indirect costs of morbidity and mortality. One of the best ways to clearly understand costs and benefits is to look at studies of specific diseases and conditions, and to attempt to link the clinical outcomes to financial outcomes. A recent paper by Fetterolf and West[7] describes one method by which this might occur. They suggest the use of medical literature to estimate the economic impact of potential quality improvement initiatives, and then suggest combining the analysis with the organizations own internal data to figure potential financial benefit. This method presents a framework for an organization to estimate ROI on any given quality initiative.

One of the barriers that has faced healthcare organizations attempting to quantify financial return on quality investments has been the lack of standards in measuring quality. Organizations such as the nonprofit National Committee for Quality Assurance (NCQA), as well as a myriad of governmental agencies have made attempts at defining standardized measures. One example of these is the relatively widely adopted HEDIS measures. These are a standard set of clinical measures that allow employers and others to "begin to quantify, in meaningful financial terms, the effects of choosing higher quality health plans."[8] Standard measures for accepted treatment of major common diseases have been developed, and providers are measured on the percent of their patient population who meet the standard criteria.

One of the problems with existing standardized measurement programs like HEDIS is that the measurement either has to be manual—requiring a search through paper-based records—or the solution has been tailored to the types of quality measurements that are already automated by large numbers of providers: namely financial measures. Using insurance information (i.e., claims data sets in an outpatient setting) means that healthcare organizations can rapidly search for the existence or absence of multiple quality measures. The drawback to measuring quality in this way is that there is a necessary attempt to use financial information as a proxy for the deeper clinical information that should be measured. These methods are then severely limited in their ability to appropriately measure real clinical effect. Automated clinical systems such as electronic health records and aggregate databases of clinical information allow for a more direct and relevant measure of quality.

Recently, there have been multiple initiatives by both the public and private sectors to tie financial incentives to adopting technology and improving quality in the healthcare setting. These so-called "pay for performance" initiatives are still in their infancy, but major employers have already decided that until providers receive direct financial compensation for the adoption of technology and improvement of quality in the provider setting, little will change. One example of these types of programs is the Bridges to Excellence program.[9] Under this program, a group of employers, physicians, health plans, and patients have come together to create programs that will realign incentives around higher quality. Programs like this appear to be the wave of the future, clear financial rewards to those that adopt technology, standardize measurement of quality, and show an improvement in care over time.

Another unique way to fund adoption of technology in quality improvement has been to search for third party commercially sponsored research opportunities. Commercial vendors such as pharmaceutical companies, medical device manufacturers, and even health plans have frequently purchased de-identified electronic data sets to study population statistics and health outcomes in a real-world setting. One such venture is the GE Healthcare Medical Quality Improvement Consortium (MQIC), which aggregates de-identified HIPAA compliant data from sites using EHR systems. The data is then scrubbed, normalized, and used for clinical quality improvement as well as in a variety of outcomes research projects. A portion of any revenue received from commercial partners is then distributed back to the providers contributing the data. Partnerships such as these can be used to subsidize the costs of initial implementation and ongoing support of IT systems needed to gather and manage information for clinical performance measurement and outcomes research.

In summary, the use of IT in making the quality case is expensive. The business case for implementing systems needs to be clear. The case can be made through a combination of quantitative proof of reduction in cost and clear financial incentives to install and maintain IT systems responsible for improvement of care. In the absence of these things it is likely that adoption rates will remain low.

Healthcare IT Infrastructure and the Physician Office

Primary care providers (PCPs), especially office-based physicians, are at the forefront of the need to deploy information technology to improve healthcare quality. As the foundation of patient care, a complete longitudinal record for each individual should reside with the PCP in stewardship with the patient: The record should show the patient's histories and risk factors, preventive care and chronic disease management interventions, and summaries of acute care episodes and care plans. In today's paper based health record-keeping system, that longitudinal record simply does not exist. Even where EHR systems have taken hold, there are silos of information scattered across inpatient and outpatient locations including specialty care centers, due to a lack of communication and interoperability among IT systems. In the future a push toward standards-based integration of healthcare IT systems using messaging protocols, common clinical vocabulary and coding systems, well-defined patient data model, and clinical document formats, will all help to break down silos and make it easier to pull together key patient information for the full longitudinal record.

Patient care information systems such as EHR and computerized physician order entry (CPOE) systems—when coupled with the appropriate re-engineering of organizational behavior in healthcare—have the potential to dramatically improve the quality of care delivery.[10] It has been shown that computerized reminders improve compliance with care guidelines both in the ambulatory[11] and inpatient[12] settings. These systems can help overcome the limits of simple human cognition, enabling the assessment and action on much more information than even the exceptional clinician can manage at a given time. For example, no fewer than twenty-two items in five categories comprise a recent "simplified" evidence-based approach to cardiovascular risk reduction.[13] The enormous task of summarizing 140 articles of literature to derive this set of guidelines illustrates the sheer volume of knowledge that could be applied to patient care; information systems providing actionable decision support for treatment guidelines are key to managing knowledge in the outpatient setting.

What are the main components of the infrastructure for longitudinal EHR in the physician office? Most physician offices that have implemented EHR have their own standalone, firewalled installations on their private local area networks. There are possibly hundreds of different EHR systems designed for the ambulatory environment; the market-leading products include Centricity® Physician Office (GE Healthcare, Waukesha, Wis.); EpiCare Ambulatory (Epic Systems, Madison Wis.), NextGen EMR (NextGen Healthcare Information Systems, Horsham, Pa.); and Healthmatics (A4 Health Systems, Cary, N.C.). The EMR database constitutes a local collection point not only for physician-entered information at the primary point of care, but also for many feeder systems across a multi-site clinical environment (see Figure 13–1). Electronic health records simplify the complex processes required for collecting and managing patient information by storing clinical information arising from laboratory results, clinical dictation, departmental data, images, text, monitoring results, and other HL7-formatted clinical information.

Electronic records assist the provider at the point of care during the individual patient encounter by making the record easily accessible, displaying clinical data in useful ways, supporting clinical documentation and communication, and providing clinical decision support.[14] Cost and implementation barriers have limited the widespread adoption of standalone EHR in the physician office, causing a mismatch between the admirable clinical value and the more pragmatic financial justification for technology. One possible solution to reduce the tremendous financial burden is the renewed interest in application service provider (ASP) models for EHR. In the ASP model, a trusted centralized service provider offers complete hosting and man-

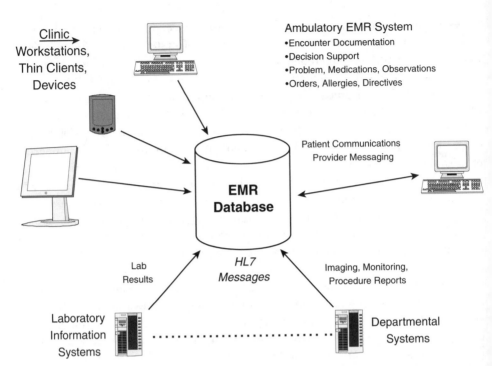

Figure 13–1 *Ambulatory EMR Architecture. Central to the system is a secure database of patient records. A variety of input devices at the point of care assist the provider to collect data on the patient encounter. HL7-standard messaging interfaces allow the integration of patient-specific information from external sources such as laboratories and imaging systems. A secure, encrypted external messaging system is key to provider-to-provider communications and patient messaging with access to the chart that involves consumers in their own care.*

Centricity® Physician Office (GE Healthcare, Waukesha, Wis.).

agement of the EHR infrastructure, effectively leasing access to the physician office by subscription thereby reducing costs, achieving an economy of scale, and pooling resources among many physician offices in a region.

Quality Measurement Enabled by IT in the Physician Office

The EMR and its underlying database are optimized for data collection and management of the individual patient encounter. However clinical quality improvement, practice benchmarking, and outcomes research also require fast retrieval of aggregated

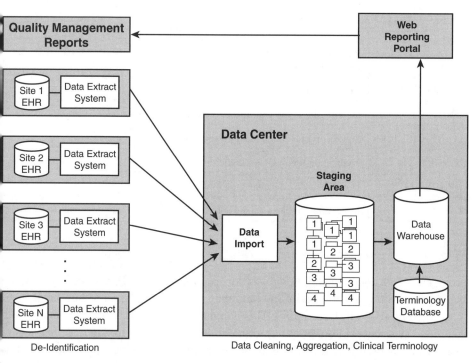

Figure 13–2 *Quality Reporting Infrastructure. After importing data into the warehouse, a process of data staging helps clean, aggregate, and structure information prior to loading it into the reporting database. EMR data requires inspection and conditioning in order to render it useful for population reporting and analysis.*

data about populations of patients. Data warehousing technology supports the queries and reports necessary for multi-site, population-based quality improvement and outcomes measurement. The data warehouse is a physically separate data store derived from the EMR and is used exclusively for reporting, analysis, and measurement. A data warehouse can aggregate EMR data from multiple locations via a secure, encrypted uplink that operates over the Internet (see Figure 13–2). Data is de-identified, extracted, transported, aggregated, and loaded into a hosted data warehouse, while preserving its location of origin.

There are some significant challenges to building an effective multi-site clinical quality reporting infrastructure. Success depends on well-understood data access and security policies, effective patient de-identification or generation of so-called "limited" data sets according to the 1996 Health Insurance Portability and Accountability Act, a financial model for sustainability of the costs of running the infrastructure, and perhaps most important, a complete, accurate, and well-coded patient chart provided by the physician office. Data entry is not always strictly controlled in the EMR, so as not to interfere with rapid documentation of the encounter. First,

Table 13–1 *Healthcare IT Standards*

HL7	Messaging standards Patient record architecture EHR standardization
SNOMED	Clinical reference terminology
UMLS	Metathesaurus integrating many vocabulary sources
LOINC, CPT, ICD9	Laboratory, procedure, and diagnosis codes
RxNORM	Medication terminology standards
DICOM	Digital Imaging documentation and communications
IHE	Integration profiles utilizing many standards applied in practical use cases

providers might enter mistaken values (for example "5 feet 10 inches" for systolic blood pressure) or additional information that is not part of the measurement itself (e.g., "120 mmHg left, large cuff"). This can make it difficult to report accurate and complete aggregate information. A clinical terminology subsystem is needed to inspect the incoming data for outliers or incongruous data and clean data of extraneous elements, leaving a pure value (e.g., "120"). Second, clinical information is usually captured at a very granular level during the patient encounter, whereas reporting and quality measurement systems require higher-level groupings of information. In order to aggregate data from patients with similar characteristics, and across multiple healthcare enterprises with different data standards, a controlled clinical vocabulary is needed in the data warehouse. The vocabulary subsystem is linked to reference terminologies from external sources. Terminology management adds significant value to raw EHR data; large amounts of information that is otherwise unusable can be salvaged with a sophisticated clinical terminology and tools. Ultimately, the adoption of standard clinical terminologies such as SNOMED® and the UMLS will reduce the burden and cost of data cleanup required to prepare clinical information for quality measurement (See Table 13–1).[15]

A Generic Model for the Facilitation of Quality Measurement Using IT

Healthcare information technology makes quality measurement possible in ways that paper-based systems fall short. Without EHR to collect data at the point of care, the barrier to population analysis of defined clinical quality metrics is high. In the absence of EHR, a quality measurement specialist must:

1. Create sampling criteria whereby a large number of patients is reduced to a small population for the purpose of analysis. The population will be driven by the minimum number of patients required to deliver a meaningful statistical analysis, due to the labor involved in subsequent steps.

2. Identify the patients of interest based on disease criteria derived from a billing system or a manual registry of some kind. This can be an error-prone process that is likely to miss many patients who would otherwise be included in the analysis.

3. Locate the paper chart or charts for each patient of interest, wherever they are located within disparate care settings. Often many incomplete charts need to be aggregated for each patient to obtain a minimal picture of the care actually delivered and the outcomes that resulted.

4. Abstract the chart(s) for each patient into a system that allows the patient characteristics to be converted into discrete, quantifiable information suitable for data analysis.

These four steps must be repeated for each measure, and the amount of labor involved scales in a linear fashion.

In contrast, EHR permits much of the data collection process to be automated, and the effort required to deploy additional quality metrics is dramatically lowered for subsequent measures, as long as the data is captured at the point of care. The architectures depicted in Figures 13–1 and 13–2 enable:

1. The sampling criteria can be as creative or comprehensive as programming logic will permit; entire populations of the EHR database are eligible to be included in the population because subsequent labor steps are relatively low.

2. Disease criteria are automated based on structured coded fields in the EHR itself, including both text-based descriptions of patient characteristics as well as numeric identifiers based on ICD9, SNOMED, LOINC, CPT standardized coding systems, and medication code bases such as GPI codes.

3. The patient's longitudinal chart is contained in the EHR, which can serve as a central data collection point for all the information about a given patient through direct provider input, lab interfaces, messaging and document exchange, and other technologies that allow information to converge on the patient record. Still, for reasons of limited adoption, poor data standards, and lack of interoperability between healthcare information systems, the EHR chart is not as complete as it should be.

4. Automated systems can abstract charts into analysis-friendly knowledge management systems such as data warehouses and their reporting subsystems. There is no need to convert EHR data into electronic format, so duplicate data entry that occurs in the paper world purely for the purpose of quality measurement disappears.

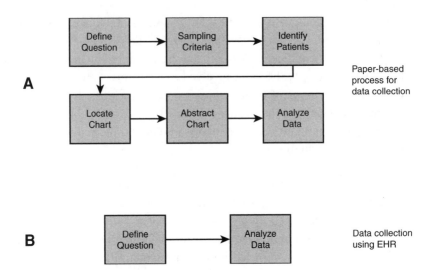

Figure 13–3. *Data Collection Methods. Data collection for quality metrics in a paper-based system (A, versus a system that uses healthcare information technology such as EHR (B).*

The contrast between these four steps in a paper-based system versus using health-care information technology allows a dramatic scaling in the breadth and depth o: quality measurement (see Figure 13–3); in other words, quality measurement o entire populations becomes more efficient and the number and types of metrics car scale due to the removal of initial barriers to data collection and conversion to analy-sis-friendly, electronic format.

Does healthcare information technology enable certain kinds of quality measures better than others? The Agency for Healthcare Research and Quality (AHRQ defined five domains of quality measurement: Access, Outcome, Patient Experi-ence, Process, and Structure.[16] Mant asserted that Process, which directly assesses the services that patients receive, is a more direct measure of quality for the pur poses of improving care delivery.[17] In contrast, Outcomes reflects the health status of a patient often assessed by a proxy such as a laboratory test or vital sign, and depends not only on the healthcare provided to the patient, but also the myriad o genetic, behavioral, lifestyle, social, and economic influences on health. Clinica and patient care information systems probably have better information on Outcome and Process than Access, Patient Experience, and Structure. Retrospective analy sis of EHR data is a relatively new undertaking but offers advantages over tradi tional sources of data from claims and billing, which are often missing key clinica information and do not always accurately reflect what took place during the physi cian–patient encounter. Not only can EHR systems discern that a particular test wa given or a procedure was performed, but also can show the actual clinical result used as quality indicators. For example, the National Committee for Quality Assur ance (NCQA) motivates providers to record the percentage of diabetes patients that have had a Hemoglobin A1c (HgbA1c) measured in the past year.[18] This is a process measure that is easily determined from either a clinical system or an administrative billing system. The lab test result for HgbA1c, which is an outcomes measure (or at least a surrogate for the outcome of well-managed diabetes), can only be obtained from a clinical system. Patient Experience or Patient Satisfaction surveys are not usually collected in clinical systems, though health status surveys, which are potential sources of outcomes measures—especially on quality of life—do have a place in the clinical record.

Privacy and Confidentiality Concerns with Healthcare IT

The healthcare industry is subject to a bewilderingly large number of governmental regulations. Information technology solutions are most significantly affected by the recently enacted Health Insurance Portability and Accountability Act of 1996 (HIPAA) with its accompanying Standards for Privacy of Individually Identifiable Health Information (Privacy Rule). Health plans and providers, as well as researchers that use and transmit information in electronic form, must be in compliance with HIPAA or face substantial civil and criminal sanctions. In the context of the sanctions that are set forth in the provisions, it is paramount that researchers have a full and complete understanding of what is permissible and what the array of options for using IT solutions and healthcare data are. While HIPAA and the privacy rule can at first glance seem draconian, there are numerous provisions within the rule that allow for sufficient flexibility in the use of the data for research and quality measurement.

The Health Insurance Portability and Accountability Act was enacted on August 21, 1996.[19] It required the secretary of Health and Human Services (HHS) to issue privacy regulations governing health information if Congress did not enact privacy regulations within three years of the passage of the act. Because Congress did not enact privacy legislation, HHS developed and published the final rule in August of 2002.[20] The Privacy Rule established, for the first time, a set of national standards for the protection of health information. Specifically, the Privacy Rule is meant to protect individual identifiable health information, while allowing the flow of health information needed to provide and promote high quality healthcare. All covered entities must be compliant with the Privacy Rule after April 14, 2003.

HIPAA and the Privacy Rule have a breathtakingly expansive application; they apply to health plans, healthcare providers, and indeed anyone that is involved in transmitting or using health information in electronic form. Every healthcare provider electronically transmitting identifiable health data, regardless of size, is covered. Researchers that use identifiable healthcare data are also covered by this rule, albeit with the following exceptions.

The Privacy Rule covers information called "protected health information" (PHI), which is defined as "all individually identifiable health information."[20] Indeed, the rule covers all such information whether it is held and transmitted in electronic form, or in paper or oral form. In essence, this provides an advantage to those using computerized solutions for storage and transmittal of information. The requirement to audit each and every time someone looks at identifiable health information means that those providers using a computer can do this automatically. Those that are still paper-based have to manually log all such encounters. This has been one of the major factors in the accelerating adoption of electronic medical record (EMR) solutions in the past few years.

Individually identifiable health information refers to any health information that either directly identifies an individual or that can reasonably be supposed to be used to identify an individual (even through indirect means).[20] Protected health information can only be used and disclosed under a very limited set of permitted circumstances. Any use or disclosure of PHI outside of these parameters constitutes a violation of HIPAA. Specifically, organizations can only disclose data containing PHI after receiving explicit consent from identified individuals to do so. Among the exceptions to this requirement for individual consent are situations that involve treatment, payment, and healthcare operations; public interest and benefit activities; public health activities; and research. The exception for research is one of the most important in the context of quality improvement and measurement. It is also one of the most problematic. The Privacy Rule defines research as "a systematic investigation, including research development, testing, and evaluation, designed to develop or contribute to generalizable knowledge."[20] With certain limitations, the Privacy Rule allows organizations to use and disclose PHI for research purposes without an individual's consent or authorization. Unfortunately, the interpretation of what is genuinely defined as research and what is not has been left up to individual researchers, or at best, institutional review boards. This has made many organizations reluctant to use PHI under these circumstances.

There are other ways that healthcare organizations and researchers can make use of data sets for research and quality improvement. One of the most popular ways is to make use of a subset of the health information with some or all of a defined set of identifiers removed. These identifiers are well-defined elements, giving an additional level of comfort to users that they will not be in violation of HIPAA or the Privacy Rule (see Table 13–2).

The first of these subsets is called a "limited data set." A limited data set is defined as a data set of protected health information with certain specified direct identifiers of individuals and their relatives, household members, and employers removed. A limited data set can be used for research and other purposes without obtaining individual patient consent. At the same time, it is not required that *all* identifiers be removed from the data set.

The second subset commonly used is a "de-identified health information" data set. When a data set is determined to be de-identified, by definition it does not

Table 13–2 *Limited and De-identified Data Sets for Use in HIPAA–Compliant Outcomes Research and Population Measures of Quality Improvement.*

Limited data set elements to be excluded	De-identified data set (safe harbor) elements to be excluded
1. names	1. names
2. postal address information other than city, state, and zip code	2. all geographic subdivisions smaller than a state, including a. street address b. city c. county d. precinct e. zip codes and their equivalent geocodes, except for the initial three digits of a zip code if, according to the current publicly available data from the Bureau of the Census, the geographic unit formed by combining all zip codes with the same three initial digits contains more than 20,000 people, and the initial three digits of a zip code for all such geographic units containing 20,000 or fewer people is changed to 000
3. telephone and fax numbers	
4. e-mail addresses	
5. social security numbers	
6. medical, health plan record, and account numbers	
7. certificate/license numbers	
8. vehicle identifiers/ license plate numbers	3. all elements of dates (except year) for dates directly related to an individual, including a. birth date b. admission date c. discharge date d. date of death e. all ages over 89 and all elements of dates (including year) indicative of such age, except that such ages and elements can be aggregated into a single category of age 90 or older
9. device identifiers	
10. URLs	
11. IP addresses	
12. biometric identifiers	
13. photographic images	4. fax and telephone numbers
	5. electronic mail addresses
	6. medical record numbers
	7. health plan beneficiary numbers, or other health plan account numbers
	8. certificate/license numbers
	9. vehicle identifiers and serial numbers, including license plate

contain protected health information (PHI). There are *no* restrictions on the use or disclosure of de-identified health information. These data sets can be used for any and all purposes, do not require individual patient consent, and are not restricted under HIPAA and the Privacy Rule. There are two ways to designate a data set as de-identified:

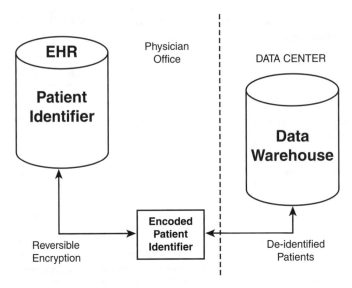

Figure 13–4 *Patient De-identification. Patient identity remains secure in the physician office. The data center for the quality reporting systems has only encoded patient identifiers, which are generated during the data extraction process. The physician office can retain the "key" to de-crypt the patient identifier in cases where individual patient follow-up is required for selected members of a population report.*

1. The removal of a set of specified identifiable data elements from the set. This is called the "safe harbor" method of de-identification when all of the specified elements have been removed *and* there is no reasonable basis to believe that the remaining information could be used to identify a person. This list is longer and more exhaustive than that required for a limited data set, but the resulting data set allows for significantly more flexibility in use.

2. Determination by a qualified statistician that a data set contains no information that could reasonably be used to increase the likelihood of re-identification of individuals. The guidelines are not specific in this case, and there are only a few statisticians who are willing to provide a formal determination that can be used.

As mentioned, the penalties for noncompliance with the regulations are substantial. HHS can impose civil fines of up to $25,000 per year. Additionally, criminal penalties can be up to ten years imprisonment and $250,000 in fines if the violation includes intent to sell, transfer, or use individually identifiable health information for commercial advantage or gain.

There are a variety of methods to safeguard patient privacy when collecting and reporting data for quality improvement and outcomes research. Figure 13–4 shows how patient information can be stripped of identifying data elements during the extraction from the EHR. Numeric database-assigned patient identifiers (keys) are encrypted. Patients are reversibly identifiable only by their providers in cases of medication recalls, disease management reporting, or other instances where it is critical to re-identify individuals.[21]

In summary, the HIPAA regulations and the Privacy Rule result in considerable restrictions around what can be done with electronic data sets. At the same time, they are useful for defining clearly to all involved the do's and don'ts of research and quality measurement with health information. As long as users have a clear understanding of permissible uses and excludable elements they can be comfortable in using these types of data sets to measure quality.

The National Health Information Network (NHIN) and the Future of IT in Healthcare

The National Health Information Network (NHIN) is intended to provide access to complete patient information where and when it is needed in order to improve the quality, safety, and efficacy of healthcare.[22] The NHIN (formerly National Health Information Infrastructure) is now managed by the Office of the National Coordinator for Health Information Technology (ONCHIT), which is part of the US Department of Health and Human Services. ONCHIT released a framework for strategic action in July 2004 that recognizes ". . . the importance of fostering the development and diffusion of technology to improve the delivery of healthcare."[23] The main goals of this strategic framework are to:

1. Inform clinical practice by promoting EHR
2. Interconnect clinicians via an interoperable technology infrastructure
3. Personalize care by giving consumers the tools to manage their own wellness and participate in care decisions
4. Improve population health through evaluating clinical information in the context of public health, research, and feedback to clinicians.

Key to this last goal are streamlined quality and health status monitoring systems enabled by the use of information technology.

The NHIN intends to support quality measurement not only by creating incentives for clinical practice to use EHR, but also by developing common IT architecture and standards for data interchange; encouraging common measurements of quality, safety, and efficacy; and providing data in a privacy-compliant fashion for population health and research. The NHIN does not propose the development of an enormous, centralized database containing the longitudinal health record for every patient. Rather, by fostering EHR adoption and data interchange, the intention is to create and share more electronic health information for both direct clinical care and the more global aim of measuring and improving quality for large populations. This will be accomplished by creating numerous regional health information organizations (RHIOs) and

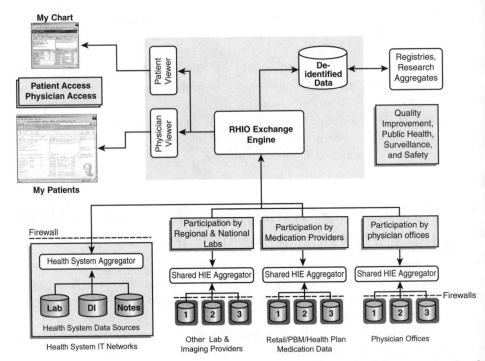

Figure 13–5 *Architecture for Regional Health Data Exchange. The RHIO Exchange is a distributed data sharing architecture. The RHIO Exchange Engine would include a request broker that allows "store and forward" of key patient data, authentication/access servers, patient authorization/consent, publish, and subscribe capabilities. An anonymous, de-identified data store would enable population-based research, public health, quality improvement, and communications with state/federal agencies involved in surveillance. Physician Viewers and Patient Viewer would allow access to data to authorized providers, patients, and family. For the health systems, the HIE Aggregators allow control over data access according to site-specific policies and network encryption.*

creating interconnections between them. There also needs to be a set of processes, policies, and technologies in place to derive aggregate, de-identified, population data for the purpose of creating quality measurements. An example schematic of an RHIO and its derived population data is shown in Figure 13–5. Two often-cited examples of successful local health data interchange are the Indianapolis Network for Patient Care[24] and the Santa Barbara Data Exchange.[25]

The NHIN has the potential to completely transform not only healthcare delivery to individuals, but also to derive enormous value by aggregating complete EHR data for entire populations to use for quality measurement and improvement. The "key actions" described in the ONCHIT framework document[23] are underway and demonstrate the high priority, profile, and momentum needed to truly address quality issues in medicine using healthcare information technology.

Conclusion

Healthcare information systems are useful tools in the hands of clinicians, enabling better documentation, decision support during the process of care, enhanced communications with all stakeholders, and assistance with managing the ballooning costs of providing high-quality, error-free care. A well-integrated network of interoperable healthcare IT systems will provide an unprecedented foundation for the collection and management of information about healthcare quality. The adoption of IT is in itself a component of some forward-looking quality measures.[9,26]

The implementation of IT solutions in healthcare will almost always require accompanying organizational changes within practice in order to be successful. Often, the technical components of an IT solution are the easiest to manage, whereas the political and human elements of practicing medicine are rarely simple to address. There can sometimes be unintended consequences of information technology if the social and group context of care is not taken into account. Successful implementations of IT will always need to address the design of human-computer interfaces, unique workflows, and collaborative nature of healthcare decision making.[27] If critical information were to become buried in an onslaught of electronic documents, test results, and messages, important steps in the care process could be omitted resulting in poor outcomes and increased provider liability. Clinical workflow and human considerations are becoming part of the everyday tool kit of IT professionals, enabling healthcare to catch up with other safety- and quality-critical industries, and are beginning to benefit from technology on a wider scale to reduce cost and improve quality.

Case Study

Norumbega Medical, a medium-sized primary care practice in Maine, implemented EHR over six years ago. The practice has approximately nine physicians and thirty allied health providers serving over 21,000 patients. With EHR and participation in the GE Medical Quality Improvement Consortium, "We can, for the first time, compare our performance to a large pool of (EHR) users" according to Frank Bragg, MD, medical director of the practice. "This is the first time we have had a true benchmark" against other practices. Against the benchmark, this practice outperformed other EMR users in metrics such as Secondary Prevention Post Myocardial Infarction (see Figure 13–6), Hyperlipidemia Management, Hypertension Management, Secondary Prevention of CHF, Secondary Prevention of Stroke, IHD and PVD, and Diabetes Mellitus. Norumbega Medical was able to validate the measures and obtain buy-in from physicians that the data accurately reflected their practice. The comparison was made worthwhile by the large patient pool across many EMR users and the fact that the majority were primary care. The quality metrics also suggested areas

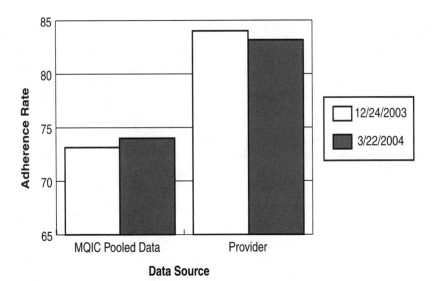

Figure 13–6 *Post-MI Patients on Beta Blocker. Quality metrics showing quarterly trends for a benchmark population (MQIC pooled data) versus a selected multi-site primary practice (provider). The graph shows compliance with a commonly accepted clinical guideline for the management of patients after a myocardial infarction.*

of improvement. Dr. Bragg notes, "For Blood Pressure control we (and the MQIC group in its entirety) do better controlling diastolic BP than systolic BP—something we have observed with our own internal audits." Norumbega Medical intends to focus on control of systolic blood pressure, which is a sizeable risk factor for myocardial infarction and stroke.[28]

Study/Discussion Questions

1. What is an electronic health record (EHR) and how has it affected the approach to quality management?

2. What is medical informatics? How has informatics shaped the practice of medicine?

3. What are some of the challenges for physician offices to adopt technology, and barriers to the adoption of EHR?

4. What are the key components of a business case for technology? Why are these so difficult to enumerate in healthcare?

5. How do privacy concerns affect the use of EHR and the application of electronic patient data to the measurement of healthcare quality?

6. What is a data warehousing technology, and how does it complement EHR for the purpose of quality measures and outcomes reporting?

7. What is the National Health Information Network (NHIN)? What are the main goals of NHIN to move healthcare IT forward?

Suggested Readings/Web Sites

American Medical Informatics Association (http://www.amia.org).

Bridges to Excellence (http://www.bridgestoexcellence.org).

Center for Information Technology Leadership (CITL) (http://www.citl.org/index.htm).

eHealth Initiative (http://www.ehealthinitiative.org).

Health Information Management Systems Society (http://www.himss.org).

Health Level 7 (http://www.hl7.org).

Logical Observation Identifiers Names and Codes (http://www.loinc.org).

National Committee for Quality Assurance (http://www.ncqa.org).

National Quality Measures Clearinghouse (http://www.qualitymeasures.ahrq.gov).

Office of the National Coordinator for Health Information Technology (ONCHIT) (http://www.os.dhhs.gov/healthit/).

RxNORM (http:/www.nlm.nih.gov/research/umls/rxnorm_main.html).

Systematized Nomenclature for Medicine (http://www.snomed.org).

The Medical Records Institute (http://www.tepr.com).

Unified Medical Language System (http://www.nlm.nih.gov/research/umls/).

References

1. Richardson W, ed. *Crossing the Quality Chasm: A New Health System for the 21st Century.* Washington, DC: National Academy Press; 2001.

2. Ricciardi TN, Masarie FE, Middleton B. *Clinical benchmarking enabled by the digital health record. Medinfo.* 2001; 10(Pt. 1):675–79.

3. Institute of Medicine. *Key Capabilities of an Electronic Health Record System.* Washington, DC: National Academy Press; 2003.

4. Hersh, W. Medical informatics: improving healthcare through information. *J Am Med Assoc.* 2002;288(16):1955–58.

5. Davis M, Galimi J. North American Healthcare IT spending forecasts to 2007. Gartner Research. Report No. M-22-6133. April 24, 2004.

6. Johnston D, Pan E, Middleton B, *Finding the Value in Healthcare Information Technologies.* Boston, Mass.: Center for IT Leadership; 2002.

7. Fetterolf D, West R. The business case for quality: Combining medical literature research with health plan data to establish value for nonclinical managers. *Am J Med Qual.* 2004; 19(2):48–55.

8. NCQA. The Business Case for Health Care Quality. Available at: http://www.ncqe.org/somc2001/BIZ_CASE/SOMC_2001_BIZ_CASE.html. Accessed on June 5, 2005.

9. NCQA. Bridges to Excellence: Rewarding Quality Across the Healthcare System. Available at: http://www.ncqa.org/Programs/bridgestoexcellence/. Accessed on June 5, 2005.

10. Bates DW, Cohen M, Leape LL, Overhage JM, Shabot MM, Sheriden T. Reducing the frequency of errors in medicine using information technology. *J Am Med Inform Assoc.* 2001; 8(4):299–308.

11. Tierney W, Overhage JM, Murray MD, et al. Effects of computerized guidelines for managing heart disease in primary care. *J Gen Intern Med.* 2003;18(12):967–76.

12. Dexter P, Perkins S, Overhage JM, et al. A computerized reminder system to increase the use of preventive care for hospitalized patients. *NEJM.* 2001;345(13):965–70.

13. Gluckman T, Baranowski B, Ashen MD, et al. A practical and evidence-based approach to cardiovascular disease risk reduction. *Arch Intern Med.* 2004;164(14):1490–1500.

14. Middleton B, Renner K, Leavitt M. Ambulatory practice clinical information management: problems and prospects. *Healthcare Inform Manage.* 1997;11(4): 97–112.

15. Brailer D. Translating ideals for health information technology into practice. *Health Affairs.* May 25, 2004. Available at: http://content.healthaffairs.org/cgi/content/full/hltaff.w4.318v1dc1. Accessed on June 4, 2004.

16. AHRQ. *Using measures.* Available at: http://www.qualitymeasures.ahrq.gov/resources/measure_use.aspx. Accessed on June 5, 2005.

17. Mant J. Process versus outcome indicators in the assessment of quality of healthcare. *Int J Qual Health Care.* 2001;13(6):475–80.

18. NCQA. Diabetes Physician Recognition Program. Available at: http://www.ncqa.org/dprp. Accessed on June 5, 2005.

19. *Health Insurance Portability and Accountability Act, in 67 CFR 53182.* 1996.

20. Standards for Privacy of Individually Identifiable Health Information, in 45 CFR Part 160 and 164. 2002.

21. Ricciardi TN, White C. Method, system, and computer product for securing patient identity. In US Patent Office, pending application. USA:General Electric Company; 2003.

22. Yasnoff, Humphreys BL, Overhage JM, et al. A consensus action agenda for achieving the national health information infrastructure. *J Amer Med Inform Assoc.* 2004;11(4):332–38.

23. Thompson T, Brailer D. The decade of health information technology: Delivering consumer-centric and information-rich health care. U.S. Department of Health and Human Services; 2004.

24. McDonald C, et al. An LHII supporting care, public health, and research in Indianapolis. 2004.

25. Brailer DJ, Evans LM, Augustinos N, Karp S. Santa Barbara County Care Data Exchange.

26. Integrated Healthcare Association. Year 2 Pay for Performance IT Investment Measure Specifications.

27. Ash J, Berg M, Coiera E. Some unintended consequences of information technology in health care: The nature of patient care information system-related errors. *J Am Med Inform Assoc.* 2004;11(2):104–12.

28. Bragg, F. Medical Quality Improvement Consortium, T. N. Ricciardi, ed. 2004.

Chapter 14

Future Research Agenda

Designing and Paying for Quality

Irene Fraser
Carolyn M. Clancy
Jan De La Mare

EXECUTIVE SUMMARY

Better quality flows from better healthcare systems. To improve quality, healthcare leaders and managers need to improve the way they organize and structure care. While improved information technology can help, major breakthroughs in quality require transformation in healthcare structure, organization, and clinical care processes. To facilitate system improvements, it will be important to change the way we pay for care—to remove perverse incentives and strengthen appropriate incentives. This chapter summarizes the kind of system design and payment changes that can improve quality; identifies holes in the knowledge needed to make these changes; and charts a course for filling those holes.

LEARNING OBJECTIVES

1. To understand how performance at multiple levels of an organization can affect quality, safety, and efficiency of healthcare.
2. To gain a better understanding of what system redesign can entail.
3. To understand how public reporting and financial incentives can affect provider behavior.
4. To understand how future research can improve use of system design and incentives.

KEYWORDS

Research

System Design

Financial Incentives

Pay-for-Performance

Evidence-Based Management

Introduction

Better quality flows from better healthcare systems. A central theme of the *Chasm Report* is that closing the quality gap will require a transformation in system design—the way we organize, structure, and deliver care. While information technology can help, major breakthroughs in quality will require substantial changes within and among the organizations that deliver care. It also will be necessary to modify the way we pay for care, specifically to remove perverse incentives and strengthen appropriate incentives. In today's competitive marketplace, it is unrealistic to expect that healthcare leaders will make quality improvements that lose money for their institutions. To plan and execute this transformation, healthcare leaders will need solid and timely information about what organizational and payment arrangements work, when, and under what circumstances. Just as improving quality at the practitioner level requires evidence-based medicine, decisions about designing and paying for quality require evidence-based management and policy making.

In mapping out its recommendations for how to close the quality chasm, the Institute of Medicine called on the Agency for Healthcare Research and Quality (AHRQ), in collaboration with others in the public and private sectors, to identify what we know and don't know about ways to improve how we organize and pay for care, and to develop an agenda for filling gaps in the evidence base and facilitating use of this evidence. The Agency's authorizing language calls on the AHRQ to improve "the quality, appropriateness, and effectiveness of health services, and access to such services, through the establishment of a broad base of scientific research and through the promotion of improvements in clinical and health system practices . . ."[1] The Agency has been a major funder of organizational, management, and payment research in the past and this work has accelerated and evolved as a result of the *Chasm* report.[2,3] This chapter summarizes what we know and don't know about the system design and payment decisions that can affect quality. It then identifies priorities for future research in these areas and some of the key activities AHRQ has taken to meet them.

System Design

What is system design and why does it matter? While it is obvious that the product of a system can be no better than the system itself, finding a way to go from that overall piece of wisdom to an improvement strategy requires looking more closely within organizations to identify the particular organizational levels and processes that would need to change, and to identify strategies for designing and implementing change. Steve Shortell identifies four levels of change: the individual, where knowledge, skills and expertise are key; the group or team, where cooperation, coordination, and shared knowledge are key; the organization, where structure and strategy are key; and the larger system or environment, where reimbursement, legal, and regulatory policy are key.[4]

Much of the research on healthcare quality improvement has focused on improvements in processes with a care team or group, but the organizational and larger system levels can be profoundly important. An example from the aviation industry illustrates this point. In the ValuJet crash of 1996, organization-wide factors were identified as prominent antecedents in the chain of errors leading to the tragedy.[5] In that case, the organization was experiencing some profound changes similar to those of today's healthcare organizations: severe cost pressures, frequent mergers and acquisitions, increased use of contract and temporary employees, and heavy reliance on outsourcing.

In healthcare, as in aviation, the structures, processes, and organizational cultures at the organizational level affect the probability of quality and safety in global ways.[6-14] The IOM estimates that 44,000 to 98,000 patients each year die as a result of inpatient errors alone, and that these deaths result from system errors.[15] If organization-wide errors remain unchanged, efforts to improve safety and quality at the team or worker level will be largely in vain.[11] Common healthcare process improvements introduced at the system level can have a tremendous advantage over the more common "condition specific" implementation schemes designed to improve processes of care for particular diagnoses. They also can have a major impact on the reduction of waste and inefficiency.

The impact of organization-level and larger system issues becomes particularly clear in the case of healthcare for people with chronic conditions, who use the system more than their healthier counterparts, and also tend to use multiple medical and nonmedical services that cross multiple organizations. Similarly, responses to bioterrorism and public health issues require collaboration across healthcare organizations, and between healthcare and other sectors.

Anyone who has spent time in the healthcare system as a professional or patient knows that the current way we organize and structure care is not ideal for achieving patient safety or good care for chronic conditions. Also lacking are timely response mechanisms to bioterrorism and public health needs. There is an undue amount of waste and inefficiency. Lost files, repeated tests, and poor linguistic skills of providers who care for non-English speaking patients are all too typical. Miscommunication during handoffs from one provider to another even within the same facility—much less between facilities—creates tremendous opportunity for safety mishaps, quality compromises, and inefficiency. At a time of rapidly rising healthcare costs, there is increasing recognition of the need to remove some of these problems from the system.

Examples of Redesign

The prospect of system redesign can be somewhat daunting, given the complexity of current systems, and the fact that good patient care often requires crossing back and forth between care sites. But in the past few years we have seen a growing body of evidence that careful measurement, coupled with attention to processes of care and the organizational units that deliver it, can yield impressive improvements in one or more process or outcome. For example:

- An Intermountain Health Care effort to improve the proportion of cardiovascular disease patients receiving appropriate discharge prescriptions for aspirin, ACE inhibitors, statins, warfarin, and beta blockers raised rates from between 40 percent and 70 percent up to an impressive 90 percent, bringing a 27 percent decrease in unadjusted absolute death rates.[16]
- Installing a computer information management system in intensive care units saved nurses almost an hour per eight-hour shift for patient care, enabling nurses to spend 40 percent of their time on patient care rather than the previous 31 percent.[17]
- Instituting "fast track" processes in the Emergency Department (ED) can shorten total cycle time from patient arrival to discharge for urgent care patients. Current performance is highly variable, but often takes several hours. Through changes in staffing, registration procedures, and faster radiology and lab return times, hospitals in the Urgent Matters collaborative, sponsored by the Robert Wood Johnson Foundation, are reducing this time substantially (see www.urgentmatters.org).
- Use of dedicated AIDS units in hospitals has been shown to increase patient satisfaction and decrease nurse burnout.[18]

There are also a few examples of efforts to do broader, organization-level changes with an eye to improving care in multiple sites and for multiple conditions at the same time. For example:

- Hospitals involved in the Urgent Matters collaborative have been trying to dramatically shorten ED boarding time—the amount of time a patient remains in the ED after orders have been issued to admit the patient. Currently, boarding time is highly variable and can reach several hours or even a full day, in large part because a patient must wait for an empty inpatient bed. Some promising models at Northwestern, Inova Farifax Hospital, and others involve changes across the hospital including earlier inpatient discharge, less complex processes for bed assignment, earlier alerts to housekeeping, among other improvements. Changes at Inova Fairfax Hospital in Virginia reduced the number of patients boarding in the ED for over eight hours by 72 percent[19] (refer to www.urgentmatters.org).

• Several years ago, the Veterans Administration launched a comprehensive reorganization and redesign of their healthcare system. The initiative included a structural reorganization into twenty-two (now twenty-one) regional networks, the movement of patients to outpatient and community providers, improvement in throughputs, new payment and incentive systems, staff reductions and reorganizations, a new quality management and accountability framework, and new information technologies incorporating an electronic health record and clinical reminders for decision support.[20,21]

Success Factors

AHRQ recently sponsored an environmental scan of redesign initiatives[22] that identifies five factors these successful efforts have in common.

1. Authentic and credible leadership. This includes management leadership, clinical leadership, and leadership of the board of trustees.
2. Visible commitment of senior management to system redesign—a commitment necessary to remove barriers and secure resources.
3. Quality-oriented culture and positive reward structure, needed to create the transparency that fosters honest and open discussion of ways to improve quality.
4. Strategic integration of projects. Successful initiatives included multiple interventions at multiple levels.
5. Deliberate incorporation of measurement and analysis into redesign efforts—to continuously benchmark, identify performance gaps, assist in clinical decision making, and facilitate knowledge sharing.

What becomes extremely clear in discussion of these and other examples of redesign is that the current incentive system discourages improvements of these sorts, because shorter inpatient stays, fewer readmissions, and other consequences from quality improvement often lead to a reduction in provider revenue. For this reason, any discussion of quality improvement through healthcare redesign is incomplete without a discussion of ways to change incentives.

Incentives

All institutions, like all individuals, are shaped by multiple motivations or incentives. Some are internally generated, while others come from outside the organization. Some are psychologic or social, while others are more clearly financial. Some are deliberate and others are unintended. Large, complex organizations such as hospitals, physician practices, and other healthcare organizations invariably have a whole host of these motivators operating at any given time, and the incentives are likely to differ within parts of the same organization.

In recent years, faced with rising costs and growing evidence of gaps in quality and patient safety, both public and private purchasers have been paying increasing attention to incentives, and in particular have been looking at ways to improve quality and efficiency through the deliberate use of incentives. This effort, which many term value-based purchasing,[23] encompasses several different activities by private employers, coalitions, and public purchasers, including collection of data on quality, partnerships for quality improvement, employee education, and finally rewarding or penalizing providers through financial and nonfinancial incentives and disincentives.[24,25] Two particular strategies have been public reporting and the use of financial incentives through pay-for-performance strategies.

Report Cards

One way purchasers and others have tried to change the incentive structure is to collect information about quality and then report it publicly. The state of New York has been collecting information on patients receiving coronary bypass surgery in New York State since the late 1980s. The Centers for Medicare & Medicaid Services (CMS) and its predecessor, the Health Care Financing Administration (HCFA), released data on hospital mortality from a broader set of procedures in the 1980s.[26] More recently, CMS has published quality data on hospitals and nursing homes (see http://www.cms.hhs.gov/quality/). Several states, including Wisconsin, Texas, and New York also have published hospital quality information.[27,28] In theory, this approach could improve quality through two paths. First, those who buy healthcare services can change their choices based on this information, thereby rewarding and moving volume to better providers based on quality scores. Second, public reporting could serve as a reputational incentive to providers, leading them to take steps to improve quality.

So far, evidence of the impact of report cards on the first path (financial incentives) has been mixed,[29] though some recent studies seem to be finding a connection in some cases. A recent PacifiCare effort to release quality scores on physician groups in California at the time of enrollment found that 30,000 enrollees chose the higher-quality physician groups,[30] and a recent analysis of the New York State data on coronary artery bypass reporting found that poor performing hospitals lost considerable volume to competing facilities.[31] In the meantime, however, it is becoming increasingly clear that publication of quality scores can have a strong impact on the providers themselves (reputational incentives). For example, in New York State, publication of CABG mortality scores led to a 41 percent decline in deaths from cardiac surgery.[32]

A recent randomized controlled trial in Wisconsin shows just how powerful this reputational incentive can be. The Alliance, a large employer-purchasing cooperative in Madison, produced and disseminated a report comparing the performance of twenty-four hospitals in south central Wisconsin. The other ninety-eight general hospitals in Wisconsin outside this area were randomly assigned to either a secondary intervention group or to a control group. Hospitals in the secondary intervention group did get a report on their own performance, but the information was not made public. In the control group, there was no report. The results were striking. Hospitals with public reporting were far more likely to engage in quality improvement efforts subsequent to publication of the report than their counterparts in the other two groups. For example, public-report hospitals reported an average of 3.4 quality improvement activities in obstetrics, compared with 2.5 for the private-report hospitals, and 2.0 activities for the no-report hospitals. There was a similar distribution among the three groups for cardiac quality improvement activities. Reputational incentives seem to have a particularly strong effect on hospitals that receive poor scores.[29]

Do Incentives Work?

Changes in payment are an explicit incentive designed to improve quality. In *Crossing the Quality Chasm*, the Institute of Medicine called attention to the fact that the present payment landscape provides strong perverse incentives.[2] That is, providers who succeed in designing and implementing system interventions to improve care for patients are often penalized for doing so because the resulting quality improvements create a loss in provider revenue. For example, because providers are paid the same amount regardless of their quality under Medicare, a facility that reduces readmissions or complication rates could experience revenue losses.[30] For this reason, any effort to bring about systemic improvements in quality must address the payment issue.

While financial incentives are not a new phenomena in the United States, the twin problems of cost and quality, coupled with advances in our ability to measure quality,[24,33] have brought a proliferation of such efforts. In the private sector, Meredith Rosenthal has identified thirty-seven separate incentive plans representing thirty-one different payers.[34] For example, Blue Cross Blue Shield of Massachusetts is using HEDIS and patient satisfaction measures to reward physicians; the Buyers Health Care Action Group gives annual awards for patient safety and clinical quality projects; and Blue Cross Blue Shield of Hawaii is using clinical metrics to award top-performing hospitals. Examples of such efforts continue to grow. The Leapfrog Group (www.leapfroggroup.org) has a Web site that captures critical information about many such efforts. These incentive programs, like the public reporting efforts, take many forms, differing substantially in terms of who is providing the incentive (employers, public purchasers, health plans); who is being given the incentives (hospitals, physicians, plans); how much is being paid and how; what the underlying payment system is; and the use of nonfinancial incentives.

The Medicare program also has accelerated its use of financial incentives through a growing number of demonstration programs. The Centers for Medicare & Medicaid Services (CMS) has two dozen programs in place, and another dozen under development,[35] and the Medicare Modernization Act[36] requires many more.

The Premier demonstration provides one large-scale example of Medicare's use of financial incentives. This demonstration, conducted with 278 hospitals belonging to the Premier, Inc. Alliance, provides financial incentives for hospital performance on five clinical conditions: acute MI, heart failure, pneumonia, coronary artery bypass graft, and hip and knee replacement. Under this demonstration, hospitals in the top deciles for each condition will be given a bonus consisting of 2 percent of their Medicare DRG payments for that condition, and those in the second decile will get a 1 percent bonus. In the third year, there is a possible penalty for those who are below the baseline threshold.[37] In addition, the top 50 percent of hospitals in each clinical area will be reported on the CMS Web site at www.cms.hhs.gov.

A recent twist on the use of financial incentives to improve care occurred when the Medicare Modernization Act was passed: To receive a payment update of 0.4 percent, hospitals must participate in the national voluntary reporting initiative, which consists of ten clinical quality measures for AMI, CHF, and community-acquired pneumonia. This starter set will be expanded.

While it seems intuitively obvious that providing incentives for quality can result in improved performance, it is also clear that many things could interfere with the success of such an attempt. For example, the incentive might be perceived as too small to motivate change. Perhaps the incentive is being offered based on behavior outside of the control of the actor. Maybe the financial reward is proffered for something the organization was going to do anyway. So what is the evidence on whether financial incentives can work and, if so, under what circumstances? First, the evidence is clear that financial incentives can and do work. For example, a large study of the use of incentives in physician group practices[38] found that the strongest predictor of the extent of evidence-based care management practices used was presence of incentives from outside the practice. An AHRQ-funded evidence review[39] on the impact of incentives reviewed all nine of the randomized controlled trials that have been completed on this question, and found clear evidence that properly designed incentives can lead to improved performance.

Factors Affecting Success of Incentives

From the perspective of a would-be designer of an incentive system, the question is not whether incentives can work, but how to make sure they work in the instance at hand. In perhaps the most useful component of the Dudley et al. evidence review,[39] the authors draw on the broader literature on organizations to identify a conceptual model for how and why a well-designed incentive system might work. In the absence of any systematic data on how successful past efforts differed from unsuccessful ones, this conceptual model can provide a framework for both designing and evaluating incentive systems in the future. The authors review three clusters of factors that can have an impact on the success of an incentive: 1) The incentive itself, 2) factors that predispose the recipient to act on the incentive, and 3) factors that enable the recipient to act.

In terms of the incentive itself, the authors posit that one is more likely to influence behavior if the incentive matches the locus of necessary action (e.g., use group incentives for group actions), if providers can predict the reward, if the reward is clearly greater than the cost of compliance, if the provider believes that achieving the performance level is within his/her control, and if the incentives themselves coincide with the values of the provider—for example, incentives to improve quality rather than reduce costs.

The second set of factors is contextual. The underlying payment systems, characteristics of the provider, and market characteristics all predispose the provider to act in certain ways. An incentive that runs counter to these will be more difficult. For example, the underlying payment system—fee-for-service, salary or budget, and capitation—provides strong incentives that can contradict or reinforce a new, targeted incentive. Many characteristics of the provider could also affect the impact of the incentive. For example, younger physicians who are accustomed to information technology might be more predisposed to using computerized physician order entry (CPOE) systems. Finally, factors such as managed care market share or community-wide provider activities can affect provider practice patterns, thereby reinforcing or counteracting the impact of a particular incentive to change practice.

Finally, even if providers are predisposed to respond to incentives as intended, they might not have the capacity to do so. Responding to incentives, like success with any other organizational decision, requires strong leadership, an organizational culture that supports change, and good IT systems. Other characteristics that typically support effective organizations will also support the organization's capacity to respond to an incentive. Provider responses to incentives will also vary depending on characteristics of their patients, and provider perceptions of what these patients might need.

For someone seeking to design an incentive system, this conceptual model provides an excellent organizing framework for making sure that critical features are reviewed. Unfortunately, past research on incentives has not captured information about most of these decision points, so there is no hard data on exactly how these factors play out. Finally, there is little information on the implementation aspect of incentives. One could hit all the right notes in Dudley's conceptual framework and still have a failed effort if the roll-out and execution of the incentive was not well implemented. Ironically, an incentive intended to improve system design could fail at the implementation stage because of the very system failures the incentive is intended to correct.

Improving System Design and Payment: An Agenda for the Future

If system design and payment are the two fatal flaws undermining safety and quality in this country, improvements will require deliberate efforts to change the way healthcare is organized and reimbursed. As system and policy leaders rise to this challenge, they will need strong evidence of what changes will work, when they will work, and how to implement them so that they work as intended. Without such evidence, ten years from now the IOM could at best be lamenting the quality impact of a different, but equally dysfunctional, organization and payment system. As previously noted, the research community has provided some solid evidence to show that organizational and payment changes have the potential to change behavior and thereby quality. But to provide the evidence base for valid decisions in these areas, research will need to move ahead more quickly, and with more concrete answers to often mundane questions about both the design and the real-world implementation of changes in the complex, rapidly changing world of healthcare.

Over the past several years, AHRQ has been holding formal and informal meetings with healthcare policy makers, public and private purchasers, health plans, hospitals, other providers, researchers, and consumers in an effort to identify their priorities in terms of both filling information gaps and getting better access to information that already exists so that they can improve the way healthcare is organized and paid for.[40–47] These discussions, and our own review of the evidence, suggest that research on organization and payment will need to meet five challenges in order to be helpful. The following sections identify these five challenges, and also identify some of the activities AHRQ is taking to help the field meet them.

Challenge No. 1. Data and Tools to Support System Redesign, Reporting, and Incentives

All of the current approaches to quality—through internal quality improvement, public reporting, or changing financial incentives—hinge on measurement and data. As the chapters in Section 2 show, one cannot improve what one cannot measure. The ability to measure, track, report on, and reward quality also will require strong, timely data at the national, state, local, and provider level. Users will need to agree on these measures and data, so that each provider is not reporting different data to different sources, and so that to the extent possible all parties are using the same data for quality improvement, reporting, pay-for-performance, and national tracking. Following are examples of several AHRQ initiatives to advance this agenda.

National Healthcare Quality and Disparities Reports

In 1999, Congress asked AHRQ to publish annual reports on the state of quality and the level of disparities in America. The National Healthcare Quality and Disparities Reports[48,49] (http://www.qualitytools.ahrq.gov/), starting with the first in 2003, summarize the leading indicators of quality and disparities, providing national data and, for some measures, state and regional data as well. The reports provide baseline information that can be tracked over time to assess where improvements have and have not occurred. They also provide a core set of national measures and data that can be used as a platform for state and local quality improvement efforts.

Measuring Experience of Care

The consumer's perspective has become an essential aspect of measuring healthcare quality, and AHRQ's CAHPS® is recognized as the industry standard for obtaining consumers' assessment of their health plans. CAHPS survey results are collected on health plans in which over 120 million Americans are enrolled, and are used for quality improvement, internal reporting, and public reporting. In recent years, CAHPS has expanded to other healthcare settings such as medical groups and behavioral health services, and to specific populations such as children with chronic conditions. New survey instruments under development are Hospital CAHPS, developed in collaboration with CMS to measure patients' perspectives on their inpatient care, and Ambulatory CAHPS, an instrument to assess patients' experiences with ambulatory care.

Using Administrative Data to Improve Quality

For many years, hospitals and other providers have used AHRQ's Inpatient Quality Indicators and Patient Safety Indicators (www.qualityindicators.ahrq.gov) to flag quality problems and track their progress in making quality improvements. These indicators, developed by AHRQ under contract with Stanford and the University of California-San Francisco, can be run against hospital administrative data, and the information can then be compared with national data from AHRQ's Healthcare Cost and Utilization Project (HCUP) on HCUPnet, an interactive Web site maintained by AHRQ. More recently, state data organizations, public payers, employers, health plans, and others seeking inexpensive and readily accessible data on outcomes that consumers care about have also begun to use these quality indicators for public reporting and pay-for-performance plans—uses not anticipated in AHRQ's original publications on the Quality Indicators. Because there was some question about how and if to use the indicators in these new ways, AHRQ recently published a "Guidance for Using the AHRQ Quality Indicators for Hospital-level Public Reporting or Payment." This document, also available on the AHRQ Web site, intends to help organizations use the best science in making and implementing their decisions via the Quality Indicators. Potential users also can contact a support contractor at AHRQ's Web site for additional help.

AHRQ is also exploring the possibility of strengthening the utility of administrative data by factoring in clinical data elements. Such a linkage could enhance the use of administrative data for individual hospital quality improvement efforts, and can also substantially strengthen its utility for public reporting and payment, particularly as organizations move toward the electronic health record. By consulting with a variety of experts, including healthcare managers, health data experts, state hospital association experts, clinicians, and others, AHRQ is learning how it can best plan for the impact of the electronic health record on administrative databases such as HCUP. Potential next steps include anticipating how clinical data from the EHR will be implemented, and testing adoption strategies. As part of this effort, AHRQ is working with the Pennsylvania Health Care Cost Containment Council (PHC4) and MediQual to learn from the PHC4 experience linking clinical to administrative data.

Measuring Efficiency

The Institute of Medicine includes efficiency as one of the six domains of quality, but so far measurement and data efforts have paid more attention to effectiveness and other domains. Rising healthcare costs have underscored the urgency of filling this gap. Identifying efficiency measures and data is a high priority for the Agency. One first step in this direction has been developing the capacity to report cost as well as charge data in the Healthcare Cost and Utilization Project (HCUP). Through a collaboration with four state partners—California, Florida, Massachusetts, and New Jersey—AHRQ developed a methodology for converting charge data to cost data, and for reporting this information in its online query system, HCUPnet (http://hcup.ahrq.gov/HCUPnet.asp). A new intramural research effort will be refining methodologies for measuring cost effectiveness in hospitals, and the Agency also will be doing a review of other provider efficiency measures.

In a related effort, RTI and Intermountain Health Care (IHC) are developing a tool that providers can use to identify and reduce inefficiency and waste. The initial phase of research activity involves abstraction of completed quality improvement projects from IHC and Providence Health System (PHS) together with results from a systematic review of the literature. This data will be used to compile a typology of waste/poor quality, which will be reviewed by an expert panel, and triangulation of the findings will direct subsequent efforts. Phase two will involve structured observations in select classes of waste, involving management engineering experts. Financial management experts will use this data to develop a financial management system to capture and assess the cost of waste/poor quality. The result of this activity will be a standardized tool that can be used to set improvement priorities among different areas of waste and/or poor quality.

Model Reporting Templates

Past research has shown that public report cards often do not have a big impact on consumer choice.[29] One potential explanation for this apparent disinterest is that many reports are published without any audience tests related to consumer interest in the measures, comprehension of information presented, or other report card attributes. To address this problem, AHRQ is currently developing and testing reporting templates for all of its Quality Indicators for a variety of audiences, including consumers, purchasers, policy makers, and healthcare providers. Findings from this project will be incorporated into the Quality Indicators software, providing users with ready access to recommended reporting templates.

Challenge No. 2. Intersection of Information Technology and System Redesign

As noted in Chapter 13, a strong electronic information infrastructure (IT) can be a tremendous asset to quality improvement, and can help strengthen the pathway for learning and acting on quality data. For this reason, improving IT has been a growing policy priority. As evidence of this priority, in May 2004, President Bush appointed Dr. David Brailer to a newly created National Health Information Technology coordinator position to help accelerate development of health information technology (http://www.hhs.gov/healthit/).

Information technology also is a growing priority for AHRQ (see http://www.ahrq.gov/research/hitfact.htm). AHRQ recently awarded several contracts and grants to promote the use of health information technology (HIT) through the development of networks for sharing clinical data as well as projects for planning, implementing, and demonstrating the value of HIT. Specifically, AHRQ awarded implementation grants to support community-wide HIT, with an emphasis on diverse and rural healthcare settings. Another part of the Agency's HIT initiative includes funding five states (Colorado, Indiana, Rhode Island, Tennessee, and Utah) to develop statewide networks allowing purchasers, public and private payers, hospitals, ambulatory care facilities, home healthcare providers, and long-term care providers to use HIT to communicate and share information. A National Health Information Technology Resource Center (National HITRC) has been established to support the work of the HIT projects funded by AHRQ and other federal partners, and will provide direct technical assistance and consulting services to individual projects during all phases of their work to develop and use HIT.

Challenge No. 3. Expanding Knowledge and Models of Effective Incentive Systems

As discussed earlier, AHRQ's evidence review of past incentive initiatives showed that incentives can work. But purchasers and others designing current initiatives need much more detail about when, and under what circumstances, incentives are effective. To get them this information, it will be important to document the trajectory and evaluate the impact of the many current pay-for-performance efforts to increase the incentives for quality.

One excellent opportunity for learning from these many "natural experiments" is the Rewarding Results program, a set of seven demonstrations funded by the Robert Wood Johnson Foundation, Commonwealth Fund, California Healthcare Foundation, and Agency for Healthcare Research and Quality. Demonstration participants include Blue Cross Blue Shield of Michigan; Blue Cross of California; Bridges to Excellence (sponsored by General Electric); California Health Care Strategies/Medi-Cal; Excellus/Rochester IPA; Integrated Healthcare Association;

Pay for Performance; and Massachusetts Health Plan Quality Partners. An evaluation team funded by the AHRQ and the Robert Wood Johnson Foundation is working with each of the Rewarding Results sites to evaluate what is working and what is not. Formal evaluations also will provide many opportunities to learn from Medicare's many payment demonstrations.

Challenge No. 4. Expanding Knowledge and Models of Effective Redesign Practices

While financial and nonfinancial incentives can increase the motivation for quality improvements, quantum leaps in quality will require knowledge about how to design and implement such changes. In 2004, AHRQ and the Centers for Medicare & Medicaid Services (CMS) convened a Roundtable on System Design to help develop a strategy and agenda for meeting these information needs. On the recommendations of this group, AHRQ commissioned an environmental scan of leading system redesign efforts and then, in partnership with CMS, The National Cancer Institute, and Project Hope, brought some of these pioneers together with national leaders in system design and payment to identify strategies to encourage similar efforts around the country.

While recognizing that national spread of effective system redesign is likely to require payment changes, the group had three recommendations about ways to encourage change in the meantime: Support development and evaluation of bold innovations to provide models for change; foster collaboratives and other peer-learning mechanisms to enable system leaders to learn from each other; and collect promising practices and disseminate them through the Web. AHRQ has been working on all three approaches and will be accelerating these efforts in the future.

The work of Denver Health provides an example of the first recommended activity. With support from AHRQ, Denver Health recently launched a comprehensive hospital redesign in which they explicitly rejected the goal of improving one particular process, component, or outcome and instead opted for complete system transformation. To begin this effort, they got input from several major service corporations from outside healthcare.[50] Denver Health is currently implementing substantial redesign of all the specialty clinics.[51]

During the past several years, the Robert Wood Johnson Foundation (www.rwjf.org), Institute for Healthcare Improvement (www.ihi.org), and others have similarly launched several national initiatives to promote redesign efforts of this sort.

Probably the most useful thing to be learned in the redesign effort is that there is no silver bullet for reforming healthcare, and that solutions to these first four challenges must be pursued in tandem. Information technology alone will not change the system, nor will new incentives or better measurement of outcomes. As shown in Figure 14–1, to close the quality gap we will need all of these, plus evidence on how to actually act on the incentives and produce the outcomes to be measured.

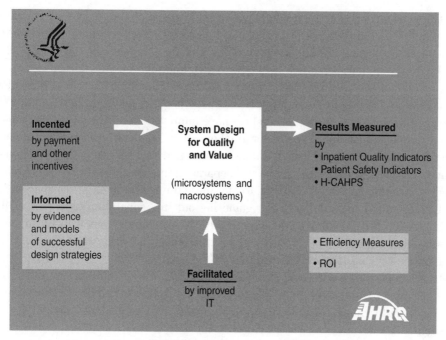

Figure 14–1 *Components of Improved System Performance.*

AHRQ, 2004.

Challenge No. 5. Redesigning Research

Our review of evidence on system design and incentives shows that closing the quality gap also is going to require meeting a fifth challenge: closing the research gap. We have made a start: Past research bolsters the common-sense assumption, underscored by the IOM and others, that real improvements in quality require changes in system design and incentives. As previously shown, there is a growing body of evidence on the kinds of system and incentive factors that can matter. It is very clear that changing organizational design and incentives operate within a world of complexity, and therefore require strong leadership, consistent messages, close attention to context, strong follow-through at the implementation end, and much attention to potential unintended consequences.

It is also clear that, faced with continuing cost increases and quality shortfalls, the field is moving very quickly to develop and implement redesign and pay-for-performance programs. These are obviously not researcher-driven efforts likely to produce randomized controlled trials of the sort reviewed by Dudley; these are field-driven innovations. For research to be useful, there will need to be a redesign of the research enterprise, and perhaps a change in incentives for researchers as well.

The traditional research paradigm is that academic and other researchers identify gaps in the literature and knowledge, and then design research studies around key hypotheses. They seek funding, conduct the research, and—if they are competent, lucky, and assiduous—publish it in a peer reviewed journal. At some point in time (an average of seventeen years, according to one estimate)[52] a fraction of this information winds its way to potential decision makers and is taken up into practice. In a search for relevance, some researchers have improved this practice, adding a user input component as they shape the original questions and a "translation" component after the work has been published. But for the most part the core part of the paradigm—that researchers do their work in a world separate from that of the users of the knowledge—has remained intact. Particularly for those trained in quantitative analysis, in fact, the methodologic rules of the game lay out this separation as a part of the requirements for objectivity and impartiality. While there is much to recommend this traditional process, the result can be knowledge that comes to light too many years after a decision has been made.

In a recent series of focus groups and other formal and informal conversations with payers, providers, system leaders, and others, AHRQ asked how organizational research could change in order to be more useful.[40–47] Respondents made five suggestions.

- Design studies that answer user questions—and bring users explicitly into the design process.
- Present findings in leaders' time and space—using their definitions of "evidence" and taking into account their needs for timeliness.
- Change the incentive system for researchers—so that findings presented to and used by decision makers (not just scholarly publications) are highly valued and rewarded.
- Build user-researcher collaborations and dialogue so that users are involved throughout the research process.
- Change the way evidence is disseminated—with greater emphasis on trade association meetings, peer-to-peer learning, and other similar nonacademic vehicles.

Based largely on the insights from these meetings, AHRQ has been doing a growing amount of its work through new researcher-user models that incorporate many of these elements and promise more immediately useful research as well as more likely implementation of the findings. In collaboratives, for example, a group of similar organizations work closely together on a related set of changes such as improving emergency department care[19] or improving care processes.[53] Under this approach, the users set the agenda and drive the process, and those with expertise in the process or content of change provide ongoing support. A new AHRQ collaborative of health plans who are working together to reduce racial and ethnic disparities follows this model.[54]

AHRQ also is doing a growing amount of work through several provider-based networks, in which researchers and providers work together directly to address problems of interest to the providers. These include the Primary Care Practice-Based Research Network (http://ahrq.gov/research/pbrnfact.htm); the HIV Research Network (http://ahrq.gov/data/hivnet.htm); and the Integrated Delivery System Research Network or IDSRN (http://ahrq.gov/research/idsrn.htm).[55,56,57] The IDSRN, for example, includes nine field-based consortia that do applied research and research implementation through short turn-around task orders. It includes both academic researchers and delivery-based researchers in some of the most sophisticated health plans, systems, hospitals, long-term care facilities, home health agencies, and other provider sites in the country. The network produces not only academic articles but also presentations to operational leadership, scalable models for implementation, tools, how-to guides, training sessions, and workbooks. As a result of strong interest and ongoing involvement by operational leadership in these organizations, promising findings and results often are taken up and implemented long before there is a publication describing them.[58]

Conclusion

Several events have combined to create a tremendous opportunity for research on organization and payment. Healthcare costs are rising rapidly, safety and quality shortfalls are becoming more apparent, and there is growing recognition that fixing either of these problems will require major changes in system design and payment. Healthcare purchasers, policy makers, consumers, and providers have a growing stake in making some of these changes. The challenge will be to provide the evidence needed—in the time frame and manner decision makers need—to enable evidence-based decisions on these issues.

Case Study

The Centers for Medicare & Medicaid Services (CMS) currently supports several efforts to improve the quality of healthcare by providing more information to the public about quality of care and through direct incentives to reward the delivery of superior quality care. Under the Premier Hospital Quality Incentive Demonstration,[37] CMS is partnering with Premier Inc., a national organization of not-for-profit hospitals, to reward participating top performing hospitals by increasing their payment for Medicare patients and reporting extensive quality data for participating hospitals on the CMS Web site. Top performing hospitals will receive bonuses for their performance on evidence-based quality measures for inpatients with specific conditions and procedures, including heart attack, heart failure, pneumonia, and hip and knee replacements. Quality measures validated through extensive research are being used to measure and report on hospital performance.

Two hundred and seventy-eight hospitals are voluntarily participating in this demonstration project. CMS will use this demonstration as a pilot test of this concept and, depending on evaluation results at the conclusion of the project, can use this as a model for additional demonstration projects.

Study/Discussion Questions

1. How does system design affect quality, safety, and efficiency of healthcare?
2. How do financial incentives affect system performance?
3. How can public reporting affect quality?
4. How can we improve availability and use of evidence in making decisions on system design and payment?

Suggested Readings/Web Sites

Hibbard JH. Does publicizing hospital performance stimulate quality improvement efforts? *Health Affairs.* 2003;22(2):84–94.

MedPAC. Using incentives to improve the quality of care in Medicare. In: *Report to the Congress: Variation and Innovation in Medicare.* June 2003.

Rosenthal MB, et al. Paying for quality: Providers' incentives for quality improvement. *Health Affairs.* Vol. 23 (2). 127–141.

AHRQ (www.ahrq.gov).

AHRQ Quality Indicators (www.qualityindicators.ahrq.gov).

AHRQ Healthcare Cost and Utilization Project (HCUP) data tool (www.hcup.ahrq.gov/HCUPnet).

Centers for Medicare & Medicaid Services (www.cms.hhs.gov).

The Institute of Healthcare Improvement (IHI) (www.ihi.org).

The Robert Wood Johnson Foundation (www.rwjf.org).

Urgent Matters (www.urgentmatters.org).

The Leapfrog Group (wwww.leapfroggroup.org).

References

1. Health Care Research and Quality Act of 1999. Agency for Healthcare Research and Quality. Available at: http://www.ahrq.gov/hrqa99a.htm. Accessed on December 2, 2004.
2. Institute of Medicine, Committee on Quality of Health Care in America. *Crossing the Quality Chasm: A New Health System for the 21st Century.* Washington, DC: National Academy Press; 2001.
3. Kovner AR, Elton JJ, Billings J. Evidence-based management. *Front Health Serv Manage* 2000;16(4):3–24.
4. Shortell SM. Increasing value: A research agenda for addressing the managerial and organizational challenges facing healthcare delivery in the United States. *Med Care Res Rev* 2004,61(3 Suppl):12S–30S.

5. Langewiesche W. The lessons of ValuJet 592. *Atlantic Monthly.* 1998;281:81–98.

6. Reason J. *Managing the Risks of Organizational Accidents.* Aldershot, UK: Ashgate Publishing Co; 1997.

7. Edmondson AC. Learning from mistakes is easier said than done: Group and organizational influences on the detection and correction of human error. *J Applied Behavioral Science.* 1996;32(1):5–28.

8. Perrow C. *Normal Accidents: Living with High-Risk Technologies.* Princeton, NJ: Princeton University Press; 1999.

9. Sagan SD. *The Limits of Safety: Organizations, Accidents, and Nuclear Weapons.* Princeton, NJ: Princeton University Press; 1993.

10. Weick KE, Sutcliffe KM, Obstfeld D. Organizing for high reliability: Processes of collective mindfulness. Proceedings of the Second Annenberg Conference on Enhancing Patient Safety and Reducing Errors in Health Care. Rancho Mirage, Calif.: National Patient Safety Foundation; 1998.

11. Vaughn D. *The Challenger Launch Decision: Risky Technology, Culture, and Deviance at NASA.* Chicago, Ill: University of Chicago Press; 1996.

12. Libuser CB, Roberts KH. Organization structure and risk mitigation. Academy of Management. San Diego, Calif.: Anderson Graduate School of Management, University of California; 1998.

13. Moray N. Error Reduction as a Systems Problem. In: Bogner MS, ed. *Human Error in Medicine.* Hillsdale, NJ: Lawrence Erlbaum Associates; 1994.

14. Gaba DM. Structural and organizational issues in patient safety: a comparison of health care to other high-hazard industries. *Calif Manage Rev.* 2000;3(1):5–28.

15. Institute of Medicine, Committee on Quality of Health Care in America. *To Err Is Human: Building a Safer Health System.* Washington, DC: National Academy Press; 2000.

16. Lappe JM, Muhlestein JB, Lappe DL. Improvements in one-year cardiovascular clinical outcomes associated with a hospital-based discharge medication program. *Ann Inter Med.* 2004;141(16):446–53.

17. Wong DH, Gallegos Y, Weinger MB, Clark S, Slagle J, Anderson CT. Changes in intensive care unit nurse task activity after installation of a third-generation intensive care unit information system. *Crit Care Med.* 2003;31(10):2488–94.

18. Aiken LH, Sloane DM, Lake ET, Sochalski J, Weber AL. Organization and outcomes of inpatient AIDS care. *Med Care.* 1999;37(8):760–72.

19. Mayer T. Innovations: Reducing ED boarder hours and volume by engaging non-ED staff. *Urgent Matters* newsletter. Available at http://www.urgentmatters.org/enewsletter/vol1_issue4/I_reducing_ED.asp. Accessed on January 5, 2005.

20. Kizer KW. The "new" VA: A national laboratory for healthcare quality management. *Amer J Med Qual.* 1999;14(1):3–20.

21. Jha AK, Perlin JB, Kizer, Dudley RA. Effect of the transformation of the Veterans Affairs healthcare system on the quality of care. *NEJM.* 2003;348(22):2218–27.

22. Wang M, Hyun J, Shortell S. Leading practices in system redesign. Presentation at AHRQ meeting, Transforming Health Systems Through Leadership, Design, and Incentives. Available at http://cms.hhs.gov/researchers/demos/mma646/1psr_draft.pdf. Accessed on June 5, 2005.

23. Meyer J, Rybowski L, Eschler R. Theory and reality of value-based purchasing: Lessons from the pioneers. Agency for Healthcare Research and Quality. Available at: http://www.ahrq.gov/qual/meyer2.htm. Accessed on June 5, 2005.

24. Fraser I, McNamara P, Lehman GO, Isaacson S, Moler K. The pursuit of quality by business coalitions: A national survey. *Health Aff.* 1999;18(6):158–65.

25. Goldfarb N, Maio N, Carter C, Pizzi L, Nash D. How does quality enter into healthcare purchasing decisions? New York: The Commonwealth Fund; 2003.

26. Gordon T, Cameron JL, eds. *Evidence-based Surgery.* Canada: DB Decker Inc; 2000. Available at: http://www.fleshandbones.com/readingroom/pdf/67.pdf. Accessed on January 19, 2005.

27. Remus D, Fraser I. Guidance for using the AHRQ Quality Indicators for hospital-level public reporting or payment. Agency for Healthcare Research and Quality. Available at: http://www.qualityindicators.ahrq.gov/documentation.htm. Accessed on December 30, 2004.

28. IPRO. 2003 review of hospital quality reports for health care consumers, purchasers and providers. Lake Success, NY: IPRO; 2003. Available at: http://company.ipro.org/dox/legFINAL10_14_03R.pdf. Accessed August 2004.

29. Hibbard JH, Stockard J, Tusler M. Does publicizing hospital performance stimulate quality improvement efforts? *Health Aff.* 2003;22(2):84–94.

30. MedPAC. Using Incentives to Improve the Quality of Care in Medicare. In: *Report to the Congress: Variation and Innovation in Medicare.* June 2003.

31. Cutler DM, et al. The role of information in medical markets: An analysis of publicly reported outcomes in cardiac surgery. Working Paper 10489. Cambridge, Mass: National Bureau of Economic Research; 2004.

32. Chassin MR. Achieving and sustaining improved quality: Lessons from New York state and cardiac surgery. *Health Aff.* 2002;21(4):40–56.

33. Fraser I, McNamara P. Employers: Quality takers or quality makers? *Med Care Res Rev.* 2000;57(Supp. 2):33–52.

34. Rosenthal MB, Fernadopulle R, Song HR, Landon B. Paying for quality: Providers' incentives for quality improvement. *Health Af.* 2004;23(2):127–41.

35. Centers for Medicare & Medicaid Services. Demonstration projects and evaluation reports. Available at: http://www.cms.hhs.gov/researchers/demos/. Accessed on January 25, 2005.

36. 108th Congress of the United States of America. Medicare Prescription Drug, Improvement, and Modernization Act of 2003. Available at: http://frwebgate.access.gpo.gov/cgi-bin/getdoc.cgi?dbname=108_cong_bills&docid=f:h1enr.txt.pdf. Accessed on December 30, 2004.

37. Centers for Medicare & Medicaid Services. Rewarding superior quality care: The Premier hospital quality incentive demonstration. Available at: http://www.cms.hhs.gov/quality/hospital/PremierFactSheet.pdf. Accessed on December 28, 2004.

38. Casalino L, Gillies RR, Shortell S, et al. External incentives, information technology, and organized processes to improve healthcare quality for patients with chronic diseases. *JAMA.* 2003;289(4):434–41.

39. Dudley RA, Frolich A, Robinowitz DL, Talavera JA, Broadhead P, Luft HS. Strategies to support quality-based purchasing: A review of the evidence. *Technical Review 10.* Rockville, Md:Agency for Healthcare Research and Quality; 2004.

40. Callahan MA. Meeting: National conference on leadership, culture and patient safety. Washington, DC: Agency for Healthcare Research and Quality; 2003.

41. Conrad DA, Christianson JB. Penetrating the "black box": Mechanisms for enhancing healthcare efficiency and clinical effectiveness. *Med Care Res Rev.* 2004;61(Suppl. 3): 37S–68S)

42. Kovner AR. Agenda setting for healthcare management research. Report of a conference. *Health Care Manage Rev.* 2003;28(4):319–22.

43. Agency for Healthcare Research and Quality. Main DS. Meeting: Assessing organizational features to improve the quality of primary care. Denver, Colo. June 12–14, 2002.

44. Agency for Healthcare Research and Quality. Wagner E. Meeting: Congress on improving chronic care: Innovations in research and practice. Seattle, Wash. September 8–10, 2002.

45. Agency for Healthcare Research and Quality. Wears RL. Meeting: Creating the organizational infrastructure for patient safety: Needs assessment, research base, and research opportunities. Ann Arbor, Mich. November 16–18, 2001.

46. Agency for Healthcare Research and Quality. User Liaison Program. Meeting: Leading health care to a new level of safety: Lessons from high hazard industries. Park City, Utah. February 6–7, 2004.

47. American College of Healthcare Executives (ACHE). 2004 ACHE Annual Meeting. ACHE/AHRQ-conducted focus group. Chicago, Il. March 1, 2004.

48. Agency for Healthcare Research and Quality. *National Healthcare Quality Report 2003.* Available at: http://www.qualitytools.ahrq.gov/qualityreport/download_report.aspx. Accessed on December 3, 2004.

49. Agency for Healthcare Research and Quality. *National Healthcare Disparities Report 2003.* Available at: http://www.qualitytools.ahrq.gov/disparitiesreport/archivdownload_report. aspx. Accessed on June 5, 2005.

50. Moore P. Outside insights: What Dr. Gabow learned from FedEx and Ritz-Carlton. *Physicians Practice: The Business Journal for Physicians.* October 2004.

51. Gabow P. Microsystem changes within hospitals and health systems. Presentation at AHRQ meeting, Transforming Health Systems Through Leadership, Design, and Incentives. Rockville, Md. October 18, 2004.

52. Balas EA, Boren SA. Managing clinical knowledge for healthcare improvement. *Yearbook of Med Informatics.* Bethesda, MD: National Library of Medicine; 2000.

53. Robert Wood Johnson Foundation. Pursuing perfection: Raising the bar for healthcare performance. Available at: http://www.ihi.org/IHI/Programs/PursuingPerfection/Pursuing Perfection.htm. Accessed on January 19, 2005.

54. Agency for Healthcare Research and Quality. Major health plans and organizations join AHRQ to reduce racial and ethnic disparities in health care. Press release. Available at: http://www.ahrq.gov/news/press/pr2004/dispcolpr.htm. Accessed on December 30, 2004.

55. Agency for Healthcare Research and Quality. Fact sheet: Primary care practice-based research networks (PBRNs). Available at: http://www.ahrq.gov/research/pbrnfact.htm. Accessed on December 30, 2004.

56. Agency for Healthcare Research and Quality. Welcome to HIVnet. Available at: http://ahrq.gov/data/hivnet.htm. Accessed on January 25, 2005.

57. Agency for Healthcare Research and Quality. Fact Sheet: Integrated Delivery System Research Network (IDSRN). Available at: http://ahrq.gov/research/idsrn.htm. Accessed on December 30, 2004.

58. Fraser I. Organizational research with impact: working backwards. *Worldviews Evid-based Nurs.* 2004;3rd QTR(Suppl. 1):S52–S59.

Chapter 15

Medical Education for Safety

Judith Owens
Alon Y. Avidan

EXECUTIVE SUMMARY

Patient safety can be considered one of the most important aspects of medical health care. There is nothing more contrary to the healthcare philosophy and mission than causing injury or harm to the patient who searches for care.[1] Striking examples that have gained considerable media attention includes a seventeen-year-old who died as a result of a blood-type mismatch in a heart-lung transplant operation and another patient who died after removal of the wrong kidney.[2,3] The Institute of Medicine (IOM) report on the quality of care titled "To Err is Human" states that errors cause between 44,000 and 98,000 deaths every year in American hospitals.[4] This equals and exceeds the number killed in traffic accidents per year[43,45] or those who die yearly from breast cancer.[42,30]

This unfortunate and unacceptable epidemic of error in healthcare, and lack of awareness of its importance, sends a clear call to educators to address the issue of patient safety.[5] This call should be heard by undergraduate and postgraduate medical educators as well as faculty, program directors, administrators, and academic personal involved in education. In fact, when it comes to patient safety, an effective and successful educational program is probably one of the most important ingredients to prevent injury. Finally, safety and quality need to be integrated into undergraduate medical school curriculum at the contextual level.[6] Students need to see the links between scientific advances and improving healthcare outcomes. Patients are a part of the problem and must be part of the solution. Patients need to play a more active role in their own medical care and need to learn about self management and how to communicate effectively with doctors.

LEARNING OBJECTIVES

1. To discuss the rationale for including education regarding patient safety at all levels of medical education.
2. To review the basic components of a patient safety curriculum for healthcare professionals.

3. To outline the various teaching methods as well as specific educational programs that have been shown to be effective in educating healthcare professionals about patient-safety issues.

4. To use resident education regarding sleep loss and fatigue to illustrate the complex interaction between medical education, science, policy, and the "culture of medicine."

5. To use resident education in sleep loss and fatigue to illustrate a model for patient safety education.

KEYWORDS

Medical Education
Medical Error Prevention Strategies
Sleep Loss
Fatigue

Introduction to Patient Safety Education

The acquisition of medical knowledge is incremental. As the new quota of information is accepted, it is added to existing dogma. Paradoxically, perhaps the greatest discovery of the last millennium was not new data but rather a latent phenomenon already imbedded within the clinical practice: medical errors. From this discovery a new and critically important discipline has emerged—the science of error prevention in healthcare. Patient safety education is currently taught by instilling a sense of deep personal responsibility in student practitioners.[7] To promote safety, medical educators will have to introduce new concepts from the safety sciences without losing the advantages that the values of commitment and responsibility have gained. There needs to be a group of safety education practitioners who can understand and implement safe practice innovations in the clinical setting and will be instrumental in changing the medical professional cultures.[7] In order to promote a successful educational initiative, there needs to be a cultural willingness to accept a change. Unfortunately, patients and physicians in the United States live and interact in an atmosphere characterized by anger, blame, guilt, fear, frustration, and distrust regarding healthcare errors.[8] Error prevention and error detection and correction before harm are paramount. Key questions such as who should be educated, what should be taught, when it should be taught, and how it should be taught need to be answered as key ingredients for a successful safety education program.[7]

Who Should Be Taught?

The students who should be taught patient safety include all those in training within the education system: medical students, nurses, pharmacists, social workers, para medics, and those in all other applicable fields. The educational initiative should extend beyond the classroom and the medical ward.[7] One of the greatest hurdles will likely be the education of our colleagues in current practice. They are a captive audience and will readily pick up attitudes and customs that we teach and adopt ourselves. However, it will be more challenging to change the attitude and belief systems of those currently in practice whose habits are ingrained and well entrenched. Old dogs take longer to learn new tricks. Considerable effort therefore will be required to socialize existing faculty into new cultures of medical error reduction.[7] The second group of students, and probably the toughest, will consist of administrators, managers, and supervisors.

What Should Be Taught?

The curriculum depends on the student targeted. The starting point of educational curriculum for those in training should be basic error theory.[7] The core curriculum should include educational initiatives directed toward individual response to error. Historically, physicians have taken the major responsibility for adverse outcomes both emotionally and legally.[7] The individual response has often been maladaptive, involving excessive self-recrimination and the use of inappropriate, counterproductive defense mechanisms. A better understanding and more open discussion of error will go a long way toward demystifying these issues. Further insights can be gained from faculty who have expertise in coping with and minimizing the impact of medical error. The educational activity in safety curriculum can fall into three areas: procedural, effective, and cognitive.[7] Each discipline has a repertoire of procedural skills that is fairly specific, although some overlap occurs. Procedural errors are often those that fall into the domain of providers who often engage in procedural skills. Errors are made primarily by all those who interact with patients, nurses, physicians, paramedics, and social workers. In part they arise from transference and attribution phenomena. The cognitive process is one that we often spend the greatest portion of our time. Another core feature is the role of feedback. It is difficult to imagine any progress being made unless we can learn from errors.

When Should Safety Education Be Taught?

The traditional approach to patient safety is reactive and stimulated by an error. Other times that capitalize on patient safety issues are just prior to an institutional review or program accreditation.[9] However, more proactive, regularly scheduled educational programs should be geared to preventing errors in the first place. For patient safety initiatives to have a meaningful impact, the "when" is now.[9]

How Should Safety Education Be Taught?

It has become abundantly clear over the last few decades that there are more ways of teaching than the traditional didactic method.

1. *Didactic sessions* remain a useful basic technique for getting information across to a large group efficiently in a short space of time and will form an integral part of most educational curriculum. Presentations can be made more effectively with visual aides such as graphics, charts, figures, cartoons, and videos.[7]

2. *Small group tutorials* were pioneered in the 1960s by McMaster University Medical College. The vehicle is problem-based learning (PBL). The tutorial-style PBL taught across North American medical schools fosters self-directed learning. PBLs are defined as learning that results from a process of working toward the understanding or the resolution of a problem and is considered more nurturing and enjoyable than traditional methods.[7]

3. *Narrative account and clinical cases.* These have long been features of clinical teachings. However, they can suffer from the typical problems associated with anecdotal accounts such as selective reminiscence, embellishment, or exaggeration; failure to take into account ambient conditions; and lack of statistical validity. Nevertheless, if these limitations are recognized they can serve as a vivid and powerful tool for gaining the attention of attendees as well as practicing physicians.[7] This is reflected in the observation that case reports are the most frequently read sections of medical journals, and supports the model that expertise is acquired only through a combination of experience and the repetition of meaningful anecdotes.[7]

4. *Workshops* share many of the features and advantages of small group learning. Through their less structured and open-ended format they allow a greater freedom of thought and creativity and encourage novelty in the search for solutions.

5. *High-fidelity simulation (HFS)* is a powerful technique and can work in several ways. It refers to artificial representation of a real-world process to achieve educational goals via experiential learning.[10] The key advantages of this educational device is that there is no risk to the patient; errors can be simulated in the clinical setting and require no immediate intervention by a supervisor; the simulation can be "frozen" at any stage to allow for a discussion of the situation; and recording, replying to, and critiquing of performance are facilitated as there are no issues of patient safety.[10] Simulation includes the techniques whereby the novice can mentally rehearse or walk through a clinical problem off-line without having experienced the real problem personally. It is a form of gaining experience without experience. An example would be the near virtual reality procedures, such as intubation, laparoscopy, and ultrasounds that can be done using sophisticated inanimate models.[7,11]

6. *Morbidity and Mortality Conferences (M & M Conferences):* The traditional format involves a review and discussion of all morbidities and mortalities that have occurred on the ward over a specified period of time. Emphasis is

placed on evaluating complications and deaths in the context of literature and experience with similar situations, with the goal of optimizing patient care to minimize future complications.[12] A culture of patient safety is strengthened when the individuals share a basic understanding of the problem. The M & M Conference is one of academic medicine's most invaluable forums for discussion of adverse events and errors.[13,14] It allows physicians to learn and prevent, rather than blame and hide. Recently McCafferty & Polk introduced a new "Near-Miss" that sets a goal of improving patient safety utilizing an internal reporting format. The cases presented introduce physicians in training to the concept of system-based learning through the evaluation of healthcare delivery as a series of interlinked processes that are best broken down into component parts and changed to effect improvement in healthcare delivery.[12]

7. *Web-based Educational Tools:* The Agency for Healthcare Research and Quality launched a monthly peer-reviewed, Web-based medical journal that showcases patient safety lessons drawn from actual cases of medical errors. Called AHRQ WebM&M (Morbidity and Mortality Rounds on the Web), the Web-based journal (http://webmm.ahrq.gov) was developed to educate healthcare providers about medical errors in a blame-free environment. Other unique features of this site include expert analysis of medical errors reported anonymously by readers, interactive learning modules on patient safety "Spotlight Cases," as well as forums for online discussion. CME credit is available.

8. *Continuing Medical Education (CME).* Continuing education and improvement of medical practice has long been a tradition in the medical profession. A key ingredient of this tradition has been a focus on recognizing and learning from medical error.[15] There are many CME safety education opportunities for physicians. A core patient safety curriculum for education of clinicians has been previously created.[15] Although a nascent science in which much remains to be learned, the applications of human factors, engineering, systems science, information science, and computer technology are widely acknowledged to hold great promise for reducing medical error and improving patient safety. These converging disciplines, combined with advances in our understanding of how continuing education can be designed to change clinical practice, offer an opportunity to effectively refocus physicians' continuing education on medical error and patient safety.

The VA National Center for Patient Safety in Ann Arbor, Michigan, has pioneered such CME activities. For example, in one program titled "Improving Patient Safety in Hospitals: Turning Ideas into Action," which took place in 2002, clinician and administrative leaders were provided practical, real-life examples of best practices to improve patient safety and reduce adverse events for hospitalized patients. The speakers and panelists included national and community leaders in the patient safety movement. The program's goals included understanding how to foster transparency and a "culture of safety" in hospitals; learning how to analyze the root causes of an adverse event, and to transform that learning into gains in quality and safety; and understanding successful implementation of practical changes that improve safety and reduce adverse events for hospitalized patients.

Another CME module addressing patient safety is the "Patient Safety: The Other Side of the Quality Equation." Its curriculum addresses seven broad domains that have been shown to exert a powerful influence on patient safety. The curriculum familiarizes participants with the key issues underlying patient safety and offers tools on how to achieve patient safety in the ambulatory care setting. This safety module curriculum targets various disciplines of patient safety. It targets "Systems" by attempting to change the culture of blame-and-shame to systems-centered problem-solving case studies illustrating how systemic breakdowns cause adverse events. It utilizes techniques for safety improvement and take-home points to help physicians apply systems-thinking in their practices. Another component of the curriculum examines "Medication Errors" describing where and how medication errors occur, illegible handwriting, look-alike and sound-alike drug names, and proven strategies to reduce these errors.

9. *Patient safety resources.* Joint Commission Resources (JCR) is a not-for-profit subsidiary of JCAHO that provides services independently and confidentially, disclosing no information about its clients to JCAHO or others. JCR offers a number of seminars, programs, publications, Web-based training, good practices, custom education, and consultation on patient safety, including: environment of care, restraint and seclusion, failure mode and effects analysis, prevention of medical errors, medication use, preventing sentinel events, risk reduction strategies, and how to conduct root-cause analyses. JCR publishes *Joint Commission Perspectives on Patient Safety,* a monthly newsletter dedicated to providing information on the prevention of errors in healthcare settings. A bimonthly newsletter, *Environment of Care News,* focuses on patient and facility safety issues. For more information or to place an order, visit JCR's Web site, www.jcrinc.com, or call the JCR toll-free customer service line at (877) 223-6866. JCAHO's Web site also provides information on sentinel events and the Sentinel Event Policy; how to complete root cause analyses; sentinel event reporting forms; and issues of *Sentinel Event Alert.*

10. *Patient Safety Awareness Week (PSAW).* PSAW is a national education and awareness-building campaign for improving patient safety at the local level. Hospitals and healthcare organizations across the country are encouraged to plan events to promote patient safety within their own organizations. Educational activities are centered on educating patients on how to become involved in their own healthcare, as well as working with hospitals to build

partnerships with their patient community. Patient Safety Awareness Week was launched in March 2002 by Ilene Corina, president of PULSE of New York and co-chair of the National Patient Safety Foundation's (NPSF) Patient and Family Advisory Council, and endorsed by the NPSF and the local Veterans Administration Hospital.

11. *National Patient Safety Foundation.* The foremost advocate of the public in regard to safety education is the National Patient Safety Foundation, which was established under the auspices of the American Medical Association in 1997 and is committed to the improvement of patient safety in the delivery of heathcare.

Who Should Be Teaching Safety Education?

Those who are currently interested in the science of error prevention in medicine and those who have brought it to its inception are by definition its first teachers.[7] Much of the pioneer work in the field of error came from diverse areas such as behavioral science, industry, and engineering. Medicine has unfortunately been a fairly late arrival, with anesthesia taking the early initiative. The faculty should develop scientific curriculum and hold regular seminars and workshops to promote and develop interdisciplinary communications and relationships.

An Educational Model: Sleep, Alertness, and Fatigue Education in Residency

In light of recent advances in circadian and sleep biology, the traditional practices regarding work hours for medical trainees have begun to raise important questions. How does sleep loss and fatigue affect learning, patient safety, medical errors, and trainees' lives? In particular, the long continuous shifts, reduced opportunities for sleep, and minimal recuperation time traditionally experienced by medical students and house staff during training—and frequently by physicians in practice as well—are likely to impact on their work, health, well-being, and the quality of their educational experience.[16,17] However, to a large extent, progress in addressing the issue of sleep loss and fatigue in medical training has been hampered both by the absence of a coordinated and comprehensive body of research, and by the potential political, professional, and economic repercussions of any proposed systemwide changes in current practices. Furthermore, it is necessary to view the existing empirical data on sleep and fatigue in medical training within the historical, political, and scientific context in which they have evolved, in order to fully understand the implications of these findings.

In particular, several separate but related series of developments have converged over the past fifteen years to provide the impetus for what is clearly now a heightened interest in and policy development regarding this issue. The first development was increasing pressure in the past several years from medical student and resident groups to institute state and federal regulation of work hours as the primary strategy to address sleep loss and fatigue in residents. New York is currently the only state to date that has enacted legislation related to resident work hours, an action that evolved from the 1989 recommendations of the Bell Commission, a task force established by the New York State Commissioner of Health to investigate the death of a young woman named Libby Zion at a New York City teaching hospital in 1988.[18] Reports of widespread violations of the New York regulations and concern about the ability of medical education and professional organizations to enforce compliance with RRC work hour standards eventually helped to prompt the filing of a petition with the Occupational Health and Safety Administration (OSHA) by several trainee groups in the spring of 2001.[19] Similar requirements were subsequently incorporated into bills introduced in the House of Representatives (HR 3236) by Representative John Conyers and in the Senate (S. 2614) by Senator Jon Corzine in 2001/2. In response to mounting pressure, in September 2001 the ACGME charged its Work Group on Resident Duty Hours and the Learning Environment with developing a set of recommendations regarding common requirements for resident duty hours across accredited programs in all medical specialties. These recommendations—which include an eighty-hour work-week; continuous duty hours limited to twenty-four hours; and one day in seven free of patient duties, went into effect on July 1, 2003.

At the same time that these political developments were occurring, public interest in the issue of sleep loss and fatigue in medical training was galvanized by the National Academy of Sciences Institute of Medicine report, "To Err is Human" released in spring of 2000,[20] which stressed the need to investigate and address human factors that are potentially involved in violations of patient safety, such as sleep deprivation. Political pressure and public concern alone, however, could not form the basis for a rational and informed discussion of the issue of sleep and fatigue in medical training without the addition of a third element, namely, an expanded understanding of the science of sleep loss and fatigue. The existence of supporting data from research regarding the effects of sleep loss and fatigue in laboratory studies of animals and humans,[21-27] from field studies in other occupations, and from studies directly addressing residency training, is obviously critical to the formulation of an empirical approach to this issue.

What Do We Know?

The consequences related to sleep loss and shift work for physicians in training, like those in any occupational setting, are potentially broad in scope and are likely to occur in a number of domains. They include personal and family consequences (mood disturbances, increased stress, ill health, negative effects on personal relationships, increased potential for alcohol and substance abuse, and increased risk of motor vehicle crashes); negative effects on cognitive and neurobehavioral function ing (attention, reaction time, vigilance, memory, as well as motivation); impact on the performance of professional duties (including procedures such as intravenous insertion, cognitive tasks such as electrocardiogram interpretation, and patient-related behavior such as communications skills); and implications for the quality of medical education (decreased retention of information, impaired information processing, and decreased motivation to learn). Finally, the net impact of potential deficits related to sleep loss and fatigue in residency training on the quality of patient care and on commission of errors in the hospital setting is of particular concern in this era of increasing accountability in healthcare.

To date, there are over fifty studies in the literature on sleep loss and fatigue in medical training, including thirty-three performance studies[28-61] that have examined specific effects on a variety of different performance and performance-related measures. These outcome variables can be broadly categorized as effects on neurocognitive and psychomotor functioning in the laboratory setting, on performance of simulated work-related tasks and of occupational tasks in actual work settings, and on mood and psychologic state. The design of most of these studies involves comparisons between pre-call ("rested") and post-call performance in a group of residents.

Although the evidence linking sleep loss and fatigue and negative outcomes in many studies is quite compelling, it is also sometimes inconsistent and inconclusive. This result is not surprising, given the wide variation in the methodology, study design, and subject characteristics employed in the studies. However, a number of conclusions can be drawn from a review of the current literature.

1. Resident physicians, particularly those at more junior levels of training and those in the surgical specialties, *routinely experience significant levels of sleep deprivation* in the work setting, and are frequently required to function under conditions that are likely to lead to compromised levels of alertness.

2. In general, the *speed or efficiency* of neurocognitive and psychomotor task completion has been found to be more affected by restricted sleep than has the quality or accuracy of performance, although increased mental effort appears to mitigate these effects in the short-term in some studies. Similar to what has been found with performance on neurobehavioral tasks in the laboratory setting, simulated tasks dependent on high and/or sustained levels of vigilance, those of longer duration, and those that involve newly learned procedural skills appear to be more vulnerable to the effects of short-term sleep loss in medical trainees. In addition, efficiency of performance on real-world tasks is often sacrificed in favor of preserving accuracy, a factor that could have significant impact in situations that require both speed and precision (intubation of a critically ill patient, for example).

3. There is little evidence in the literature on the effects of sleep loss on performance to support *adaptation* to or development of increased tolerance for the effects of sleep loss over time in human beings. In particular, those studies of medical trainees that have examined the relative impact of

fatigue in different populations have failed to demonstrate any attenuation of impairment with increasing level of training.

4. Although the data is rather sparse, *clinical performance* in actual medical settings, particularly in surgery and anesthesia, appear to be significantly compromised by degrees of sleep loss typically experienced by residents during training.

5. Negative effects of sleep loss on *mood* in medical trainees is one of the most consistent findings in the literature on this topic, paralleling what is known about the effects of sleep deprivation in humans in general.

6. Residents commonly report negative effects of sleep loss on their *physical health,* including increased somatic complaints; changes in weight; and self-reported increases in stress level; accidents and injuries; and alcohol and stimulant use.[62] An increase in a number of *pregnancy-related complications*—pregnancy-induced hypertension, abruptio placenta and pre-term labor, and adverse fetal outcomes such as low birth weight and intrauterine growth retardation—has also been reported among trainees.[63] An increased risk of morbidity and mortality related to *drowsy driving accidents* in medical trainees, is also supported by a number of studies.[64,65]

7. Although there are only a handful of studies that have examined the impact of sleep loss and fatigue on learning and on *medical education,* the data suggests that residents are able to compensate on tests of factual knowledge for the negative effects of sleep loss and fatigue and that they are appropriately confident about their performance, but the same trainees' motivation to learn appears to be significantly impacted by inadequate sleep.

Finally, for a number of reasons, including the difficulties inherent in proving a direct causal relationship between fatigue and adverse medical events, and the lack of systems for reporting various types of adverse events and errors, there have been few studies to date that have examined the specific *contribution of sleep deprivation to actual medical errors.* Several recent studies, in attempting to unravel this relationship, have employed a number of different methodologies to assess prevalence, type, and risk factors for medical errors,[66–69] but no study to date has conclusively demonstrated a direct causal relationship between fatigue and medical errors in the healthcare. However, given the fact that most of the studies cited here show some adverse affects of sleep loss and fatigue in medical trainees on neurocognitive function and performance of occupational tasks, it is logical to postulate that sleep loss in medical trainees has significant potential to compromise the margin of safety in the delivery of patient care. In addition, fatigued residents might be less likely to seek out additional information after an incident, thereby potentially reducing the opportunity to avoid future similar errors. Furthermore, the almost universal effects on affective domains (e.g., mood, motivation) and the many negative effects on performance outcomes would naturally be expected to have some impact on communication and interaction with patients and on professionalism. Thus, fatigue affects the quality of the provider-patient relationship.

The Case for Sleep Education

Given the accumulation of evidence cited, which supports the existence of a significant negative impact of sleep loss and fatigue on patient care and on trainees themselves, regulation of work hours and other operational changes such as scheduling adjustments would seem to be a necessary and perhaps sufficient step in addressing these concerns. However, there is both anecdotal and empirical evidence to suggest that operational or system changes in and of themselves do not guarantee well-rested and optimally functioning residents. There are a number of reasons for this observation. First, it is clear from recent experience that system changes can be very difficult to implement and maintain. Second, it is unlikely that work hour regulations alone could counteract the pervasive influence of the culture of medical training that requires and even encourages physicians, in the interest of patient care, to survive and function on little or no sleep; nor are regulations alone likely to eliminate resistance to change in the current system on the part of the medical profession itself. Third, work hour regulations and other system changes cannot by definition govern residents' behavior outside of the workplace (e.g., moonlighting activities) or establish their personal priorities regarding adequate sleep, and thus cannot ensure that residents are adequately rested. In a striking illustration of the complexity and challenges involved in implementing system changes to address sleep and fatigue, one study that examined the impact of a "night float" on-call coverage system on resident performance found that, counter to expectations, the "covered" residents who had protected time for sleep actually obtained *less* sleep overall than the residents who were relieved by the night float.[52] The authors concluded that the covered residents used their protected time to catch up on work, not sleep.

In addition to scheduling and other systems changes, industries such as transportation and aviation that face similar challenges in fatigue management have also examined the impact of personal fatigue management strategies, or countermeasures, in mitigating the effects of sleep deprivation on workers. The most effective countermeasure for sleepiness is clearly sleep; thus, the efficacy of napping in combating the effects of fatigue has been an active area of research in the laboratory as well as in other occupational settings. Other sleep-related behavioral strategies to enhance alertness in occupational settings have included use of a variety of sleep schedules (including anchor and split-sleep periods); judicious and appropriately timed use of caffeine; timed manipulation of light exposure; and education regarding principles of sleep hygiene.[70,71] One review article examining the impact of shift work in emergency medicine[72] proposed the use of both operational and personal strategies to optimize alertness. The program included: an educational component on sleep physiology, circadian rhythms, and sleep hygiene that was based on a fatigue countermeasure program developed by NASA; institution of a shift rotation schedule that adhered to accepted chronobiologic principles (i.e., rotating shifts in a clockwise direction, limiting consecutive night shifts); and use of a variety of countermeasure strategies by the physicians (use of caffeine, napping).

The overriding goal of any recommendations or policies regarding sleep and fatigue in medical training should be to ensure that medical trainees receive adequate rest to enable them to perform and learn at their optimal level on a consistent basis. Educational interventions regarding the antecedents and consequences of sleep loss and fatigue and alertness management strategies that are targeted at faculty, medical students, and hospital administrators (and other hospital personnel), as well as resident physicians, are a necessary part of any comprehensive and integrated approach to this issue. Education is a necessary part of affecting any substantial and sustained behavioral change on the individual level (i.e., the individual needs to understand the rationale for the changes in order to "buy into" them), and also accepts personal responsibility for instituting them. Education at the systems-wide level is also a critical part of affecting change; from a social dynamic perspective, one of the most powerful identified barriers to adherence to work-hour regulations is the culture of the workplace and, on a pragmatic level, systems-wide changes need to support and complement the changes in individuals. Furthermore, education is the only vehicle for affecting changes in lifestyle or personal behaviors that impact on fatigue and alertness, but is not likely to be amenable to external regulation.

However, medical students and house officers typically receive little or no education about normal sleep and circadian rhythms, or the essential role of sleep in maintaining adequate health and performance. Therefore, the content of a sleep education curriculum should include basic principles of sleep and chronobiology; the impact of sleep deprivation in experimental settings, occupational settings, and medical settings; common myths and misconceptions about sleep loss and fatigue; principles of sleep hygiene; use of countermeasures; and operational changes. Furthermore, because current medical education standards require application of rigorous methodologic criteria for outcome measures and demonstration of efficacy of teaching methods and tools, changes in knowledge, competence, and behavior in residents, faculty (including residency and program directors), and hospital administration as well as measures of organizational/cultural change at these institutions across time must also be systematically examined.

Case Study

The SAFER Program

The SAFER (Sleep, Alertness, and Fatigue Education in Residency) program was developed under the auspices of the American Academy of Sleep Medicine (AASM) in 2003 to address the knowledge gap that exists in regard to the impact of sleep loss and fatigue in medical training, and potential management strategies. The goal of the SAFER program is to increase knowledge and awareness about sleep and fatigue among medical students and residents, and to help create a learning environment that maintains optimal performance and alertness. The first specific objective in achieving that goal was to develop an educational curriculum module for medical professionals on sleep, fatigue, and alertness management and to make it available to every residency program in the country; the module was also designed to be easily adaptable to a variety of target audiences including medical students, residents, residency directors, hospital administrators, and support staff (other healthcare professionals who work with medical trainees as well as for residents' families). The SAFER curriculum was developed by a task force of individuals with diverse backgrounds and expertise in sleep medicine, medical education/curriculum development, and residency training programs headed by members of the AASM Board and AASM Medical School Education Committee, as well as resident representatives, and representatives from ACGME and the AMA. The SAFER program also stresses the importance of supporting balanced, evidence-based, and socially responsible policies regarding sleep, and sleep loss and fatigue in medical education settings, and provides standardized and empirically based information, including strategies that have already been developed in other industries facing similar needs (transportation, aeronautics).

SAFER Curriculum Content

The basic content areas of the SAFER curriculum include:

- Principles of sleep and chronobiology
- Impact of sleep loss and fatigue on medical trainees (mood, health and safety, work performance, medical education, medical errors)
- Myths and misconceptions about sleep loss and fatigue
- Framework for developing strategies at the systems levels and at the individual level for addressing and managing sleep loss and fatigue.

The fifty-minute PowerPoint presentation is designed to be given by non-sleep as well as sleep medicine faculty to a variety of target audiences, and to present an educational overview of the issues that is both accessible and pragmatic. Most of the key educational points are contained in the content of the slides themselves; the accompanying speaker's syllabus was developed to provide users with the empirical basis for the slide presentation content, and to supplement the information contained herein. The syllabus also contains a pre- and post-test evaluation tool for assessment of educational goals and objectives.

Study/Discussion Questions

1. What are the appropriate target audiences for patient safety education efforts?

2. Describe barriers that currently exist in the development of adequate patient safety education programs for medical professionals.

3. Describe and discuss the relative advantages and disadvantages of different formats (didactic lectures, case discussion, high fidelity simulation, M&M conferences, etc.) for teaching healthcare professionals and trainees about patient safety.

4. Discuss the historical, political, and scientific context in which the 2003 ACGME work-hour regulations for medical residents evolved.

5. Summarize the key findings in the literature regarding the impact of sleep loss and fatigue on performance in medical trainees.

6. Describe the key components of a sleep loss and fatigue educational program for residents.

Suggested Readings/Web Sites

AHRQ Morbidity and Mortality Rounds on the Web, also known as WebM&M (http://webmm.ahrq.gov).

Joint Commission Perspectives on Patient Safety (http://www.jcrinc.com).

National Patient Safety Foundation (http://www.npsf.org).

American Academy of Sleep Medicine, The SAFER Program (http://www.aasmnet.org).

The Association of Perioperative Nursing (AORN) has developed a site devoted to patient safety in the OR with support from Sandel Medical Industries. It provides numerous resources news, and an educational module on patient safety (http://www.patientsafetyfirst.org).

APIC Association of Professionals in Infection Control and Epidemiology (APIC) provides a series of topics for continuing education credit including a full-length module on Patien Safety (http://www.apic.org).

ASHRM American Society of Healthcare Risk Management (ASHRM) provides a number of pub lications and videos for minimal fees. Disclosure of Medical Errors: Demonstrated Strategy to Enhance Communication, a one-hour video produced by ASHRM, focuses on risk man agement strategies to approach disclosure (www.ahaonlinestore.com/).

Pearls for Medication Error Reduction is a pocket guide to medication error reduction. It covers issues such as the five most common medication errors, system errors, high risk drugs problematic devices, training, and effective communication (www.ahaonlinestore.com).

Patient Safety Program: A free Patient Safety Training Resource from Healthcare Quality Special ist. Brown-Spath & Associates, Forest Grove, Oregon. (http://www.brownspath.com).

VA National Center for Patient Safety (www.patientsafety.gov).

References

1. Marin HF. Improving patient safety with technology. *Int J Med Inf.* 2004;73(7–8):543–46.
2. Campion EW. A death at Duke. *NEJM.* 2003;348(12):1083–84.
3. Dyer C. Doctors go on trial for manslaughter after removing wrong kidney. *BM.* 2002;324:1476

4. Institute of Medicine. *To Err Is Human: Building a Safer Health System.* Washington, DC: National Academy Press; 1999.

5. Holmes JH, Balas EA, Boren SA. A guide for developing patient safety curricula for undergraduate medical education. *J Am Med Inform Assoc.* 2002;9(6 Suppl):S124–27.

6. Goode LD, Clancy CM, Kimball HR, Meyer G, Eisenberg JM. When is "good enough"? The role and responsibility of physicians to improve patient safety. *Acad Med.* 2002; 77(10):947–52.

7. Croskerry P, Wears RL, Binder LS. Setting the educational agenda and curriculum for error prevention in emergency medicine. *Acad Emerg Med.* 2000;7(11):1194–1200.

8. Leape LL, Woods DD, Hatlie MJ, Kizer KW, Schroeder SA, Lundberg GD. Promoting patient safety by preventing medical error. *JAMA.* 1998;280(16):1444–47.

9. Cook DJ, Montori VM, McMullin JP, Finfer SR, Rocker GM. Improving patients' safety locally: Changing clinician behavior. *Lancet.* 2004;363(9416):1224–30.

10. Flanagan B, Nestel D, Joseph M. Making patient safety the focus: Crisis resource management in the undergraduate curriculum. *Med Educ.* 2004;38(1):56–66.

11. Seymour NE, Gallagher AG, Roman SA, et al. Virtual reality training improves operating room performance: Results of a randomized, double-blinded study. *Ann Surg.* 2002; 236(4):458–63.

12. McCafferty MH, Polk HC. Addition of "near-miss" cases enhances a quality improvement conference. *Arch Surg.* 2004;139(2):216–17.

13. Harbison SP, Regehr G. Faculty and resident opinions regarding the role of morbidity and mortality conference. *Am J Surg.* 1999;177(2):136–39.

14. Orlander JD, Barber TW, Fincke BG. The morbidity and mortality conference: The delicate nature of learning from error. *Acad Med.* 2002;77(10):1001–6.

15. Elkin PL, Gorman PN. Continuing medical education and patient safety: An agenda for lifelong learning. *J Am Med Inform Assoc.* 2002;9(6 Suppl):S128–32.

16. Veasey S, Rosen R, Barzansky B, Rosen I, Owens J. Sleep loss and fatigue in residency training: A reappraisal. *JAMA.* 2002;288:1116–24.

17. Howard SK, Gaba DM, Rosekind MR, Zarcone VP. The risks and implications of excessive daytime sleepiness in resident physicians. *Acad Med.* 2002;77(10):1019–25.

18. Asch D, Parker R. The Libby Zion case: One step forward or two steps backward? *NEJM.* 1988;318:771–75.

19. Petition to the Occupational Safety and Health Administration requesting that limits be placed on hours worked by medical residents. (HRG publication #1570). Washington DC: Public Citizen Health Research Group: 2002. Available at http://www.citizen.org/publications/release.cfm?ID=6771. Accessed on September 24, 2002.

20. Institute of Medicine of the National Academies of Science Report. *To Err Is Human: Building a Safer Health System.* Washington, DC: National Academy Press; 2000.

21. Doran SM, Van Dongen HPA, Dinges DF. Sustained attention performance during sleep deprivation: Evidence of state instability. *Arch Itali Biol.* 2001;139:253–67.

22. Williams HL, Lubin A, Goodnow JJ. Impaired performance with acute sleep loss. *Psychol Monographs: Gen Appl.* 1959;73:1–26.

23. Pilcher JJ, Huffcutt AI. Effects of sleep deprivation on performance: A meta-analysis. *Sleep.* 1996;19:318–26.

24. Carskadon M, Dement WC. Cumulative effects of sleep restriction on daytime sleepiness. *Psychophysiol.* 1981;18:107–13.

25. Blagrove M, Alexander C, Horne JA. The effects of chronic sleep reduction on the performance of cognitive tasks sensitive to sleep deprivation. *Appl Cogn Psychol.* 1994;9:21–40.

26. Dinges DF, Pack F, Williams K, et al. Cumulative sleepiness, mood disturbance, and psychomotor vigilance performance decrements during a week of sleep restricted to 4–5 hours per night. *Sleep.* 1997;20:267–77.

27. Anderson CM, Maislin G, Van Dongen HP, et al. Effect of chronically reduced nocturnal sleep, with and without daytime naps, on neurobehavioral performance. *Sleep.* 2000;23:A74.

28. Hart RP, Buchsbaum DG, Wade JB, Hamer RM, Kwentus JA. Effect of sleep deprivation on first-year residents' response times, memory, and mood. *J Med Educ.* 1987;52:940–42.

29. Hawkins MR, Vichick DA, Silsby HD, Kruzich DJ, Butler R. Sleep deprivation and performance of house officers. *J Med Educ.* 1985;60:530–35.

30. Poulton EC, Hunt GM, Carpenter A, Edwards RS. The performance of junior hospital doctors following reduced sleep and long hours of work. *Ergonomics.* 1978;21:279–95.

31. Leonard C, Fanning N, Attwood J, Buckley M. The effect of fatigue, sleep deprivation and onerous working hours on the physical and mental wellbeing of pre-registration house officers. *Ir J Med Sci.* 1998;167:22–25.

32. Nelson CS, Dell'Angela K, Jellish WS, Brown IE, Skaredoff M. Residents' performance before and after night call as evaluated by an indicator of creative thought. *J Am Osteo Assoc.* 1995;95:600–3.

33. Deaconson TF, O'Hair DP, Levy MF, Lee MB, Schueneman AL, Codon RE. Sleep deprivation and resident performance. *JAMA.* 1988;260:1721–27.

34. Bartle EJ, Sun JH, Thompson L, Light AI, McCool C, Heaton S. The effects of acute sleep deprivation during residency training. *Surg.* 1988;104:311–16.

35. Reznick RK, Folse JR. Effect of sleep deprivation on the performance of surgical residents. *Am J Surg.* 1987;154:520–25.

36. Ford CV, Wentz DK. The internship year: A study of sleep, mood states, and psychophysiologic parameters. *South Med J.* 1984;77:1435–42.

37. Friedman RC, Bigger JT, Kornfeld DS. The intern and sleep loss. *NEJM.* 1971;285:201–3.

38. Lingenfelser T, Kaschel R, Weber A, Zaiser-Kaschel H, Jakober B, Kuber J. Young hospital doctors after night duty: Their task specific cognitive status and emotional condition. *Med Educ.* 1994;28:566–72.

39. Storer JS, Floyd HH, Gill WL, Giusti CW, Ginsberg H. Effects of sleep deprivation on cognitive ability and skills of pediatrics residents. *Acad Med.* 1989;64:29–32.

40. Smith-Coggins R, Rosekind MR, Hurd S, Buccino KR. Relationship of day versus night sleep to physician performance and mood. *Ann Emer Med.* 1994;24:928–34.

41. Engel W, Seime R, Powell V, D'Alessandri R. Clinical performance of interns after being on call. *South Med J.* 1987;80:761–63.

42. Christensen EE, Dietz GW, Murry RC, Moore JG. The effect of fatigue on resident performance. *Radiology.* 1977;125:103–5.

43. Gottlieb DJ, Parenti CM, Peterson CA, Lofgren RP. Effect of a change in housestaff work schedule on resource utilization and patient care. *Arch Int Med.* 1991;151:2065–70.

44. Goldman LI, McDonough MT, Rosemond GP. Stresses affecting surgical performance and learning: Correlation of heart rate, electrocardiogram and operation simultaneously recorded on videotapes. *J Surg Res.* 1972;12:83–86.

45. Haynes DF, Schwedler M, Dyslin DC, Rice JC, Kerstein MD. Are postoperative complications related to resident sleep deprivation? *S Med J.* 1995;88:283–89.

46. Taffinder NJ, McManus IC, Gul Y, Russell RC, Darzi A. Effect of sleep deprivation on surgeons' dexterity on laparoscopy simulator. *Lancet.* 1998;352:1191.

47. Grantcharov TP, Bardram L. Funch-Jensen P, Rosenberg J. Laparoscopic performance after one night on call in a surgical department: Prospective study. *BMJ.* 2001;323:1222–23.

48. Browne BJ, Van Susteren T, Onsager DR, Simpson D, Salaymeh B, Condon RE. Influence of sleep deprivation on learning among surgical house staff and medical students. *Surg.* 1994;115:604–10.

49. Godellas CV, Huang R. Factors affecting performance on the American Board of Surgery in-training examination. *Am J Surg.* 2001;181:294–96.

50. Jacques CH, Lynch JC, Samkoff JS. The effects of sleep loss on cognitive performance of resident physicians. *J Fam Pract.* 1990;30:223–29.

51. Robbins J, Gotlieb F. Sleep deprivation and cognitive testing in internal medicine house staff. *West J Med.* 1990;12:82–86.

52. Richardson GS, Wyatt JK, Sullivan JP, et al. Objective assessment of sleep and alertness in medical house staff and the impact of protected time for sleep. *Sleep.* 1996;19:718–26.

53. Light AI, Sun JH, McCool C, Thompson L, Heaton S, Bartle EJ. The effects of acute sleep deprivation on the level of resident training. *Curr Surg.* 1989;46:29–30.

54. Bertram DA. Characteristics of shifts and second-year resident performance in an emergency department. *NY State J Med.* 1988;88:10–15.

55. Klose JK, Wallace-Barnhill GL, Craythorne MWS. Performance test results for anesthesia residents over a five-day week including on-call duty. *Anesthesiol.* 1985;63;A485.

56. Denisco RA, Drummond JN, Gravenstein JS. The effect of fatigue on the performance of a simulated anesthetic monitoring task. *J Clin Monit.* 1987;3:22–24.

57. Orton DI, Gruzelier JH. Adverse changes in mood and cognitive performance of house officers after night duty. *Br Med J.* 1989;298:21–23.

58. Rubin R, Orris P, Lau SL, Hryhorczuk DO, Furner S, Letz R. Neurobehavioral effects of the on-call experience in housestaff physicians. *J Occup Med.* 1991;33:13–18.

59. Deary IJ, Tait QR. Effects of sleep disruption on cognitive performance and mood in medical house officers. *Brit Med J Clin Res Ed.* 1987;295:1513–16.

60. Parker JB. The effects of fatigue on physician performance—an underestimated cause of physician impairment and increased patient risk. *Can J Anaesth.* 1987;34:489–95.

61. Smith-Coggins R, Rosekind MR, Buccino KR, Dinges DF, Moser RP. Rotating shiftwork schedules: Can we enhance physician adaptation to night shifts? *Acad Emerg Med.* 1997;4:951–61.

62. Daugherty SR, Baldwin DC, Rowley BD. Learning, satisfaction, and mistreatment during medical internship: A national survey of working conditions. *JAMA.* 1998;279(15):1194–99.

63. Klebanoff MA, Shiono PH, Rhoads GG. Outcomes of pregnancy in a national sample of resident physicians. *NEJM.* 1990;323(15):1040–45.

64. Marcus CL, Loughlin GM. Effect of sleep deprivation on driving safety in housestaff. *Sleep.* 1996;19(10):763–66.

65. Kowalenko T, Hass-Kowalenko J, Rabinovich A, Grzybowski M. Emergency medicine residency related MVC's—is sleep deprivation a risk factor? *Acad Emerg Med.* 2000;7(5):451.

66. Jha AK, Duncan BW, Bates DW. Fatigue, sleepiness, and medical errors. In: Shojania KG, Duncan BW, McDonald KM, Wachter RM, eds. *Making healthcare safer: A critical analysis of patient safety practices.* Rockville, Md: Agency for Healthcare Research and Quality; 2001.

67. Gander PH, Merry A, Millar MM, Wellers J. Hours of work and fatigue-related error: A survey of New Zealand anaesthetists. *Anaesth Intensive Care.* 2000;28:178–83.

68. Lewittes LR, Marshall VW. Fatigue and concerns about quality of care among Ontario interns and residents. *CMAJ.* 1989;140(1):21–24.

69. Morris GP, Morris RW. Anaesthesia and fatigue: An analysis of the first 10 years of the Australian incident monitoring study 1987–1997. *Anaesth Invensive Care.* 2000;28:300–4.

70. Rosekind MR, Gander PH, Gregory KB, et al. Managing fatigue in operational settings 1: Physiological considerations and countermeasures. *Behavioral Medicine.* 1996;21:157–65.

71. Rosekind MR, Gander PH, Gregory KB, et al. Managing fatigue in operational settings: An integrated approach. *Behavioral Medicine.* 1996;21:166–70.

72. Whitehead DC, Thomas H, Slapper DR. A rational approach to shift work in emergency medicine. *Ann Emerg Med.* 1992;21:1250–58.

Chapter 16

Visions of the Future

Stephen C. Schoenbaum
Karen Davis
Annie-Marie J. Audet

EXECUTIVE SUMMARY

As has been seen in earlier chapters, America's healthcare system is the world's most expensive and complex; yet, its effectiveness is far from optimal.[1] It is neither the best nor the worst on clinical quality indicators among five English-speaking countries.[2] Care is inefficient: The cost and effectiveness of care are often not related or even can be inversely related.[3,4,5] The patient-centeredness of care could be improved, as could timeliness of provision of services, such as obtaining same-day appointments, when a patient feels s/he needs one; or spending minutes rather than hours waiting for care in emergency rooms.[6,7] Our system of care is not safe for patients who, when hospitalized, have about a 4 percent likelihood of sustaining an adverse event caused by medical management,[8,9] and neither is it safe for healthcare workers.[10]

Perhaps the greatest failing of the American healthcare system is that care in this country is more inequitable than in any other highly developed country.[11,12,13] Indeed, despite the fact that we spend more of our gross domestic product (GDP) on healthcare than any other of the OECD (Organization for Economic Cooperation and Development) countries, the United States is the only major industrialized nation that does not cover its population under a health financing system.[14] Contrary to myth, uninsured Americans do not get all the care they need;[15,16,17] and 18,000 deaths can be attributed to the inequities in care for the uninsured. There is also evidence of inequitable provision of care to minorities, including care to minority Medicare beneficiaries.[18,19] These problems are pervasive. They exist across each type of care delivered in the United States—preventive, acute, chronic, and end-of-life.

It would be easy to think that with all these problems the future of healthcare for Americans must be bleak. Yet, there is reason for optimism. National polls show that Americans support completely rebuilding the health system or at least making fundamental changes to it.[6] Healthcare leaders in the private sector increasingly conclude that a laissez-faire market strategy is not capable of achieving fundamental goals for the health system.[20] Physicians are frequently frustrated by the current system, especially in regard to rising malpractice costs; burdensome administrative costs from the proliferation of private insurance payment methods and rules; and in some cases, reduced real-net incomes.[21] There is a growing recognition that federal leadership is required to tackle fundamental problems in the system, including health insurance coverage for all. Enactment of some Medicare prescription drug coverage, after an admittedly fractious debate, at least demonstrated that Congress can act on health legislation. Other factors that bode well for the future include the inevitable improvement in the standard of living as economic growth continues to "raise all boats," and the high value that Americans place on healthcare. Major obstacles include federal budget deficits and tax cuts that impair the ability of the federal government to fulfill its commitments to Social Security and Medicare as the baby boom generation retires. These obstacles also make major new initiatives almost impossible.

LEARNING OBJECTIVES

1. To identify the factors that will shape healthcare in the future.
2. To develop knowledge of the steps involved to improve healthcare in the future.
3. To understand the critical roles of federal legislation and leadership on improving healthcare.

KEYWORDS

Health Insurance
Patient-Centeredness
Cultural Competency
Continuous Improvement
Future Design

Introduction

Healthcare for Americans can be significantly better in the future than it has been in the past. A number of individuals and organizations are responding to the challenge of envisioning a health system worthy of the twenty-first century. The Institute of Medicine has produced major reports on improving quality and health insurance coverage.[17,22,23] The House of Representatives has established a Caucus on Twenty-first Century Health Care, and numerous Congressional leaders across a broad political spectrum have set forth thoughtful ideas for the future.[24–29] While there is a major leap from ideas to action, these are promising signs on the horizon.

In 2000, Davis et al. published "A 2020 Vision for American Health Care."[28] Its components included automatic and affordable health insurance coverage for all; access to healthcare for all; patient-responsive healthcare; information-driven healthcare including care that is based on scientific evidence and supported by clinical information systems; and a commitment by each provider of healthcare and provider organization to continuous improvement of care and to betterment of health outcomes. Since then, two components to the vision have been added—having a satisfied healthcare workforce and a willingness to learn from and share lessons with other countries so that American healthcare can cross the quality chasm. The clock is ticking: In this chapter, we discuss this vision and what would need to be done to achieve it by 2020 or sooner.

Affordable Health Insurance Coverage for All

Equity is one of the six dimensions of quality-of-care outlined in 2001 by the Institute of Medicine in *Crossing the Quality Chasm.*[22] Because the lack of insurance coverage is the single most important contributor to inequitable care and subsequent poor outcomes, one cannot have a vision of crossing the quality chasm without addressing the need for adequate health insurance coverage for all Americans.

Approximately 44 million Americans were uninsured at any given time in 2002. Although this is "only" 16 percent of the population of the United States uninsured, the instability of coverage as people switch jobs or family circumstances change substantially increases the number of Americans at risk. One-quarter of all adults under age 65 in the United States are uninsured at some point during the year.[29] In addition, 85 million Americans were uninsured at some point over the four years from 1996 to 1999, representing 38 percent of Americans under age 65, and 68 percent of those with low incomes.[30] Many Americans have health insurance but benefits are so limited or cost-sharing so high that they are effectively underinsured—either unable to obtain needed care because of costs or subject to burdensome medical bills.

The consequences of being uninsured or underinsured are relatively well known.[31] The uninsured are more likely to report going without needed care; not filling prescriptions; not getting a recommended test or procedure; and not scheduling a specialist visit or follow-up visit because of cost. They are much less likely to receive preventive services, and less likely to have chronic conditions appropriately maintained. They also perceive that the quality of care they receive is less good than that received by insured patients. They also are at risk of incurring burdensome medical bills, or facing bankruptcy as a result of incurred medical debts. The result is both an economic and health toll—an estimated 18,000 lives lost per year and lost economic productivity amounting to $65 billion to $130 billion per year.[17]

Our vision for addressing this gap in coverage would be to build on existing sources of group coverage to make coverage automatic and affordable for all.[32] The tax system would be used to verify insurance coverage annually, with all uninsured individuals automatically enrolled in a source of coverage tailored to their circumstances. Tax credits would ensure that no individual or family faced a premium in excess of 5 percent of income (for those in the lowest tax brackets and

10 percent of income for those in higher tax brackets). It would be a mixed public-private system of insurance including: employer-sponsored health insurance; a new group insurance pool modeled on the Federal Employees Health Benefits Plan that we call a Congressional Health Plan; expansion of the Children's Health Insurance Program to low-income individuals with incomes below 150 percent of poverty; and expanding Medicare by eliminating the two-year waiting period for coverage of the disabled and the option of buying coverage for uninsured adults age 60 and over who do not have access to employer coverage. Coverage would be financed through a combination of savings from current sources of charity care and a 1 percent marginal income tax on all tax brackets. It is estimated that this plan would cost about $70 billion annually and would cover about forty million uninsured individuals.

Numerous political leaders have advanced plans to expand health insurance coverage.[33] While proposals differ in the extent to which they rely on expansion of private insurance coverage or public programs and the magnitude of funds committed to addressing the problem, there are areas of consensus. Public programs are generally favored for those with low incomes, while private insurance is favored for higher income individuals. Subsidies are gradated with income, providing the greatest protection to low-income uninsured. Most proposals would retain employer-sponsored coverage, and some would make that coverage more affordable by reinsuring coverage for individuals with high expenses.

Several states have also mounted pragmatic efforts to expand health insurance coverage. Maine has implemented a Dirigo Health Plan to make coverage affordable for small businesses and uninsured individuals.[34] California has enacted an employer mandate law to require larger businesses to cover employees. Minnesota has integrated five separate programs to achieve near universal coverage.[35] Rhode Island has expanded its RIte Care program to cover low-income children and their parents, and has provided standards and financial incentives to encourage managed care plans participating in the program to improve quality of care.[36]

Achieving automatic and affordable health insurance for all requires shared responsibility among patients, providers, purchasers, and payers. A recent survey finds broad support among Americans for a shared responsibility among government, employers, and individuals.[29] Patients will contribute a portion of their insurance premiums and direct out-of-pocket cost-sharing—but be guaranteed that their premium contribution will not exceed 5 percent of income (for those in the lowest tax brackets). Employers will be required to either provide insurance to employees—meeting standards on benefits and contributing at least 75 percent of the premium—or contribute either $1 per hour or 5 percent of earnings into a pool to finance coverage for workers. Government, and ultimately taxpayers, would subsidize care for low-income individuals up to 150 percent of poverty; provide tax credits; and finance reinsurance of a new group option for small businesses and uninsured individuals. Government would largely be responsible for low-income and the sickest individuals, while private insurers would provide coverage to healthier working families. Insurers would be subject to the same rules that apply to the current Federal Employees Health Benefits Plan with regard to community rating and accepting all enrollees regardless of pre-existing health conditions (after a six-month wait). Providers would also make a contribution by foregoing current subsidies for uncompensated care.

Access to Healthcare for All

There are multiple problems in accessing the American healthcare system or its components. One is cost-related lack of access to care. High out-of-pocket costs for the uninsured leads to many Americans being unable to fill a prescription; skipping doses of medications; not taking recommended tests or procedures; or being unable to see a specialist.[29,37] Another access problem is long wait times for appointments. Unduly long waits for primary care appointments or inconvenient office hours can drive Americans to seek care in emergency rooms.[38] In many care settings, but especially emergency rooms, waits for service can be long. At a minimum this creates inconvenience for the patient. At its worst, it leads to patients sustaining unnecessary pain and suffering, or to patients leaving without receiving care.

Emergency rooms merit specific mention because when their beds are crowded they tend to "go on diversion" and refuse access to all patients. This can lead to patients not being able to be seen at the nearest emergency room when time is of the essence. It can also lead to patients being seen in a healthcare system that does not include their usual physician.

Problems with access to care include the fact that 23 percent of adults do not have a regular physician, and 43 percent of adults have been with the same physician for less than five years.[39] The uninsured are particularly unlikely to have a long-term relationship with a physician; almost half have no regular physician and another third have been with a physician for less than five years. But even among insured adults 65 percent either have no regular physician or have been with the same physician for less than five years. Having a regular source of care is key as to whether individuals obtain regular preventive care and is central to a 2020 vision of healthcare that guarantees access to care. Public and private insurers should require that all enrollees enlist with a personal clinician who will assume the responsibility of a medical home—and to ensure that patients receive needed preventive, primary, and specialized services.

Successfully reducing access problems can help address a variety of quality-of-care dimensions including equity and patient-centeredness, as well as timeliness of care. Reducing the problem of cost-related access requires assuring that all Americans are adequately and stably insured, and that benefits are sufficiently comprehensive to avoid financial barriers to care. At a minimum, benefits should include preventive care, acute and chronic care, mental health, prescription drugs, and emergency dental care.

Reducing wait times requires very different approaches. For example, evidence indicates that the most likely source of emergency room congestion is not excess demand but rather inefficient operations management elsewhere in the hospital, leading to back-up or pooling of patients in the emergency room.[40] Failure to discharge hospitalized patients and prepare the beds for new arrivals can lead to unavailability of needed hospital beds for patients in the emergency room. Congestion in the emergency room can also be due to inefficient scheduling of elective surgical procedures.[41] These problems can be remedied by applying systems engineering principles and techniques.[42] Interestingly, although many hospitals consider enlarging their emergency room, this approach is less promising. Indeed, a result of increased emergency room capacity without solving the basic operations engineering problems in the hospital can simply be to increase the pool of people waiting for inpatient care in the emergency room, which is a suboptimal setting for delivering the care that regular hospital admissions need.

Physician appointment access can be shortened considerably by using the methods of "advanced access" (or "open access"), another systems engineering approach.[43,44] In the United States and United Kingdom, teams from physicians' offices, working in formal quality improvement collaboratives, have been able to shorten waits for appointments and provide many, if not most, appointments on the same day that the patient calls for one.[45,46,47]

Our vision is that insurance access for all—or increased benefits where necessary—will allow all Americans to receive care from the physicians and specialists whom they need to see. In turn, Americans will be able to receive the tests, procedures, and medications they need. By being able to avail themselves of, and adhere to, the advice of physicians and other care providers, outcomes will improve. Our vision is also that all providers will be motivated to deliver more timely care, which will require their learning and applying systems or operations engineering approaches to their organizations and practices. Less wait time for appointments and within healthcare settings is also an aspect of patient-centered care.

Ensuring access to care is also a shared responsibility. Patients need to select a personal clinician in whom they trust, and work with that physician to assure their health: obtaining recommended preventive care and adhering to medical advice and jointly agreed on treatment plans. Physicians who are selected as personal clinicians need to adopt practices, processes, and systems that guarantee care will be accessible in a way that works for patients. Insurers need to "take all comers" and provide a scientific-based package of benefits that ensures financial access to beneficial care. Employers need to ensure that worker contributions to coverage and care are affordable, given the wages of their employees. Government needs to set standards and provide financial subsidies for those unable to afford care. Public programs for low-income populations especially need to guarantee comprehensive benefits and an adequate supply of providers willing to provide care to low-income people.

Patient Responsive Healthcare

As noted by Margaret Mahoney, "By the mid-1980s, public opinion polls began to reflect patients' dissatisfaction with the way in which care is delivered in hospitals."[48] She stated further, "Medical professionals observe that patients are becoming not only less passive but downright aggressive about their own care. Responding positively to them can only help medical professionals and institutions survive and grow . . . Sharing knowledge with patients on treatment options and risks, also increases the likelihood of attracting and holding patients. Moreover, it may well decrease the possibility of later legal action by patients on the grounds of inadequate information."[48]

Patient-centeredness was listed as one of the six major elements of quality of care by the Institute of Medicine in *Crossing the Quality Chasm,* which noted that similar terms include care that is "person-centered, consumer-centered, personalized, and individualized." Research by the Picker Institute has delineated eight dimensions of patient-centered care. These include the following: 1) respecting a patient's values, preferences, and expressed needs; 2) providing information and education; 3) access to care; 4) emotional support to relieve fear and anxiety; 5) involvement of family and friends; 6) continuity and transition securely between healthcare settings; 7) physical comfort; and 8) coordination of care.[49]

In 1998, attendees at a conference in Salzburg, Austria, developed a self-described "Utopian" vision for a patient-centered healthcare system.[50] In this ideal world, the clinician-patient relationship is enhanced by "computer-based guidance and communications systems"; medical records that are Internet-based and available to the appropriate party when needed; and patients who regularly complete surveys on their experiences, which are fed back to the clinicians as "real time" information for improving care. Other attributes of this system include the following. Patients and their clinicians have contracts about quality of care, setting out individual and joint goals appropriate for the patients and their condition(s). Performance is then measured against those goals and aggregated for both clinicians and patients. Community leaders work with clinicians to integrate community resources with clinical care; and patient advocates are represented in the healthcare legislative, regulatory, and financing processes.

Although, as previously stated, there are multiple dimensions to patient-centered care, we concentrate here on two that are key: clinician-patient communication and shared decision making. Clearly, patients' comprehension and being involved in decision making *to the extent they feel is appropriate* is an essential aspect of patient-centered care. It requires clinicians who can communicate well in ways the patient can understand, currently a major deficit in American healthcare. Indeed, in the *2001 Commonwealth Fund Survey on Quality of Care,* one in five adult Americans surveyed reported that in the prior two years they had a problem understanding the doctor; felt the doctor had not listened; or reported leaving the office with unasked questions. And minorities—close to one-fourth of African Americans and up to one-third of Hispanics—were more likely to report these problems.[39]

"Cultural competency" can be considered a special case of patient-centered communication as it can hinder efforts to deal with patients of limited English proficiency and low-health literacy. These problems are beginning to be addressed at several levels and settings including medical schools and organizations such as the American Medical Association and the American College of Physicians.[51] Reducing these problems will not only make care more patient-centered but also more equitable.

Overall, it is hard to picture a patient-centered care system that does not consider and design each of its key processes from the perspective of its patients. Without considering the patient perspective, care is unlikely to be timely; but it also is less likely to be safe, equitable, and effective.

We believe that it is both possible and necessary for healthcare in the United States to become more patient-centered. The fact that there is now regular input to health plans from their members about their experiences is a very positive sign. This required the development of Consumer Assessment of Health Plans Survey (CAHPS), a public-domain survey instrument developed by the Agency for Healthcare Research and Quality (AHRQ) and required by both the Centers for Medicare & Medicaid Services for Medicare Advantage (formerly Medicare + Choice) health plans and by the National Committee for Quality Assurance (NCQA) as part of its health plan accreditation process. AHRQ is now developing a family of CAHPS surveys that will obtain standardized information on patient experiences in hospital, nursing home, and ambulatory care settings and for diverse population groups. Because feedback of performance information usually leads to performance improvement, it is likely that surveys will lead to improved patient-centered care in each of these settings—especially if coupled with tools to help physicians and their practices solve problems that patients report experiencing.[52]

Information-driven Healthcare

We live in the Information Age. Yet, the healthcare delivery industry has been slow to embrace the opportunities that information technology (IT) can offer for the improvement of care. IT can facilitate storage and retrieval of clinical data, measurement of the population served, and parameters of the care delivered. Even the most basic electronic medical records (EMR) can support these functions.[53] IT can provide support for integration of care including transfer of information as a patient moves from place to place or service to service in the course of an episode of care; it produces legible information; it can reduce the numbers of times that data is re-entered and thus reduce transcription errors; and it can reduce the likelihood that information will be lost, thus eliminating waste or the duplication of tests. Logic pathways can be built into IT systems to provide decision support or check for incompatibilities, such as medications that might cause adverse interactions. These features have allowed the development of computerized physician order entry (CPOE) systems, which have been shown to reduce adverse drug events in hospitals.[54] In this Information Age it should be a given to have IT-driven healthcare. Instead, we are at a rudimentary state of adoption. Almost all physicians' practices use computers, but primarily for administrative functions such as billing. Only one-fourth of physicians regularly or sometimes use an EMR; and less than 20 percent of physicians regularly or sometimes exchange e-mail with patients.[55] Hospitals also have computers, not only for administrative functions such as billing but also in support of hi-tech medical equipment (e.g., imaging); however, they too have been very slow to adopt clinical IT systems such as CPOE,[56] EMRs, or ones that would provide decision support for their staff.

As if this were not enough, we need more than simple IT-driven healthcare. We need information-driven healthcare, care that is based on information about individual patients and the best evidence about how to manage them, their medical problems, and their health and healthcare issues. As intelligent as those who work in healthcare are, they cannot possibly keep up with all the advances in medicine and healthcare—hence the recent emphasis on technology transfer from the research setting into practice. Even technology transfer is not sufficient, because much research looks at relatively narrow problems or patient populations and needs to be integrated into a form that can be used in the day-to-day healthcare setting. Thus, to have information-driven healthcare, we must first have the right information and then get it to the right people in the right way at the right time. Having the right information requires that appropriate information be developed and aggregated, which in turn requires the implicit or explicit development of clinical guidelines. Getting information to people who need it in a way it can be used requires translation of the aggregated information or guidelines into a variety of presentations or formats, often extracting just the portion that is likely to be needed and assuring that it is easily usable. In the past, textbooks have included much of the appropriate information. Today, this information is often out-of-date, hard to access, and not in the format that might be most suitable for the clinician or patient. Facilitating the availability of the appropriate presentation in the clinical setting is a process that IT can support. Finally, determining that the right thing was done requires measurement, another process that IT can support.

The healthcare professions have demonstrated significant resistance to this entire sequence of needed steps. In the early 1990s, the federal government supported the development of clinical guidelines through the Agency for Health Care Policy and Research (AHCPR). A guideline on the management of back pain was extremely controversial and led to the near dissolution of AHCPR.[57] Under the skillful leadership of John Eisenberg, the Agency was reconstituted as the Agency for Healthcare Research and Quality (AHRQ), but the function of developing clinical guidelines was dropped. In order to move forward on developing information-driven healthcare in the United States, it will be necessary to have national priorities or aims that can then drive the process of developing guidelines to meet those aims.

Major barriers to adoption of clinical IT systems have been a lack of standards for these systems—a problem that is beginning to be addressed at the federal level— and cost. The standards are needed to assure interoperability of different systems and to assure that information is available in forms that can be aggregated across the diverse components of the US healthcare system. With standardization, there will be less fear among those who purchase new systems that the systems will become obsolete in a short time. Also, clinical IT systems represent a major capital expenditure. Unlike other new technologies (e.g., imaging), clinical IT is not directly reimbursed by public and private payers and insurers. Raising large amounts of capital is difficult for nonprofit organizations dependent on the bond market and is almost impossible for individual physicians and partnerships. Having a well-developed clinical IT infrastructure is virtually necessary, albeit not sufficient, for making quantum leaps in improvement of clinical care. Thus, it is critically important that all payers help support its implementation.

Continuous Improvement

It is over fifteen years since Donald M. Berwick published the landmark article, "Continuous Improvement as an Ideal in Health Care."[58] Although there are now thousands of people in hospitals and group practices working on quality improvement, there is no evidence that healthcare is improving at a faster rate now than in the past. Indeed, we do not even have the basic measures for assessing progress in the United States on improving healthcare, and we know that problems in quality of care abound.[59,60] It is one thing for accreditors, such as NCQA and JCAHO, to mandate that each organization they accredit, including health plans, hospitals, and other healthcare delivery organizations, have a quality improvement program in place, and another thing to have a commitment in each institution to cross the quality chasm. Nonetheless, the seeds are planted for continuous improvement to grow as a driving principle for all healthcare organizations, and there are promising local models that could spread nationally.

For example, the Northern New England Cardiovascular Disease Study Group has systematically improved mortality rates for cardiovascular surgery across a set of collaborating hospitals.[61] At Allegheny General Hospital, in Pittsburgh, using the principles of the Toyota Production System, rates of central line-associated bloodstream infections (CLABS) were reduced in two intensive-care units by 90 percent in ninety days, to near zero, and have been maintained at very low rates over the next year—a dramatic breakthrough in control of this type of nosocomial infection and improvement in patient safety.[62]

To improve care continuously it is necessary to have appropriate information, motivation, and the knowledge, skills, and capacity to improve. Information is necessary to understand what is currently being done, so that priorities for improvement can be set, and to monitor the improvement process itself. This information will be much easier to achieve when healthcare providers in the United States adopt clinical information technologies.

Although information will be needed at every level of the healthcare system, initially much could be done with a multi-payer claims database, which could come from a collaboration among Medicare, Medicaid, and private insurers. Government could take the lead and make the database widely available to researchers and providers. After improving the accuracy and validity of the data, public information on provider quality and efficiency could be a very strong motivator for improvement.[63]

Incentives

If the United States healthcare delivery system were motivated to improve, it undoubtedly would be performing better than it currently is. One often hears that there needs to be a business case for quality improvement—in short, that quality improvement must pay a net return to those who institute improvements. It has been difficult to make such a case.[64,65] Payment for healthcare has been related to the quantity of services delivered (fee-for-service) or units of service (capitation, DRG payments), not to the quality of care delivered. There are even instances in which current payment practices appear to reward poorer care. For example, when the profit on inpatient care for a condition, such as asthma, exceeds the profit attainable on outpatient care for the same condition, there is no incentive to reach out to patients with asthma to provide them optimal ambulatory care and reduce the likelihood that they will be admitted for asthma or its complications. Or, when an inpatient complication, such as urinary tract infection, leads to a higher DRG payment, there is no incentive to avoid the complication. Or, when inpatient care is paid for at a flat rate, irrespective of length of stay, and readmissions are also paid for, there is no incentive to assure that the patient has been treated optimally at the time of discharge to avoid post-hospital complications and subsequent readmission.[66]

These problems of misaligned incentives and lack of incentives for better performance are beginning to be addressed. Insurer- or employer-initiated pay-for-performance programs are beginning to proliferate.[67] Disease management programs and case-management programs, developed by providers, insurers, or third-party disease management or case-management companies, are also attracting greater attention. Each of these programs has the potential to integrate care across traditional boundaries, such as hospital/home or physician-provided services/nonphysician-provided services (e.g., physical therapy, nutrition counseling, health education). Each is likely to be sustained when it is profitable for its sponsor, that is, there is a "business case" for the program.

Negative incentives, punishment, or threat of punishment, can also be important. These include regulations that must be met for licensure and standards that are required for accreditation. The Medicare Modernization Act of 2003 contains an interesting provision that can be thought of as either a negative or positive incentive:

The Centers for Medicare & Medicaid Services has been maintaining a database for voluntary hospital reporting of performance on a set of measures that have been endorsed by the National Quality Forum. Very few hospitals had enrolled prior to the passage of the Act. In the eight months after passage of the Act, most hospitals in the United States indicated their willingness to report on the measures, undoubtedly owing to a provision of the Act that ties Medicare payments to hospital reporting on the measures. Hospitals that choose not to report would receive 0.4 percent for each hospital admission less than hospitals that do.

There are many different types of incentives that could be developed. It is likely, given constant concerns in the United States about the cost of care, that much effort in the near future will be directed toward developing payment systems that reward a combination of higher quality or quality improvement, and better efficiency. Some incentives might need to supply operating or capital dollars, possibly as bonuses (as in most pay-for-performance systems) or as loans. Some incentives for improving patient safety could also be tied to physicians' and hospitals' expenditures on liability insurance.[68] Some could stimulate reporting of information, not only by tying these reports to payment as in the Medicare Modernization Act, but also by protecting the person who reports—a desirable way to enhance reports of medical error so that systematic approaches to improving patient safety can be devised and implemented. Some might offer a nonfinancial "carrot" by recognizing providers for exemplary performance, for example, National Committee on Quality Assurance's recognition programs for physicians who meet or exceed certain standards of care for diabetics; patients with cardiac conditions or strokes; or physician practices that use up-to-date information and systems to enhance patient care.[69]

The notion that persons engaged in the altruistic practice of healthcare delivery should need incentives troubles some critics of pay-for-performance. It is natural, however, that people generally do what is best for their customers, clients, or patients, when it is at least reasonable for themselves. It should be possible to devise incentives that help all who provide healthcare in the United States to provide the best possible care. We will know that we have a proper system of incentives when those who provide care are eager to know their own performance, are following their results regularly, can take pride in their improvement, and are setting targets for performance at the level of perfection.

Capacity to Improve

One can be motivated to improve, but not have the wherewithal to do it. Despite the fact that since the mid-1980s most healthcare providers have heard about quality improvement and many participate in quality improvement activities, most are not formally trained or skilled in quality improvement methods.

Change of habits begins with intellectual inquiry. Traditionally, much of the intellectual inquiry in medicine and medical care has come from academia. Quality improvement, however, is a field not yet fully recognized in the context of an academic achievement in medicine, nursing, or other health professions. Quality improvement interventions occur in real-time through action projects in operating organizations; and only infrequently will it be possible for serious quality improvement efforts to adopt the controlled conditions of a laboratory or clinical trial.[70] No new model of academic achievement has yet emerged that values team activities versus individual achievement and fosters or rewards the evaluation of nonrandomized quality improvement interventions and their dissemination to and adoption by others.

Here again is some reason to be optimistic. A lot is known about methods of improvement, including methods for improving quality of care. There are the original methods of Deming and Juran, and now Six Sigma, Lean Thinking, and the Toyota Production System. There is also a potential driver for improvement embedded in the Accreditation Committee on Graduate Medical Education's (ACGME) six competencies that must be achieved as part of postgraduate residencies.[71] Three of the competencies are particularly relevant to stimulating education about quality improvement. They are "practice-based learning and improvement that involves investigation and evaluation of their own patient care, appraisal and assimilation of scientific evidence, and improvements in patient care" and "systems-based practice, as manifested by actions that demonstrate an awareness of and responsiveness to the larger context and system of healthcare and the ability to effectively call on system resources to provide care that is of optimal value." Another, on interpersonal and communications skills, fosters "teaming," not only with patients and their families, but also with other health professionals. Training residents to be competent in these areas is being built into the accreditation process for residency programs. It is leading to activity at the level of undergraduate medical education; and undoubtedly, it will lead to a cadre of more skilled medical professionals. Another trend in medical education that is likely to enhance the abilities of graduates to participate successfully in quality improvement activities is the proliferation of combined MD-MPH and MD-MBA programs. Thus, more medical school graduates are learning about population-based approaches to care and about management. Finally, there appears to be more interest in cross-education of physicians, nurses, and other health professionals.

A Satisfied Healthcare Workforce

It is difficult to picture effective, patient-centered, healthcare delivered by a demoralized workforce. Yet, an Aon survey of the US healthcare workers shows that very low percentages of the workforce plan to stay with their employer or are willing to recommend the place they work to other people as a place to work or as a place to get care.[72] In addition, in the United States, many physicians have been disillusioned first by the administrative hassles that they associate with managed care and, more recently, by markedly increased malpractice premiums. The primary care fields of general internal medicine, pediatrics, and family medicine are having difficulty attracting new trainees because practitioners in these fields tend to have long hours, global responsibilities, and relatively low compensation, compared to procedural specialists.

Furthermore, in recent years, there has been a serious shortage of nurses in many developed countries. In a recent international survey of five countries, 30 percent of hospital CEOs in the United States and Canada reported serious shortages, versus 22 percent to 23 percent of CEOs in Australia and the United Kingdom, and 11 percent in New Zealand.[73] This problem, clearly not unique to the United States, reflects the relative unattractiveness of front-line nursing positions in many hospitals. It must be solved because there is evidence that hospital nurse staffing is related to patient outcomes.[74,75,76]

The solution to these problems for physicians and nurses requires an understanding of the root causes of their dissatisfaction and then addressing those causes.[77] For example, in several hospitals observation of nurses has shown that they spend much of their time problem solving; but there usually is no management process within the hospital to aggregate the information about these problems and to address them systematically so that the same problem does not need to be solved over and over again. This failure of organizational learning leads to front-line frustration and burnout.[78]

Nonetheless, there are hospitals that are well known for their nursing care. The "magnet hospitals," which have applied for and achieved accreditation from the American Nurses Credentialing Center, actually serve as a "magnet" by attracting and retaining nurses. It is likely that these institutions also support other front-line staff better than the average hospital, and it is likely that there are lessons that can be learned from them and applied elsewhere.

Willingness to Learn from Others

Quality improvement in the United States is likely to proceed faster if healthcare organizations "walk the talk" and learn from best practices. Without comparative data, it is not possible to know what level of performance has already been attained by others. Without easy access to best practices associated with better performance, it is necessary to fabricate one's own solutions. Unfortunately, the tendency has been to resist providing or receiving information that can be used comparatively, for example, about physician or hospital competencies. The first response to comparative data is usually "these findings must be flawed," rather than "what can we learn from these findings?"

There are few, if any, formal mechanisms for gathering best practices. Even when information on best practices is available to organizations, there is a tendency to reject the practice due to a not-invented-here attitude. Those who deliver healthcare should welcome comparative improvement data from outside their own practice or organization; and those who regulate healthcare should facilitate provision of these types of comparative facts and information. Ideally, an attitude of "stealing shamelessly" should be encouraged, rather than not-invented-here attitudes. In addition, those who develop better ways of delivering care should not think that their ways are proprietary. There is little competitive advantage to having achieved any given level of performance, because as soon as others know that a certain goal can be achieved (e.g., a 90 percent reduction in central line associated bloodstream infections to near zero)[62] it will not take long for others to catch up. If there is any competitive advantage to be gained for organizations that provide high quality care, it should be through developing a track record of leadership in achieving high targets first. Thus, it is possible to picture a future in which all healthcare is delivered at a much better level of quality than today and in which certain providers are recognized for their zealousness in finding new targets for improvement, achieving those targets, and then helping their peers do likewise.

The US healthcare delivery system is so diverse that it is a boundless source of innovation. Nonetheless, it is not only parochial but dangerous to think that there are no lessons to be learned from other countries. Because the US healthcare system is not demonstrably better than those of other developed countries, based on all parameters of quality, it is important that lessons from abroad be sought and adapted.

For example, the United Kingdom, in its general practitioner (GP) contract implemented on April 1, 2004, has taken on pay-for-performance and performance assessment for GPs at a level unprecedented in the United States.[79] Practices, depending on performance, can receive up to 30 percent more compensation than before the contract. This large sum can lead to very different results than programs in the United States that seek to provide incentives for similar performance, but try to do so with much smaller sums. On the other hand, the money in the United Kingdom is, at first, an amount that is being added to compensation; whereas, in the United States, an adaptation might not be able to add any, or as much, new money and might have different results. Another example is the experience of New Zealand and several Scandinavian countries with various versions of no-fault compensation for malpractice or adverse events in healthcare.[80] Given the malpractice crisis in the United States and the deleterious effects of defensive medicine on quality of care, it is reasonable to explore the attributes of these approaches from abroad. A third example is the public reporting of information about hospital performance that occurs regularly in the United Kingdom. Both government and private sources of information about hospitals are made public.[81,82]

Important Next Steps for Achieving the Vision

The vision outlined in this chapter has seven components: 1) automatic and affordable health insurance coverage for all; 2) access to healthcare for all; 3) patient responsive healthcare; 4) information-driven healthcare; 5) continuous improvement stimulated throughout the healthcare system by appropriate incentives and facilitated by a workforce that is knowledgeable about and skilled in the methods of quality improvement; 6) a satisfied workforce; and 7) willingness, at all levels of the healthcare system, to learn from others at home and abroad.

Although the United States is far from achieving this vision, we believe it is possible to achieve. For each component, we have not only pointed out the current problems, but also examples of positive work or possibilities for change. There are a relative handful of changes that must occur if the vision is to be achieved, particularly by 2020. These include: 1) a more proactive stance to health insurance coverage by the federal government or, failing that, by more state governments; 2) a more proactive stance to improvement of quality of care by the federal government; 3) serious changes in the education of all health professionals; 4) activation of consumers to understand that they could receive, and must demand, considerably better care—care that is safer, more effective, more efficient, more timely, more equitable, and better designed around the needs of its customers not its providers; and 5) all-payer coalitions to support the financing of quality improvement activities, at least in the short run.

1. A more proactive stance to health insurance coverage by the federal government or, failing that, by more state governments is the only way all Americans will have insurance coverage. There are now several states with relatively low rates of uninsurance owing to various types of state-specific legislation. States offer an important opportunity to experiment with different approaches to covering the entire population and gather data on the pluses and minuses of these various approaches. As previously indicated, we believe there is already sufficient information to design federal legislation that would either guarantee coverage for all Americans or would require all states to develop appropriate state-specific approaches. Missing, at this writing, is a mandate from the American people to embolden Congress to enact and the President to sign such legislation.

2. A more proactive stance to improvement of quality of care by the federal government is essential to put some order into the chaos of the American healthcare system, or "nonsystem" as some consider it to be. There are many things that the federal government could and must do—and some are beginning to be done. We believe these include developing a dedicated federal agency for setting of national priorities for improvement, development or ratification of clinical guidelines, performance measures, and standards of care; leading initiatives for public reporting of performance; further support for the development and adoption of clinical information technology; developing the capability to provide technical assistance in quality improvement to all parts of the healthcare system; heading the effort to align incentives so that quality improvement is stimulated and rewarded; and funding key demonstration projects that explore new ways of coordinating care and paying for improved care.[83]

3. Serious changes in the education of all health professionals is essential; but this will require a change in academia's approach to quality improvement. Just as in the late nineteenth century, with the opening of Johns Hopkins' medical school, medical education began to be more scientific, a process that accelerated in the early twentieth century thanks to the Flexner Report that highlighted the poor scientific quality of most schools, now medical education and the education of other health professionals must become oriented to putting the patient/person and his/her health, and not the scientific aspects of disease, at the center of the universe. Academic health centers must become leaders in patient-centered care and quality improvement. The ACGME's competencies seem to be the catalyst for this change and could serve as the twenty-first century equivalent of the Flexner Report.

4. Activation of patients to understand that they can receive, and must demand, considerably better care—care that is safer, more effective, more efficient, more timely, more equitable, and better designed around the needs of consumers, not providers. This is easier said than done. For the most part, consumers/patients are not organized as a lobby in the United States and, unfortunately, have depended on the chaotic healthcare system to give them "the best care in the world." Public concern about quality of care in the United Kingdom has led to the public's willingness, indeed demand, to expend more national resources on health. This is another lesson from abroad that the United States could profit from importing. Public activation is likely to come in response to problems highlighted in the media or by politicians who are leaders, not more reactors. The more information the public receives, the more likely consumers will become activists. Accordingly, we strongly favor public reporting of information about quality of care.

5. All-payer coalitions are needed to support the financing of quality improvement activities, at least in the short run. Ultimately, all quality improvement activities should either benefit providers by being more efficient or yielding performance-based payments, or benefit society as a whole by creating a healthier, more productive country. Initially, adoption of information technology and training the workforce in quality improvement methods are likely to be seen as net expenditures by those who must invest in and implement them. The federal government, as the single largest payer for healthcare in the United States, can take the lead, but ideally would bring together all payers so that there is broad-based financial support for creating rapid change in the healthcare delivery system.

The "perfect storm" is known to happen and cause unspeakable disasters. We believe the time is ripe for the "perfect opportunity." It is appropriate to be hopeful that we are reaching a tipping point. Major progress in the five areas outlined would allow the seven components of our vision to be achieved. This would produce a vastly improved healthcare system for all Americans and a healthier and more productive country.

Study/Discussion Questions

1. What are some obstacles to the process of improving healthcare? What are the roles of medical students and physicians?
2. What are the consequences of an increasing uninsured population? How can physicians participate in reducing the uninsured population?
3. What is the significance of the development of the Consumer Assessment of Health Plans Survey (CAHPS)? What are the most important changes in the way care is designed and delivered that would have to occur for it to be patient-centered?

Suggested Readings/Web Sites

The Commonwealth Fund (*www.cmwf.org*).

Davis K, Schoen C, Schoenbaum SC. A 2020 vision for American health care. *Arch Intern Med.* 2000;160:3357–62.

Schoenbaum SC, Audet A-M, Davis K. Obtaining greater value from healthcare: The roles of the U.S. government. *Health Affairs.* 2003;22(5):183–90.

References

1. McGlynn EA, Asch SM, Adams J, et al. The quality of health care delivered to adults in the United States. *NEJM.* 2003;348:2635–45.
2. The Commonwealth Fund. *First Report and Recommendations of The Commonwealth Fund's International Working Group on Quality Indicators.* New York: The Commonwealth Fund; 2004. (Fund Publication #752) Available at: www.cmwf.org. Accessed on June 6, 2005.
3. Baicker K, Chandra A. Medicare spending, the physician workforce, and beneficiaries' quality of care. *Health Aff.* Web exclusive. 2004;W-4:184–97. Available at: http://content.healthaffairs.org/webexclusives/index.dtl?year=2004. Accessed on July 30, 2004.
4. Fisher ES, Wennberg DE, Stukel TA, Gottlieb DJ, Lucas FL, Pinder EL. The implications of regional variations in Medicare spending. Part 1: the content, quality, and accessibility of care. *Ann Intern Med.* 2003;138(4):273–87.
5. Fisher ES, Wennberg DE, Stukel TA, Gottlieb DJ, Lucas FL, Pinder EL. The implications of regional variations in Medicare spending. Part 2: Health outcomes and satisfaction with care. *Ann Intern Med.* 2003;138(4):288–98.
6. Blendon RJ, Schoen C, DesRoches C, Osborn R, Zapert K. Common concerns amid diverse systems: Healthcare experiences in five countries. *Health Aff.* 2003;22(3): 106–21.
7. Davis K, Schoen C, Schoenbaum SC, Audet A-M, Doty MM, Tenney K. *Mirror Mirror on the Wall: The quality of American Health Care Through the Patients' Lens.* New York: The Commonwealth Fund; 2004. (Fund Publication #683) Available at: www.cmwf.org. Accessed on June 11, 2005.

8. Kohn LT, Corrigan JM, Donaldson MS, eds. *To Err Is Human: Building a Safer Health System.* Washington, DC: National Academies Press; 1999.

9. Brennan TA, Leape LL, Laird NM, et al. Incidence of adverse events and negligence in hospitalized patients: Results of the Harvard Medical Practice Study I. *NEJM.* 1991: 324:370–76.

10. O'Neill P. Keynote Address from Secretary of the Treasury, Paul O'Neill. The Summit with Joseph M. Juran, University of Minnesota's Carlson School of Management—Juran Center for Leadership in Quality. June 25, 2002. Available at: http://www.csom.umn.edu/Page 1306.aspx. Accessed on July 28, 2004.

11. World Health Organization. *World Health Report, 2000: Health Systems, Improving Performance.* Geneva: World Health Organization; 2000.

12. Schoen C, Doty MM. Inequities in access to medical care in five countries: Findings from the 2001 Commonwealth Fund International Health Policy Survey. *Health Policy.* 2004; 67(3):309–22.

13. Schoen C, Davis K, DesRoches C, Donelan K, Blendon R. Health insurance markets and income inequality: Findings from an International Health Policy Survey. *Health Policy.* 2000;52(2):67–85.

14. Anderson GF, Petrosyan V, Hussey PS. *Multinational Comparisons of Health Systems Data, 2002.* New York: The Commonwealth Fund; 2002. Available at: www.cmwf.org. Accessed on June 11, 2005.

15. Samuelson RJ. Myths of the uninsured. *Newsweek.* November 8, 1999.

16. Ayanian JZ, Weissman JS, Schneider EC, Ginsburg JA, Zaslavsky AM. Unmet Health Needs of uninsured adults in the United States. *JAMA.* 2000;284:2061–69.

17. Institute of Medicine. *Insuring America's Health: Principles and Recommendations.* Washington, DC: National Academy Press; 2004.

18. Gornick ME. *Vulnerable Populations and Medicare Services: Why Do Disparities Exist?* New York: Century Foundation Press; 2000.

19. Schneider EC, Zaslavsky AM, Epstein AM. Racial disparities in the quality of care for enrollees in medicare managed care. *JAMA.* 2002;287(10):1288–94.

20. Nichols LM, Ginsburg PB, Berenson RA, Christianson J, Hurley RE. Are market forces strong enough to deliver efficient health care systems? Confidence is waning. *Health Aff.* 2004;23(3):8–21.

21. Sandy LG, Schroeder SA. Primary care in a new era: Disillusion and dissolution? *Ann Intern Med.* 2003;138(3):262–67.

22. Institute of Medicine. Committee on Quality of Health Care in America. *Crossing the Quality Chasm: A New Health System for the 21ˢᵗ Century.* Washington, DC: National Academy Press; 2001.

23. Institute of Medicine. *Care Without Coverage. Too Little, Too Late.* Washington, DC: National Academy Press; 2002.

24. Clinton HR. Now can we talk about health care? *The New York Times Magazine.* April 28, 2004.

25. Gingrich N, Kennedy P. Operating in a vacuum. *The New York Times.* May 3, 2004: A23.

26. Connolly C. Frist proposes health insurance reform. *The Washington Post.* July 13, 2004: A4.

27. Broder DS. Our broken health care system. *The Washington Post.* July 15, 2004: A21.

28. Davis K, Schoen C, Schoenbaum SC. A 2020 vision for American healthcare. *Arch Intern Med.* 2000;160:3357–62.

29. Collins SR, Doty MM, Davis K, Schoen C, Holmgren AL, Ho A. *The Affordability Crisis in US Health Care: Findings from the Commonwealth Fund Biennial Health Insurance Survey.* New York: The Commonwealth Fund; 2004. Available at: www.cmwf.org. Accessed on June 11, 2005.

30. Short PF, Graefe DR, Schoen C. *Churn, Churn, Churn: How Instability of Health Insurance Shapes America's Uninsured Problem.* New York: The Commonwealth Fund, 2003. Available at: www.cmwf.org. Accessed on June 11, 2005.

31. Davis K. Commentary: The consequences of being uninsured. *Med Care Res Rev.* 2003;60(2):89S–99S.

32. Davis K, Schoen C. Creating consensus on coverage choices. *Health Aff.* Web exclusive. 2003;W3:199–211.

33. Collins SR, Davis K, Lambrew JM. *Health Care Reform Returns to the National Agenda: 2004 Presidential Candidates' Proposals.* New York: The Commonwealth Fund; 2004. (Fund Publication #671) Available at: www.cmwf.org. Accessed on June 11, 2005.

34. Rosenthal J, Pernice C. *Dirigo Health Reform Act: Addressing Health Care Costs, Quality, and Access in Maine.* Portland, Maine: National Academy for State Health Policy; 2004.

35. Chollet D, Achman L. *Approaching Universal Coverage: Minnesota's Health Insurance Programs.* New York: The Commonwealth Fund; 2003. (Fund Publication #566) Available at: www.cmwf.org. Accessed June 11, 2005.

36. Silow-Carroll S. *Building Quality into RIte Care: How Rhode Island is Improving Health Care for Its Low-Income Populations.* New York: The Commonwealth Fund; 2003. (Fund Publication #566) Available at: www.cmwf.org. Accessed on June 11, 2005.

37. Gusmano MK, Fairbrother G, Park H. Exploring the limits of the safety net: Community health centers and care for the uninsured. *Health Aff.* 2002;21(6):188–94.

38. Billings J, Parikh N, Mijanovich T. *Emergency Department Use in New York City: A Substitute for Primary Care?* New York: The Commonwealth Fund; 2000. (Fund Publication #433) Available at: www.cmwf.org. Accessed on June 11, 2005.

39. Davis K, Schoenbaum SC, Scott Collins K, Tenney K, Hughes DL, Audet AM. *Room for Improvement: Patients Report on the Quality of Their Health Care.* New York: The Commonwealth Fund; 2002. (Fund Publication #534) Available at: www.cmwf.org. Accessed on June 11, 2005.

40. Rozich JD, Resar RK. Using a unit assessment tool to optimize patient flow and staffing in a community hospital. *Jt Comm J Qual Improv.* 2002;28(1):31–41.

41. McManus ML, Long MC, Cooper A, et al. Variability in surgical caseload and access to intensive care services. *Anesthesiology.* 2003;98(6):1491–96.

42. Espinosa JA, Case R, Kosnik LK. Emergency department structure and operations. *Emerg Med Clin North Am.* 2004;22(1):73–85.

43. Murray M, Berwick DM. Advanced access: Reducing waiting and delays in primary care. *JAMA.* 2003;289(8):1035–40.

44. Murray M, Bodenheimer T, Rittenhouse D, Grumbach K. Improving timely access to primary care: Case studies of the advanced access model. *JAMA.* 2003;289(8):1042–46.

45. Chin M. *Sustainability and the Second Law of Thermodynamics.* New York: The Commonwealth Fund; 2003. (Fund Publication #674) Available at: *www.cmwf.org.* Accessed on June 11, 2005

46. Gordon P, Chin M. *Achieving a New Standard in Primary Care for Low-Income Populations: Case Studies of Redesign and Change Through a Learning Collaborative.* New York: The Commonwealth Fund; 2004. Available at: www.cmwf.org. Accessed on June 11, 2005.

47. National Primary Care Development Team (UK). Available at: www.npdt.org. Accessed on June 11, 2005.

48. Mahoney ME. Innovative mind-set: revitalize or dismantle when there's something more suitable. *Hospitals & Health Networks.* 1994;68:74,76–7.

49. Edgman-Levitan S, Cleary PD. What information do consumers want and need? *Health Aff.* 1996;15(4):42–56.

50. Delbanco TL, Berwick DM, Boufford JL, et al. Healthcare in a land called PeoplePower: Nothing about me without me. *Health Expect.* 2001;4:144–50.

51. American Medical Association. Cultural Competence Compendium. Available at: http://www.ama-assn.org/ama/pub/category/4848.html. Accessed on July 28, 2004.

52. Schoenbaum SC. Feedback of clinical performance information. *HMO Practice.* 1993;7:5–11.

53. Schoenbaum SC, Barnet GO. Automated ambulatory medical records systems: An orphan technology. *International J Techn Assess Health Care.* 1992;8(4):598–609.

54. Bates DW, Leape LL, Cullen DJ, et al. Effect of computerized physician order entry and a team intervention on prevention of serious medication errors. *JAMA.* 1998;280(15):1360–61.

55. Audet A-M, Doty MM, Peugh J, Shamasdin J, Zapert K, Schoenbaum S. Information technologies: When will they make it into physicians' black bags? *Medscape Gen Med.* 2004;6(4).

56. Poon EG, Blumenthal D, Jaggi T, Honour MM, Bates DW, Kaushal R. Overcoming barriers to adopting and implementing computerized physician order entry systems in U.S. hospitals. *Health Aff.* 2004;23(4):184–90.

57. Gray BH, Gusmano MK, Collins SR. AHCPR and the changing politics of health services research. *Health Aff.* Web exclusive. 2003;W-3:283–307.

58. Berwick DM. Continuous improvement as an ideal in health care. *NEJM.* 1989;320(1):1424–25.

59. Leatherman S, McCarthy D. *Quality of Health Care in the United States: A Chartbook.* New York: The Commonwealth Fund; 2002. (Fund Publication #520) Available at: www.cmwf.org. Accessed on June 11, 2005.

60. Leatherman S, McCarthy D. *Quality of Health Care for Children and Adolescents: A Chartbook.* New York: The Commonwealth Fund; 2004. (Fund Publication #700) Available at: www.cmwf.org. Accessed on June 11, 2005.

61. O'Connor GT, Plume SK, Olmstead EM, et al. A regional intervention to improve the hospital mortality associated with coronary artery bypass graft surgery: The Northern New England Cardiovascular Disease Study Group. *JAMA.* 1996;275(11):841–46.

62. Pittsburgh Regional Healthcare Initiative. PRHI Executive Summary, April 2004. Available at: www.prhi.org/newsletters.cfm. Accessed on August 1, 2004.

63. Lee TH, Meyer GS, Brennan TA. A middle ground on public accountability. *NEJM.* 2004;350(23):2409–12.

64. Leatherman S, Berwick D, Iles D, et al. The business case for quality: Case studies and an analysis. *Health Aff.* 2003;22(2):17–30.

65. The Child Health Business Case Working Group. Exploring the business case for improving the quality of health care for children. *Health Aff.* 2004;23(4):159–66.

66. Pittsburgh Regional Healthcare Initiative. PRHI Executive Summary, June 2004 and July 2004. Available at: www.prhi.org/newsletters.cfm. Accessed on August 1, 2004.

67. The Leapfrog Group. Leapfrog Incentive and Reward Compendium. Available at: www.leapfroggroup.org/ircompendium.htm. Accessed on July 30, 2004.

68. Schoenbaum SC, Bovbjerg RR. Malpractice reform must include steps to prevent medical injury. *Ann Intern Med.* 2004;140:51–53.

69. NCQA Recognized Physician Directory. Available at: www.ncqa.org/PhysicianQuality Reports.htm. Accessed on July 30, 2004.

70. Berwick DM. Harvesting knowledge from improvement. *JAMA.* 1996;275(11):877–78.

71. ACGME Outcome Project. General competencies. Available at: http://www.acgme.org/outcome/comp/compMin.asp. Accessed on July 29, 2004.

72. American Hospital Association, Commission on Workforce for Hospitals and Health Systems. *In Our Hands: How Hospital Leaders Can Build a Thriving Workforce.* Chicago, Ill: American Hospital Association; 2002.

73. Blendon RJ, Schoen C, DesRoches CM, Osborn R, Zapert K, Raleigh E. Confronting competing demands to improve quality: A five-country hospital survey. *Health Aff.* 2004; 23(3):119–35.

74. Needleman J, Buerhaus P, Mattke S, Stewart M, Zevlinsky K. Nurse-staffing levels and the quality of care in hospitals. *NEJM.* 2002;346(22):1757–66.

75. Aitkin L. Hospital nurse staffing and patient mortality, nurse burnout, and job dissatisfaction. *JAMA.* 2002;288(16):1987–93.

76. Person SC, Allison JJ, Kiefe CI, et al. Nurse staffing and mortality for Medicare patients with acute myocardial infarction. *Med Care.* 2004;42(1):4–12.

77. Keenan P. *The Nursing Workforce Shortage: Causes, Consequences, Proposed Solutions.* New York: The Commonwealth Fund; 2003. (Fund publication #619) Available at: www.cmwf.org. Accessed on June 11, 2005.

78. Tucker AL, Edmondson AC, Spear S. *J Organizational Change Manage.* 2003; 15(2):122–37.

79. Smith PC, York N. Quality incentives: The case of UK general practitioners. *Health Aff.* 2004;23(3):112–18.

80. Studdert DM, Mello MM, Brennan TA. Medical malpractice. *NEJM.* 2004; 350(3):283–92.

81. Healthcare Commission. Acute trust overview. Available at: http://ratings2004.healthcare commission.org.uk/Trust/Overview/acute_overview.asp. Accessed August 1, 2004.

82. Dr. Foster. Available at: www.drfoster.co.uk. Accessed on August 1, 2004.

83. Schoenbaum SC, Audet A-M, Davis K. Obtaining greater value from healthcare: The roles of the U.S. government. *Health Aff.* 2003;22(5):183–90.

Index